PLASTIC SURGERY ORALS

A Suggested Plan of Attack

Wellington J. Davis III, M.D., F.A.C.S.
Assistant Professor of Surgery and Pediatrics
Drexel University College of Medicine
Section of Plastic & Reconstructive Surgery
St. Christopher's Hospital for Children
Philadelphia, Pennsylvania

Editor

John D. Pemberton D.O., M.B.A.
Assistant Professor of Ophthalmology
University of Arkansas College of Medicine
Oculoplastics & Orbital Reconstructive Surgery
Harvey and Bernice Jones Eye Institute
Little Rock, Arkansas

Illustrations by Debra Lynn Basso

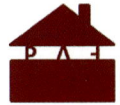

Crimson House Publishing LLC
224 Valmar, Little Rock, Arkansas 72205

PLASTIC SURGERY: ORAL EXAM STUDY GUIDE © **2014**

No part of this book may be reproduced or transmitted in any form or by any means, electronic or mechanical, including photocopying, recording, or any information storage and retrieval system, without permission in writing from the publisher or authors. Permission may be sought directly from Crimson House Publishing LLC website: ophthalmology.oralboardprep.com

Notice

Plastic Surgery is a constantly changing profession. Standard precautions must be followed as new research and clinical findings widen the knowledge base, changes in treatment may be necessary. Readers should check current information for medications and management of cases and not use this book as a therapeutic reference guide. It is the responsibility of the licensed practitioner to determine the best treatment of their patients. Neither the publisher nor the authors assume any liability for any injury and/or damage to individuals or property arising from this publication.

Disclaimer

This book has been written based on public information gathered from the American Board of Plastic Surgery website, printed policies, and the authors own personal and clinical experience. No Board material has been replicated, recalled, or taken from the actual examination. Clinical cases and material in this book that seems to be similar is coincidental as it is impossible to know what specific material will be covered on any given exam day. It is against board rules to divulge specific information regarding prior or future examination content.

The Publisher

Library of Congress Control Number: 2014948810

ISBN 978-0-692-27730-0

Table of Contents

- **Dedication** 9
- **Foreword** 10
- **How to Use the Book** 11
- **Material to Master** 15
- **Study Sheet Template** 23
- **Presentation Tips** 25
- **Game Day Strategy** 27
- **Core References** 29

TORSO 31

- **Section 1: General Breast** 33
  - Chapter 1 Overview 35
  - Chapter 2 Breast Reduction 41
  - Chapter 3 Breast Augmentation 51
  - Chapter 4 Mastopexy 65
  - Chapter 5 Gynecomastia 73
  - Chapter 6 Poland Syndrome 81
  - Chapter 7 Tuberous Breast Deformity 89
- **Section 2: Breast Reconstruction** 97
  - Chapter 8 Overview 99
  - Chapter 9 Breast Reconstruction 103
- **Section 3: Trunk Reconstruction** 127
  - Chapter 10 Overview 129
  - Chapter 11 Abdominal Wall Recon 133
  - Chapter 12 Chest Wall Reconstruction ... 141
  - Chapter 13 Pressure Sores 153
  - Chapter 14 Abd. Compart. Syndrome ... 169
  - Chapter 15 Bariatric Reconstruction 173

- Chapter 16 Abdominoplasty 191

FACE 205

- **Section 4: Facial Reconstruction** 207
  - Chapter 17 Overview 209
  - Chapter 18 Scalp & Calvarial Recon 213
  - Chapter 19 Upper Eyelid 225
  - Chapter 20 Lower Eyelid 235
  - Chapter 21 Ectropion 245
  - Chapter 22 Nasal 257
  - Chapter 23 Ear 269
  - Chapter 24 Upper Lip 279
  - Chapter 25 Lower Lip 291
  - Chapter 26 Cheek 301
- **Section 5: Facial Fractures** 311
  - Chapter 27 Overview 313
  - Chapter 28 Facial Fractures 319
- **Section 6: Facial Paralysis** 343
  - Chapter 29 Overview 345
  - Chapter 30 Facial Paralysis 349
- **Section 7: Cosmetic Face** 363
  - Chapter 31 Overview 365
  - Chapter 32 Non-operative Rejuvenation 369
  - Chapter 33 Facial Rejuvenation 379
  - Chapter 34 Forehead Rejuvenation 395
  - Chapter 35 Eyelid and Blepharoplasty 405
  - Chapter 36 Rhytid. and Cervicoplasty 417
  - Chapter 37 Facelift Principles 433
- **Section 8: Rhinoplasty** 445
  - Chapter 38 Overview 447
  - Chapter 39 Rhinoplasty 453
  - Chapter 40 Genioplasty 479
  - Chapter 41 Secondary Rhinoplasty 489

EXTREMITIES 495

- **Section 9: Lower Extremity** 497
    - Chapter 42 Overview 499
    - Chapter 43 Lower Extremity Trauma 503
    - Chapter 44 Diabetic and Chronic Wound 519
- **Section 10: Hand** 523
    - Chapter 45 Overview 525
    - Chapter 46 Flexor Tendon Injury 531
    - Chapter 47 Extensor Tendon Injury 543
    - Chapter 48 Boutonniere Deformity 561
    - Chapter 49 Swan Neck Deformity 569
    - Chapter 50 Extensor Mechanism 577
    - Chapter 51 Tendon Reconstruction 585
    - Chapter 52 Tendon Transfers 591
    - Chapter 53 General Hand Fracture 605
    - Chapter 54 Specifics of Hand Fractures 611
    - Chapter 55 Thumb Amputation 627
    - Chapter 56 Fingertip Injury 643
    - Chapter 57 Compartment Syndrome 649
    - Chapter 58 Mutilating Hand Injury 657
    - Chapter 59 Ulnar Collateral Ligament 671
    - Chapter 60 Ulnar Nerve Palsy 677
    - Chapter 61 Finger Mass 685
    - Chapter 62 Dupuytren's 691
    - Chapter 63 Syndactyly 697
    - Chapter 64 Thumb Hypoplasia 705
    - Chapter 65 Thumb Duplication 713

PEDIATRIC PLASTIC SURGERY 719

- **Section 11: Congenital/Pediatric** 721
    - Chapter 66 Overview 723

- Chapter 67 Cleft Lip and Palate 729
- Chapter 68 Cleft Palate 745
- Chapter 69 Pierre Robin Sequence 753
- Chapter 70 Velopharyngeal Insufficiency..... 763
- Chapter 71 Cleft Lip and Nasal Deformity.... 771
- Chapter 72 Giant Congenital Nevus 785
- Chapter 73 Syndactyly (refer Ch. 63).......... 795
- Chapter 74 Hemangioma/Vasc Malf. 797
- Chapter 75 Prominent Ear Deformity 813
- Chapter 76 Gynecomastia (refer Ch. 5) 825
- Chapter 77 Meningomyelocele 827
- Chapter 78 Ptosis 835
- Chapter 79 Microtia-Hemifacial Microsomia. 843
- Chapter 80 Treacher Collins Syndrome 855

BURNS 863

- **Section 12: Burns** 865
  - Chapter 81 Overview 867
  - Chapter 82 Burns 871
  - Chapter 83 Burn Reconstruction.................. 883
  - Chapter 84 Hand (Burn and Frostbite).......... 897
  - Chapter 85 Keloids, Hypertrophic Scars 907

Dedication

This book is dedicated to my loving wife, Debra. For loving and supporting me through my medical training and far beyond. For standing by me through the best and the worst of times. You are my favorite person, you are my heart.

It is also dedicated to all of the candidates who have struggled with this exam. To all of my colleagues who have passed on invaluable pearls and inspired me to write this book. Most especially, Dr. Diane V. Dado, my pediatric plastic surgery mentor, guru, jedi master.

-Wellington

Foreword

The process of board certification is a true rite of passage in the medical field that is time honored and a mark of distinction. It marks the culmination of years of testing, loans, and effort that is both hard earned while at the same time humbling. Safe Answers for the Oral Examination in Plastic Surgery, by Dr. Wellington Davis, is a wonderful resource that is the product of years of collective experience and dedication. Wellington told me of his project years ago, and it is a testament of his follow-through and dedication to the field that this project is now completed.

In plastic surgery, there may not be one exact correct procedure of choice, but there exist correct principles of management with each setting in the care of plastic surgery patients. Few medical fields are more technically demanding, and in plastic surgery our results are frequently evaluated by our patients, patients' families and friends, and potentially acquaintances alike.

Plastic surgery represents the balanced combination of technical skill, creative problem solving, and "doing the right thing" for the patient. Plastic surgeons draw upon a breadth of skillset from skin grafting and local tissue rearrangement to vascular composite transplantation in the form of hand and face transplantation.

It is an honor and privilege to contribute to the education of future leaders in plastic surgery, and the preparation and passage of oral boards is one huge step!

All the best in your preparation and good luck!

Samuel J. Lin, MD FACS

How to Use the Book

This book is intended for use as a guide for preparation for the American Board of Plastic Surgery oral examination. There is no one correct way to prepare for the exam. This books lays out a suggested plan of attack, which I believe was critical in assisting me in successfully passing the exam.

I wrote this book because I felt there is a lack of resources that focus purely on plastic surgery oral board examination. I did not encounter any resource that simply details the core of you what you need to know and how to present that information in an organized fashion that is plastic surgery oral board oriented.

With the current pace of clinical practice at many plastic surgery residency programs residents are exposed to the full gambit of plastic surgery problems, learn many operations and get a solid clinical experience. The problem is that there is often little time spent on teaching residents how to synthesize the information, understand the thought process of the work-up and teach the broad wide stroke principles that are applied to general clinical problems, i.e. the method to the madness. Exactly how did the attending come up with that specific intervention before walking into the operating room? Often it is left to the residents in the end to ultimately "put it together" and make their own way through the examination process.

An educational gap at many programs is too little time spent in giving focused and stream-lined preparation for the oral examination. The reality is, in spite of focused attention on board preparation at the best of training programs, there will be the occasional seemingly bright, brilliant candidate who may fail the oral boards with no clear understanding of what went wrong. For those with minimal appropriate preparation chances of successful navigation through the process may be equivalent to a coin toss.

While one can probably manage many routine problems by the seat of their pants, operation by operation, as demonstrated by other specialists doing plastic surgical procedures, it is the thought process that really matters. That is the difference between the plastic surgeon and another specialist doing the same procedure. This is what the board wants to know. Do you know the thought process behind the operation? Believe it or not there really is one. All board examiners know this, unfortunately all the exam candidates do not.

This book presents the broad categories which are bread and butter topics that are "fair game" on the ABPS oral examination.

Included are common sub-topics a general plastic surgeon should be expected to be able to manage. Plastic surgery is a very broad clinical specialty. The types of problems plastic surgeons manage can fill volumes upon volumes. Sub-specialty topics can also fill volumes upon volumes. When considering the oral examination trying to get one's head around the amount of information that must be mastered is a formidable, intimidating task. Fortunately, the board can only ask a finite number of questions. They tend to ask about "routine, non-controversial, basic" topics. The goal: test the candidates on the principles. They want to know if you "the basics", not if you are the slickest plastic surgeon in the country.

The unknown portion of the exam is approximately 90 minutes. Only a finite amount of information can be tested. With a total of 12 unknown topics you only have approximately 6 and 1/2 minutes to discuss everything you know about each of those topics. If your presentation is not focused on the highlights, core problems and relevant issues, then your chances of failure increase exponentially. You will miss the opportunity to demonstrate what you know about the most relevant aspects of the topic. It is important to stick to basics.

This book presents a finite but comprehensive list of topics. I've complied them from topic lists at review courses and the main general plastic surgery texts. I've also given a suggested format for preparation as well as a skeletal framework for presentation and organization of thoughts to help keep one on track. Cruising through an oral presentation is not natural for everyone. Having a foundation to work from will hopefully be quite helpful.

Unfortunately, I can by no means guarantee anyone's success by just reading this book alone. As we know there are no magic bullets. Besides this is just a suggested plan of attack. That being said I do believe it will be very helpful to most, probably most helpful to candidates taking the exam a second or third time. It is quite disturbing how many seemingly bright candidates manage to fail this particular exam. My suggestion is to use this text as a ground work for preparation for the exam.

Other suggestions for success:

1) Read Guyuron and study it cover to cover during residency, take notes. Then read it again while preparing for the orals. It is an invaluable text.
2) Give yourself plenty of time to prepare for the exam. I believe a period of 3 months is the minimum needed to prepare for this

exam. Start preparing the day you get the letter of notification that you may sit for the exam.
3) Take the time to prepare your own organized "Stanford" style short study sheets for each of the listed topics in addition to studying them from this text.
4) You will need to prepare short cards of the key 5 steps of any relevant surgical procedure independently from this book. Surgical procedures and surgical anatomy are the one area not covered in intense detail in this text. Although the key steps of any operation may be the same, the technical approach, intraoperative details and post-op management can vary surgeon to surgeon. Note any key anatomical landmarks as well as additional maneuvers to make the procedure safer or optimize the goal of the procedure.
5) The last weeks before the exam streamline and memorize, just study cards and review this text.
6) Try to streamline study materials
7) Follow the ABPS bible to the letter for case-preparation and finish casebooks early so you can study them. Preparation should be as for a malignant general surgery M&M or legal deposition

This text focuses primarily on preparation of the unknown section of the exam. It is an important 60% of the exam. It may be helpful for the preparation of case books as well. I have heard it said that the casebooks should be the easier part of the exam and you have the most control over this section. Personally, I disagree with this. It is hard to know what the board is looking for in the case book section of the exam. I believe all you can do is thoroughly prepare the cases, code appropriately, have ethical practice patterns, stick to "standard" algorithms and hope for the best. Not very encouraging. I do believe though if you are very well prepared for the unknowns, orient your study by what is going to be tested from what is in the ABPS bible, you may have more control over this portion of the exam than you expect. I believe more so than the case books.

What does the board want to know on the unknowns? In a nutshell, your ability to do the following:

1. Identify General Problem/Make a Diagnosis/Surgical Planning
2. Consider reasonable goals in diagnosis and management
3. Select appropriate options in diagnosis and management

4. Understand risks and benefits of various approaches
5. Address complications and unexpected problems adequately
6. Demonstrate ability to structure alternative plan

That's direct from the "bible".

Prepare well young Jedi. "May the force be with you" and may this text help you on your journey.

Material to Master

1. These broad topics WILL be on the exam!
    - General Breast (1 question)
    - Breast Reconstruction (1 question)
    - Trunk Reconstruction (1 question)
    - Facial Reconstruction (1 question)
    - Facial Fractures (0 or 1 question)
    - Facial Paralysis (0 or 1 question)
    - Cosmetic Face (1 question)
    - Rhinoplasty (1 question)
    - Lower Extremity Reconstruction (1 question)
    - Hand (1 or 2 questions)
    - Pediatric Plastic Surgery (1 or 2 questions)
    - Burns (1 question)
2. Multiple areas in one broad topic may be combined in one question.
    - E.g. Mangled hand covers management of:
        - Soft tissue
        - Tendon reconstruction
        - Hand fractures
        - Nerve injury
        - Rehab and PT issues
3. Broad topics may be combined.
    - Syndactyly (Hand & Pediatric)
    - Pediatric Burn (Facial recon, Pediatric, Hand, Burn)
    - Poland (Breast, Hand)
    - Giant congenital nevus of face (Facial recon, Pediatric)
    - Isolated hand electrical injury (Burn, Hand)
    - Bariatric recon (Breast, Trunk Recon)
    - If you know the following topics you should be well prepared for any type of question that you may be asked.
4. Prepare and organize your own 1-2 page study sheets or cards on all of the listed topics. The most important core topics are covered in this book.
5. Focus on brushing up on your weakest areas.
6. On the exam weekend you can predict which topics will be tested the second day based on what was covered in the unknowns the first day.
    - GENERAL BREAST AND BREAST RECONSTRUCTION

- Breast reconstruction
  - Radiation
  - Flaps
  - Implants
  - Immediate vs. delayed
  - Previous surgery
  - Body habitus considerations
- Breast augmentation
  - Complications
  - Saline vs. silicone
  - Placement
  - Indications
  - Severe capsular contracture
  - Breast reduction
  - Juvenile or massive macromastia
  - Vertical reduction techniques
  - Incidental cancer management
- Tuberous breast deformity
- Poland sequence
- Gynecomastia
- Asymmetric breast

- **TRUNK**
  - Body Contouring
  - Liposuction
  - Abdominoplasty
    - Options
    - Indications
  - Brachioplasty
  - Buttock and calf implants
  - Thigh lift
  - Buttock lift
  - Bariatric reconstruction
    - Flanks
    - Breast
    - Trunk
    - Buttocks
    - Thighs
    - Arms
  - Chest wall reconstruction
  - Sternotomy wounds
  - Pressure sores
    - Sacral

- Ischial
- Trochanteric
- Heel
- Occipital
- Posterior trunk
      - Perineum
      - Chronic wounds
      - Abdominal wall reconstruction
      - Abdominal compartment syndrome
  - FACIAL RECONSTRUCTION
      - Skin cancer management
          - Basal cell
          - Squamous cell
          - Melanoma
          - Merkel Cell
      - Eyelid Reconstruction
          - Classification
          - Partial vs. full thickness
          - Upper and lower
          - Medial canthal recon
      - Nasal reconstruction
      - Lip reconstruction
          - Vermilion reconstruction
      - Scalp reconstruction
      - Ear reconstruction
          - Local flaps and total reconstruction
      - Forehead reconstruction
      - Cheek reconstruction
      - Mandible/Midface Reconstruction
      - Parotid mass
      - Tongue reconstruction
  - FACIAL FRACTURES
      - Acute trauma management
      - Facial fractures
      - Panfacial trauma
      - Shotgun wound to face "mangled face"
      - Mandible
      - Orbital Floor
      - ZMC and zygomatic arch
      - Maxillary fractures
      - Parotid gland injury
      - Frontal sinus fractures

- o NOE fractures
- o Calvarial reconstruction
- o Scalp and forehead reconstruction
- o Pediatric facial fractures
- o Complications
  - Enophthalmos
  - Nonunion
  - Malunion
  - Ectropion
  - Loose hardware
- FACIAL PARALYSIS
  - o Etiology
    - Trauma
    - Congenital
    - Tumor
  - o Management options
    - Static vs. dynamic
    - Based on time, age and etiology
  - o Issues based on age of patient
    - Indications and operations
  - o Timing and interventions
  - o Anatomy
    - Upper face- brow, eyelids, ptosis
    - Midface- nose, cheek
    - Lower face- lip droop, drooling, speech
  - o Complications of paralysis
  - o Algorithm of management of nerve injury
    - Parotid tumors
    - Facial Reconstruction
    - Iatrogenic or Traumatic injury
- COSMETIC FACE
  - o Forehead
  - o Brow
  - o Eyelids
  - o Nose
  - o Midface
  - o Chin
  - o Face
  - o Neck
  - o Complications
    - Ectropion/Entropion
    - Extra ocular muscle injury

- Skin slough
- Management of ptosis
- Surgical options
  - Brow lift
  - Rhytidectomy
  - Cervicoplasty
  - Bleph
  - Chin implants
  - Contouring
- Non-surgical options
  - Botox
  - Fillers
  - Laser

- **RHINOPLASTY**
  - Nasal tip deformity
  - Nostril show deformity
  - Nasal airway obstruction
  - Nasal septum deformities
  - Anatomic deformity by region
  - Male vs. female
  - Skin type
  - Nasal supra-tip deformities
  - Crooked nose
  - Bulbous vs. Boxy tip
  - Saddle Nose
  - Secondary rhinoplasty
  - Genioplasty indications
  - Orthognatic surgery indications
  - Complications

- **LOWER EXTREMITY**
  - Trauma
  - Chronic wound
  - Ischemic limb
  - Diabetic wounds
  - Heel
  - Foot
  - Distal third
  - Middle third
  - Upper third
  - Indications for amputations
  - Orthopedic management

- **HAND**

- Tendon Reconstruction
- Flexor tendon injury
- Extensor tendon injury
- Extensor mechanism:
  - Swan Neck
  - Boutonnière
  - Sagittal Band
- Ulnar collateral ligament injury
- Dupuytren's Disease
- Hand fractures
- Thumb metacarpal fractures
  - Bennett
  - Rolando
- Phalanx fractures
- Ulnar Nerve Palsy
- Tendon transfers
- Enchondromas
- Brachial Plexus
- Compartment syndrome
- Mutilating hand trauma
- Replant
- Amputations indications
- Limb salvage
- Nerve repair
- Dorsal hand defects
- Contraction deformities
- Melanoma
- 1st Web space contracture
- Syndactyly (acquired, congenital)
- Thumb duplication
- Thumb reconstruction
- Scaphoid fractures
- Soft tissue reconstruction
  - Fingertips to shoulder
- Local flaps & indications
  - Moberg
  - Kite flap
  - Littler
  - Cross finger

- PEDIATRIC PLASTIC SURGERY
  - Cleft lip
    - Unilateral

- - - Bilateral
  - Cleft palate
    - Isolated
    - Submucous cleft palate
  - Velopharyngeal insufficiency (VPI)
  - Cleft Secondary Revisions
  - Myelomeningocele
  - Microtia/Hemifacial microsomia
  - Facial paralysis
  - Gynecomastia
  - Prominent ear deformity
  - Treacher Collins
  - Macrostomia
  - Syndactyly
  - Brachysyndactyly
  - Macrodactyly
  - Giant congenital nevus
  - Hemangioma
  - Vascular malformations
    - Facial reconstruction
    - Trunk reconstruction
    - Extremity reconstruction
    - Scalp reconstruction
    - Hand soft tissue reconstruction
  - Tissue Expansion
- BURNS
  - Acute injury >30% TBSA
  - Scar management
  - Hand reconstruction
  - Facial reconstruction
    - Ear
    - Eyelid
    - Nose
    - Lips
    - Neck
  - Pediatric burn
  - Keloids/Hypertrophic scar
  - Electrical injuries
  - Chemical Injuries
  - Contracture management
  - General burn reconstruction
    - Scalp

- Neck
- Trunk
- Extremity
- Axilla
- Breast
- Oral commissure
- SPECIAL TOPICS
  - Common flaps in any category
  - Microsurgical principles and management
  - Failed free flap
  - Common complications in any category
  - Healing of grafts (skin, fat, bone)
  - Fat Injections
  - Know classification systems
  - Body dysmorphic syndrome
  - Toxic shock syndrome
  - Necrotizing fasciitis
  - Radiation injury
  - Wide tumor resection any category
  - Maxillofacial prosthesis
  - Palliative care
  - Hand infections
  - Safety issues any category

Study Sheet Template

[Topic]

1. Identify General Problem/Diagnosis/Planning: (Describe photo, working diagnosis, key problems, evaluates patient)

2. Consider reasonable goals in diagnosis and management: (Management and treatment, surgical indications, operative procedures and anesthesia)

3. Select appropriate options in diagnosis and management

4. Understand risks and benefits of various approaches

5. Address complications and unexpected problems adequately

6. Demonstrate ability to structure alternative plan

Presentation Tips
The Formula: Things to Think About When Presenting

1. Identify general problem/diagnosis/planning:
   - List pertinent positives and negatives of history and PE
   - Information that might influence treatment options, choice of operation
   - Your diagnosis will come from your analysis of the given photo.
   - Clinical findings/features of diagnosis

2. Consider reasonable goals in diagnosis and management.
   - Having identified the general problem
   - List if further work-up is necessary
   - Consultants needed?
   - What further work-up you would want or information you would want prior to proceeding with surgery or other management
   - What would you like to achieve, what needs to be addressed

3. Select appropriate options in diagnosis and management.
   - Be able to list the available treatment options
   - Detail the reconstructive ladder
   - Detail the whys and why not's, this demonstrates understanding of the principles.
   - Detail the most appropriate option, explain why
   - Detail timing, operation, post op care

4. Understand the risks and benefits of various approaches.
   - Detail the potential complications & downsides of any approach
   - Some overlap with the selection of options in diagnosis and management
   - Relate the specifics of your chosen procedure
     - Morbidity of donor sites
     - Long-term monitoring
     - Risk of further surgery
   - Anticipated patient satisfaction.

5. Address complications and unexpected problems adequately.
    - Be aware of procedure and condition related complications short-term and long-term
    - Detail your worries (potential for relapse, recurrence, PT requirements)
    - List the most common complications
    - Detail the management of all common complications including timing of management
    - Be prepared for unexpected problems
        - Patient refusing payment
        - Illegal immigrant
        - Angry patient
        - Difficult or noncompliant patient
    - Requesting surgery but unwilling to follow through with post-op care.

6. Demonstrate ability to structure alternative plan.
    - Have multiple reasonable life-boats
    - Detail alternative therapy even if it may not be something "that you do"
    - Anticipate and manage all common complications.
    - Work with or around patient expectations or desires even if not concurrent with your own
    - Be able to work around adverse patient social situations
    - Know when enough is enough or when to reassess

Game Day Strategy

1. Always clearly identify the general problem:
   - Spend some time giving a detailed oral analysis of the photo
     - This establishes your working diagnosis
     - It also demonstrates to the examiner how you evaluate a problem, your thought process and understanding of algorithms
     - It should direct you to your surgical management
     - Will lead you to the next step

2. Consider reasonable goals in diagnosis and management.
   - Quickly mention pertinent medical work-up and history questions you would want to know
   - History related considerations
   - Previous surgeries, identify potential barriers to surgical options
   - Discuss safety issues barriers, things to avoid, goals of
   - reconstruction

3. Select appropriate options in diagnosis and management.
   - Discuss specifically what you think are the key points of managing the presented problem
   - Mention reasonable options for management then choose one
   - Go with the most "standard" first
   - Verbalize the reasons for your decision
   - Climb the ladder one rung at a time

4. Understand the risks and benefits of various approaches.
   - Discuss your informed consent
   - Anticipate complications and interventions to minimize or avoid them
   - Discuss potential benefits of one intervention over another

5. Address complications and unexpected problems adequately.
   - Verbalize complications
   - Be ready to address the most common complications of standard therapies.
   - Etiology and treatment of complications, timing of intervention.

- Know when to ask other disciplines for help including social work, PT, OT

6. Demonstrate ability to structure alternative plan.
    - Have your life-boats prepared and ready before you walk in the room!
    - Address timing
    - Staging of procedures

Run through all of the above in your head with each presented scenario with the 10 minutes given before you walk into the exam room. Cue up your horse and pony show. You should be able to predict the core material to discuss on each scenario before you walk into the room.

Core References

1. Plastic Surgery: Indications and Practice. Guyuron, Eriksson, Persing. Saunders, 2009. ISBN: 978-1-4160-4081-1.

   -Most comprehensive text for oral exam preparation.

2. Plastic and Reconstructive Surgery (Oxford Specialist Handbooks in Surgery). Giele and Cassell. Oxford University Press, 2008. ISBN 978-0-19-263222-7.

   -Particularly excellent for reviewing flaps and surgical procedures. Great short, detailed summaries of all topics.

3. Grabb and Smith's Plastic Surgery. Thorne. Wolters Kluwer Lippincott Williams & Wilkins, 2013. ISBN 978-1-4511-0955-9.

   -Good for cross-checking sources and reviewing basics.

4. Soft-Tissue Surgery of the Craniofacial Region. Persing. CRC Press, 2007. ISBN: 978-0824728939.

   -In particular best chapter on facial paralysis. Great for all facial plastic surgery topics.

5. Plastic Surgery: Clinical Problem Solving. Taub and Koch. McGraw Hill, 2009. ISBN 978-0-07-148150-2.

   -Excellent photos for practicing analysis of scenario pictures.

6. Principles and Practice of Pediatric Plastic Surgery. Bentz, Bauer, Zuker. CRC Press, 2007. ISBN 978-1576262252.

   -Best reference for pediatric plastic surgery topics.

7. The White Journal (PRS) CME articles on any core topic.

   -Generally follows board presentation format, the broad wide strokes of management.

8. Emedicine and Wikipedia

   -Good review for most topics.

TORSO

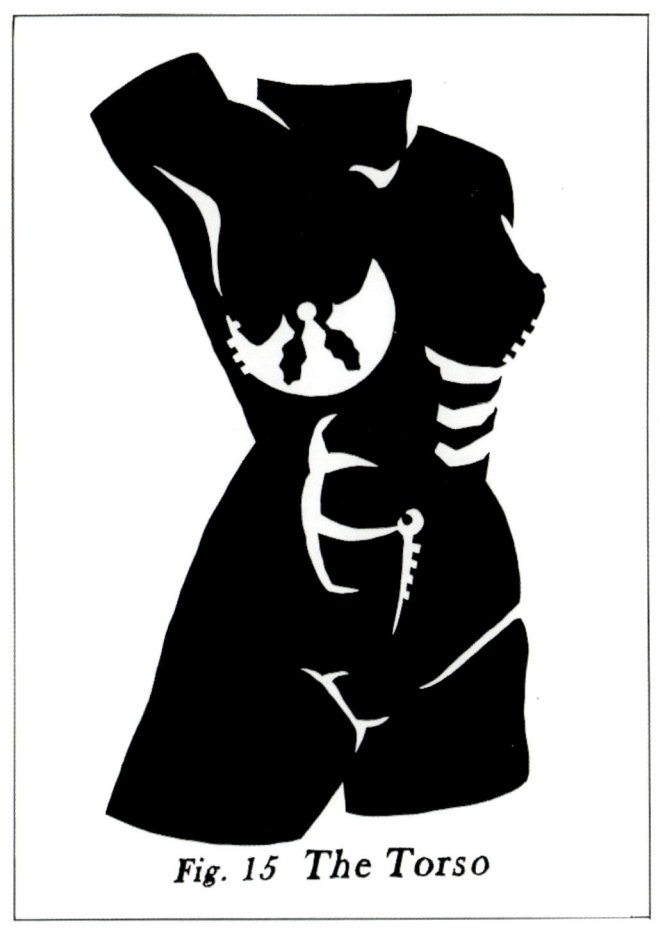

Fig. 15 The Torso

Section One
General Breast

Chapter One

General Breast Overview

———

1
General Breast Overview

1. Identify General Problem

   - Describe photo
   - Give working diagnosis
   - Key problems
   - Evaluate patient
   - Classify deformity, specific diagnosis, grade deformity (Tuberous breast, Poland, Baker's classification, grade ptosis)
   - Note pertinent positives and negatives in H&P
     - Medications: Anticoagulants/steroids/natural supplements
     - Birth control- DVT risk?
     - History of depression? Suicide risk in breast augmentation candidates
     - Brachysyndactyly/upper short limb
     - Examine for pectoralis and latissimus on affected side
     - Scoliosis
     - Sternal deformity
     - If patient is obese (when do you operate? Specific BMI?)
   - Okay to make global statement:
   - "If the patient is a healthy, non-smoker, no DM, CAD, HTN, anticoagulants, steroids, "normal" BMI, not on birth control, no history of depression I would proceed with........"
   - Important to briefly note to examiners you know the relevant potential medical issues prior to proceeding with surgery.
   - Note concerns based on patient age
     - Need for staged reconstruction
     - Plans for child bearing/breast feeding impact
     - Risk of breast cancer
       - Personal history
       - Family history
       - Testing
       - BRCA criteria and interpretation
   - Previous surgeries

- Pre-op work-up
    - B-HCG
    - Imaging? (Mammogram/U/S/MRI) At what age?
    - CXR and EKG over 50ys?
    - Lab work
    - Gynecology work-up? Based on patient age? Other?
        - Endocrine consult
        - Ultrasound
        - Testicular exam
        - Lab work
            - LFT, FSH, LH, Testosterone, TSH
        - Drugs (H2-blockers, marijuana)
        - Tumor (liver, testicular, other)
- What is your pre-op evaluation of patients for breast augmentation?
- Ptosis evaluation
- How do you decide on implant and placement?
- Common conditions to consider
    - Tuberous breast
    - Poland Syndrome
    - Implant Contracture
    - Asymmetric breast
    - Micromastia
    - Macromastia
    - Gynecomastia
- Need for additional work-up for operative planning?

2. Consider reasonable goals in diagnosis and management

    - Individualize, management and treatment
    - Surgical indications
    - Operative procedures and anesthesia
    - Age of patient may affect implant choice
    - Mention all reasonable surgical options

3. Select appropriate options in diagnosis and management

    - Choose and commit to your plan
    - Specify your surgical approach and why?
    - Your timing (staging?)
    - Would you do simultaneous mastopexy and augmentation?
        - Why or why not?

- Clinical concerns
- How do you do your surgery?
  - Incisions
  - Dissection plane of choice
  - Drains?
  - Sutures
  - Skin closure
- What is your post-op management?
  - Antibiotics?
  - Time to return of full activity
  - Bra-support
  - Implant massage
- How is procedure performed?
- Key steps of surgery
- Markings and relevant anatomy

4. Understand risks and benefits of various approaches

- Surgical approaches and differences
- Consider staging procedures
- Discuss all relevant potential complications
- Effect on nipple sensitivity
- Effect on breast feeding
- Scars
- Need for revision or implant exchange
- Saline vs. silicone
- Infected implant
- Nipple necrosis
- Future breast cancer screening
- Eklund views, MRI

5. Address complications and unexpected problems adequately

- Be able to manage all aforementioned complications.
  - Infected implant
  - Loss of nipple sensation
  - Nipple necrosis
  - Cancer in specimen/intraop tumor
  - Wound breakdown
  - Hematoma
  - Inadequate correction/residual deformity

- - - o Double bubble deformities (inferior, superior)
  - Discuss ways to prevent them in your surgical plan or in your post-operative management.
  - Know rates of contracture by implant type
  - % risk of any complication

6. Demonstrate ability to structure alternative plan

    - Patient doesn't agree with your plan.
    - Wants refund after complication.
    - Complications after your initial operation (infected implant, ruptured implant)
    - Nipple reconstruction
    - Scar management
    - Persistent pain post-reduction
    - Inadequate correction
        - o Why?
        - o Your solution?

Chapter Two

Breast Reduction

2
Breast Reduction

1. Identify General Problem/ Diagnosis/Planning
   (Describe photo, working diagnosis, key problems, evaluate patient)

   - Describe physical findings:
     o Breast size, approximate cup size
     o Ptosis
     o Shoulder grooving
     o Nipple areolar complex size
     o Approximate pedicle length
     o Skin changes
     o Any asymmetry?
   - History/Elicit Symptoms:
     o When did enlargement begin, time of problem?
     o Back pain or shoulder pain
     o Musculoskeletal symptoms may be numerous
     o Any previous physical therapy?
     o Skin rashes, dermatitis, and fungal infections
     o Ask about intertrigo
     o SMOKER- potential negative impact on flap survival/nipple areolar complex
     o Plan for future breast-feeding?
     o In juvenile virginal breast hypertrophy not as important, will still proceed with surgery
     o Family history of breast disease/cancer
     o Interference with activity of daily living/psychosocial impact
   - Breast exam
     o Breasts are heavy, solid, difficult to examine
     o Skin under tension
     o Current bra size, usually > D-cup
     o Masses?
     o Check axilla for lymphadenopathy
     o Shoulder grooving
     o Sensory changes?
       - Superior breast *(Supraclavicular n. C3, C4)*

- Medial breast *(anterior cutaneous, 2nd to 7th Thoracic intercostals)*
- Nipple *(lateral cutaneous 4th Thoracic intercostal)*
  - Note skin changes, striae
    - Nipple discharge? (Bloody discharge may indicate tumor)
  - Previous surgical scars
  - OBESITY- Height and Weight- Body Mass Index
    - BMI (kg/m^2) Categories
      - Underweight   <18.5
      - Normal Weight   18.5-24.9
      - Overweight   25-29.9
      - Obesity   >30
      - Severe Obesity   >35
      - Morbid Obesity   >40
      - Super Obesity   >50
- Work-up
  - Suspicious lesions- biopsy
  - Mammography is difficult- dense glandular tissue
  - Mammography not indicated in under age 35.
  - Juvenile Virginal Breast Hypertrophy (JVBH) (gynecomastia)
    - Rapid bilateral change in breast size
    - Interferes with activities of daily living
    - Etiology multifactorial
    - Body weight not a significant role
    - Surgical treatment indicated EARLY
    - Exact etiology unknown
      - Abnormal end organ response to normal levels or systemic hormones
    - Histopathology: no proliferative change, mild hyperplasia

2. Consider reasonable goals in diagnosis and management *(Management and treatment, surgical indications, operative procedures and anesthesia)*

- INDICATIONS FOR SURGERY
- Symptoms associated with large breasts
  - Back pain
  - Neck pain

- o Shoulder grooving
- o Breast pain
- o Rashes
- o Headaches
- o Reduced ability to exercise
- o Numbness and tingling in fingers and hands
- o Impaired psychological wellbeing
- If obese
  - o Start weight loss program- weight watchers, etc.
  - o Loss of breast volume may occur
  - o Decreases morbidity of surgery
  - o In JVBH weight loss will not affect breast volume
- Recommendation for surgery based on:
  - o Severity of problem for patient
  - o Rapidity of breast enlargement
  - o Patient maturity
  - o Patient expectations (scarring, loss of sensation, inability to breast feed)
  - o May be urgent in some cases
  - o TIMING OF SURGERY IMPORTANT
    - JVBH can recur
    - Best timing dictated on case by case basis
- Hormone manipulation no benefit, consider if postop recurrence
- CHALLENGES OF BREAST REDUCTION
  - o Moving nipple-areolar complex to higher position while maintaining blood supply, sensation, breast feeding
  - o Resecting parenchyma without damaging blood supply
  - o Designing skin flaps to preserve blood supply, while excising redundant skin.
  - o Redundant skin will require excision.
- BLOOD SUPPLY
  - o Primarily superficial except for perforators through pectoralis muscle:
  - o Perforator- 4th or 5th interspace from internal mammary artery (IMA) with venae comitantes, several branches
  - o Superficial arteries
  - o 2nd or 3rd interspace from IMA system
  - o Medial branches of IMA
    - o Superficial thoracic vessel
    - o Veins: Found separately, do not accompany arteries, just beneath dermis
- PEDICLE CHOICES:

- Inferior
  - Workhorse, excellent blood supply
  - Good preservation of breast-feeding ability
  - Must accept long-scars and bottoming out
  - Relies on perforator and venae comitantes for blood supply
  - Enters breast just medial to breast meridian about 4-6cm above Inframammary fold (IMF)
  - Safe, reliable
  - Skin used as a brassiere to maintain shape
  - Down side- long scars and bottoming out
- Central
  - Not as reliable as inferior pedicle in regard to blood supply. Relies on perforator
- Superior
  - Supplied by long branch of internal mammary system from 2nd or 3rd interspace
  - Good choice for mastopexy
  - Requires thinning for inset
- Medial
  - Medial vessels, Good sensation
- Lateral
  - Superficial thoracic artery (Problem: it rests in region requiring resection)

Inferior pedicle must be full thickness dermatoglandular to survive, all others except central, may be dermal due to superficial blood supply. In theory innervation and ductal system is preserved only by full thickness pedicle.

- CHOICE OF OPERATION
  - Personal preference
  - All have comparable postop sensibility
  - Lateral 4th intercostal main sensation to nipple areolar complex (NAC)
  - Choice is skin resection pattern and pedicle pattern
- SKIN RESECTION PATTERNS
  - Determined by amount and quality of excess skin:
  - Full inverted-T
    - Most common pattern
    - If significant excess skin or poor quality skin present

- Horizontal and vertical scars
  - Vertical
    - Ideal for small to medium reductions
    - Minimizes scarring
    - Shorter scars
    - Improved shape
    - Less bottoming out
    - Uses breast parenchyma for reshaping
  - Periareolar
    - Small breast reductions
    - Little skin excess
    - Useful in constricted lower pole
      - Tuberous breast deformity

3. Select appropriate options in diagnosis and management

   - Present your proposed operative plan based on surgical options.
   - Address:
     - Parenchymal reduction
     - Skin reduction
     - Preservation of nipple-areolar complex viability
     - Creation of natural shape
   - Breast blood supply:
     - IMA through perforators
     - Lateral thoracic artery (lateral breast)
     - Anterior and lateral branches of intercostals
   - OPTIONS:
   - Liposuction-only
     - Addresses parenchyma only
     - Relies on skin contraction
     - Not an option in JVBH
     - Option in older patients with high adipose content
     - Poor option for glandular breasts
     - Can be used if only small nipple elevation needed
   - Circumareolar technique
     - Addresses skin envelope
     - Useful in small reductions
     - May flatten breast shape
   - Vertical Reduction Mammoplasty
     - Mosque shaped skin incision
     - Scar placement

- Around areola
  - Vertically down breast to IMF
- NAC preserved on skin based pedicle
- Pedicle choices (superior, inferior, medial)
  - Lateral less common, area where tissue excised
- Full thickness pedicle better preserves sensation and breast-feeding ability
- Medial pedicle, tendency superior and inferior dog-ears
  - Superior dog-ear disappears into areola
  - Inferior one disappears with time
- 5% revision rate
- Effects of vertical reduction mammoplasty
  - Cones the breast
  - Narrows the base
  - More projection

- Steps of Vertical Reduction Mammoplasty
  - Mark with patient standing
  - Symmetry for what is left behind
  - IMF level
  - Breast meridian (ignores nipple position)
  - New nipple position (at most projected part of breast)
    - 2cm lower than inverted T
    - Important to determine preop
  - Areolar opening
    - End as circle when closed
  - Skin resection pattern
    - Shape determined by resection and closure of breast pillars
  - Avoid bringing pattern down to IMF
  - Pedicle design
    - Half below and half above areolar opening
    - Keep a vein in design
  - Infiltrate
  - Create pedicle
  - Tissue resection
    - En bloc, beveled medially and laterally
    - Leave wise pattern of breast parenchyma not skin
  - Pillar closure/Skin closure

- Inverted-T skin incision (Wise pattern)
    - Addresses skin and parenchymal excess
    - Useful in large volume reductions
    - Marked with patient standing
    - Sternum/Breast meridian
    - Critical determine-level of nipple areola complex
        - AVOID TOO HIGH- hard to correct
    - IMF acceptable level for NAC placement
    - In asymmetric breast use the higher position
    - Mark keyhole
        - Increase width to increase skin excision
    - Inferior pedicle
        - Horizontal excision
        - Medial and lateral dog-ears
        - Inferior pedicle must be: Full thickness dermoglandular pedicle to survive
- Steps of Inverted-T Breast Reduction
    - Markings with patient standing
    - IMF level
    - Breast meridian
    - New nipple position (at most projecting portion of breast)
    - Areolar opening
    - Skin resection pattern- vertical limbs 5-6cm
    - Pedicle design 8-10cm wide at base
        - Perforator enters just medial to meridian 4-6cm above IMF
        - Leave tissue over pectoralis fascia to preserve nerve
    - Infiltration
    - Pedicle creation
    - Tissue resection within keyhole pattern
    - Flap closure/Skin closure
        - Postop: Drains (+/-, your choice), Sports bra
    - Inverted T with free nipple grafting
        - For larger breast
        - Patients with poor skin quality
        - Free nipple graft may be required
        - May need to convert to free nipple if nipple appears significantly compromised during surgery
    - What is your postop management protocol?

- o What is your deep vein thrombosis protocol?

4. Understand risks and benefits of various approaches

    - Review above discussion under OPTIONS.

5. Address complications and unexpected problems adequately

    - Unsightly scarring
    - Loss of sensation- nipple and/or breast skin
    - Inability to breast-feed
    - Sensation 85% for all pedicles (normal to near normal)
    - Complete symmetry is NOT possible
    - Risk of nipple necrosis 1 in 300
    - Early surgical complications (generally <5% of cases)
        - o Hematoma
        - o Impending nipple compromise
        - o Early dusky or engorged nipple (venous congestion)
            - Remove sutures
            - No improvement return to OR
            - Check for kinking of pedicle
        - o Deep vein thrombosis
    - Late complications
        - o Infection, poor wound healing, seroma
    - Compromised nipple
        - o Topical antibiotics until healed, reconstruction delayed for 3 months after complete healing
    - Nipple necrosis
        - o Allow demarcation
        - o Debride
        - o Topical antibiotics
        - o Healing by secondary intention
        - o Reconstruct

6. Demonstrate ability to structure alternative plan

    - Your management of complications
    - Manage patient expectations
    - How would to manage?
        - o Cancer in pathology specimen
        - o Early wound dehiscence
        - o Recurrent hypertrophy
        - o Dissatisfied patient

Chapter Three

Breast Augmentation

3
Breast Augmentation

1. Identify General Problem/Diagnosis/Planning
   (Describe photo, working diagnosis, key problems, evaluate patient)

   - Most important consideration:
     - Patient motives for augmentation
     - Reasonable expectations
   - General indication/clinical scenario:
     - Subjective hypomastia
     - Post pregnancy glandular ptosis
   - History (Hx):
   - Pertinent Positives:
     - Family Hx breast cancer
     - Associated congenital anomalies
     - Medical Hx
       - Birth control- deep venous thrombosis risk
       - Coagulation disorders
       - Steroids
       - Diabetes mellitus
       - Other
   - Physical Exam (PE)
   - Note what you will look for:
     - Chest wall asymmetries (scoliosis)
     - Differences in breast volumes and dimensions
     - Degree of breast ptosis
     - Size of nipple areola complex (NAC)
     - Skin quality
       - Tone, Elasticity
       - Presence or absence of striae
     - Signs of malignancy:
       - Check for unusual masses in breast/axilla
       - Skin dimpling
       - Nipple discharge
     - Specifically note:
       - Sternal width
       - Inframammary fold (IMF) location

- o In unilateral micromastia note extremities for brachysyndactyly, check for chest wall deformity
- Identify and communicate all preoperative asymmetries to patient prior to procedure
  - o Any asymmetry will persist and may be amplified postoperatively
- Breast measurements
  - o Used to determine implant size and shape:
  - o Sternal notch to nipple distance
  - o Nipple to IMF fold distance
  - o **Base diameter (width) of breast (most important parameter)**
  - o **Exception tubular breast deformity, narrow base width**
  - o N:IMF length should correspond to implant volume
    - 7cm at 250ml
    - 8cm at 300ml
    - 8.5cm at 350ml
    - 9cm at 375ml
    - 9.5cm at 400ml
  - o Areola to IMF distance should approximate radius of implant and half of breast base width.
  - o Intra-nipple distance
  - o Amount of forward mobility of nipple when traction applied anteriorly
  - o Pinch test- tells about parenchymal coverage- superior and lower poles
  - o Parenchymal coverage:
  - o Greater the projection and parenchymal coverage
  - o The less projection needed in underlying implant.
- Work Up
  - o IS PREOP MAMMOGRAM NEEDED?
  - o American cancer society now recommends baseline mammogram at age 50, up from age 40.
  - o Not necessary in young patient (20's) and no family history
  - o At 50 baseline mammogram recommended
  - o Over 40 and family history of breast cancer get baseline mammogram
  - o GET SCREENING MAMMOGRAM IF AGE 35 or OLDER AND PLANING TO OPERATE ON BREAST.

- Consider screening ultrasound in patients under 35 with strong family history of breast cancer.
- Mammogram is **not** indicated in patients under 35.
- No specific consultations needed.
  - Psychiatry consult
    - If body dysmorphic syndrome, depression or suicidal ideation suspected & don't operate
- PATIENT DISCUSSION
  - Desired breast size
  - Types of implants available
  - Surface (smooth, textured)
    - Smooth- less palpable
    - Textured- less capsular contracture
      - More propensity to show dimpling or waviness
  - Shape (round, anatomic)
    - Anatomic treats superior pole deficiency
    - Problems: potential to rotate and cause asymmetry
    - Round
      - Low profile
      - Moderate profile
      - High profile
      - Other profiles
    - Profile
      - Refers to increased projection for given base width
      - HIGH profile preferred in tuberous breast deformity
  - Filler (silicone, saline)
    - Saline
      - Traditionally lower capsular contracture rates, today's silicone has similar contracture rates to saline.
      - Can be placed through smaller incisions
      - Higher rupture risk especially if not overfilled
      - Requires 3-4 cm incision

- Silicone
    - Feels more natural
    - Rupture more difficult to diagnose
    - Requires intermittent MRI f/u
    - Does not adjust to body temp changes quickly (cool after swimming)
    - Requires 4.5- 6.0 cm incision
    - Current generation- thicker shell, cohesive gel filler
        - Maintains integrity after rupture
- All implants are a lifetime commitment- not permanent!
    - Modern implants likely to last 10-20 years
- Re-operation will be necessary at some point in time!
    - Exchange minimum intervention that will be needed
    - Revision may be necessary
- On-going surveillance needed especially with silicone.
- Ecklund view added to standard mammogram for cancer surveillance
- No increase in cancer risk or increase in poor outcomes in breast cancer.
- No reports of higher stage breast cancer at time of diagnosis in breast augmentation patients vs. patients without breast augmentation.
- Increased suicide rate in patients that undergo breast augmentation.
- Suspicion of psychiatric issues or unreasonable expectations refer for counseling.

2. Consider reasonable goals in diagnosis and management *(Management and treatment, surgical indications, operative procedures and anesthesia)*

- INDICATIONS

- Hypomastia
- Glandular ptosis
- Grade I Breast ptosis
- Congenital breast issues (tuberous breast deformity, Poland syndrome, volumetric asymmetry)
- Involutional breast deformity (weight loss or pregnancy and breast feeding)
- Normal breast volume in patients who desire more youthful appearance
- Can give appearance of breast lift and increased cleavage
- Implants may augment mastopexy in area of superior pole fullness

- **CONTRAINDICATIONS**
  - Unrealistic expectations
  - Body dysmorphic disorder
  - Presence of untreated breast oncologic disease
  - Unstable weight
  - Ongoing breast-feeding
  - Grade 2 or 3 ptosis without mastopexy
  - Response to peer, spousal, parental pressure
  - Under age 18, controversial

- **RELATIVE CONTRAINDICATION**
  - Smoking
  - Diabetes Mellitus
  - Radiation therapy
  - Preop breast shape:
  - If constricted base
    - Periareolar or transaxillary approach beneficial
  - Small areola:
    - Not a candidate for silicone implant through periareolar approach
    - Must use inframammary approach in this situation
  - Base diameter dictates upper limit of implant volume.
  - Higher incidence of asymmetry and revision in >350ml augmentation.

- **IMPLANT SELECTION**
  - Based on:
    - Patient desire

- Width of existing glandular tissue, desired breast width
- Thorax shape
- Envelope characteristics
- Amount and shape of glandular tissue
- Digital imaging
- Photos of other women
          - To increase one cup size 125-150 ml needed
          - Larger body frame larger implant needed
    - Breast measurements
          - Used to determine implant size and shape:
          - Sternal notch to nipple distance
          - Nipple to IMF fold distance
          - **Base diameter (width) of breast (most important parameter)**
              - **Exception tubular breast deformity, narrow base width**
          - N:IMF length should correspond to implant volume
              - 7cm at 250ml
              - 8cm at 300ml
              - 8.5cm at 350ml
              - 9cm at 375ml
              - 9.5cm at 400ml
          - Areola to IMF distance should approximate radius of implant and half of breast base width
          - Intra-nipple distance
          - Amount of forward mobility of nipple when traction applied anteriorly
          - Pinch test- tells about parenchymal coverage- superior and lower poles
          - Parenchymal coverage:
          - Greater the projection and parenchymal coverage
          - The less projection needed in underlying implant.
          - Use intraop breast sizer to assist implant selection.
    - Access incisions:
          - Inframammary
          - Periareolar
              - Widely used, well-hidden scar
              - Can affect sensory nerve and more contamination than inframammary approach
          - Transaxillary
              - Requires specialized equipment

- Incision at vertex or 1-2cm medial to vertex of axilla
- Follow skin creases, perpendicular to length of axilla
- Subglandular or submuscular implant placement
- Blind dissection
- Hard to divide inferior medial muscle
- Cannot do dual plane
- Difficult to control implant folds and rotation
- Less lower pole control
            - Transumbilical
                - Requires specialized equipment
                - More amenable to saline implant
                - More difficult to control placement
                - Remote incisions
        - Tissue pocket planes:
            - Subglandular- increased capsular contracture
            - Subfascial
            - Submuscular
            - Dual plane- below pectoralis superiorly, below breast parenchyma inferiorly

3. Select appropriate options in diagnosis and management

    - Present your proposed operative plan.
    - Implant placement
        - Triple antibiotic solution
            - 50,000 bacitracin, 80mg gentamicin, 1gm cefazolin in 500ml NS
        - Betadine okay for extraluminal use
        - Respect medial border of pocket (cleavage definition)
        - Respect Inframammary fold
            - Determines implant location on the chest
        - Lateral dissection depends on diameter of implant
            - Minimize to avoid lateral migration of implant
        - Avoid blunt dissection
            - Less risk of hematoma

- - - o Leave tissue on ribs in submuscular implant placement
    - o Position is always under glandular tissue
    - o Consider vertical location of implant on chest wall
      - ▪ Too high- NAC will point down
      - ▪ Too low- breast too full in lower pole
    - o Ideal nipple position central on implant
      - ▪ Half above and half below
  - ▪ In subpectoralis pocket
    - o Critical to release muscle inferiorly
    - o No touch technique to minimize contamination
      - ▪ Glove change
      - ▪ Only surgeon touches implant
      - ▪ Antibiotic irrigation
  - ▪ Subglandular vs. submuscular based on pinch test
    - o Pinch below 2-3 cm + 1-1.5cm tissue cover
      - ▪ Generally place submuscularly
    - o Pinch > 4cm
      - ▪ Subglandular may be favorable
      - ▪ Submuscular can be used
  - ▪ Subglandular
    - o More natural aging with gradual ptosis
    - o Favored position in tuberous breast deformity.
  - ▪ Submuscular
    - o Better soft tissue cover
    - o Less visibility
    - o Less soft tissue atrophy
    - o Better long-term results
    - o Incise and close pectoralis fascia
    - o Subcuticular closure
  - ▪ Postop Care
    - o +/- drains through axilla
    - o Prophylactic antibiotics
      - ▪ Postop antibiotics 3 days: Common practice
    - o Perioperative antibiotics
      - ▪ Keflex or Clindamycin
    - o Arm elevation directly after procedure
    - o Implant massage
    - o Stretch pectoralis muscle once per hour; first 24 hrs
    - o Sports and vigorous activity 3 weeks
    - o Sports that exert tension on scar or too much implant movement tennis, trampoline bouncing 3 months.

4. Understand risks and benefits of various approaches

    - Saline vs. Silicone
    - Incision choices
    - Subglandular vs. submuscular placement
    - Breast cancer risk
    - Breast screening issues

5. Address complications and unexpected problems adequately

    - Oversized implants higher complication rate (larger than 350-400ml)
        o Stretch and stress tissues
        o Atrophy and thinning of parenchymal and skin
        o Increased palpability
        o Traction rippling
    - Avoid patients who expect exact results
    - Caution in severe asymmetry cases
    - Capsular contracture (10%)
        o Baker Classification (I-IV)
        o I- soft and natural
        o II- firm
        o III- firm with visible deformity
        o IV- cool, hard, visible deformity and pain
        o Cause-subclinical infection Staph. epidermidis
        o Treatment
            - Implant removal
            - Capsulectomy
            - Implant replacement
        o Most contractures occur within 1 year
    - Leak or rupture (1%/year)
        o May require MRI for workup for silicone (linguine sign)
        o Saline- days to weeks leak will be clinically evident
        o Treat as soon as possible to prevent further distortion
    - Increased areolar diameter
        o Treatment: mastopexy, potential for scarring
            - Use purse string with permanent suture- Gortex first choice
    - Change in nipple sensation

- - - - - Permanent in 15%
    - 5% loss of some nipple sensation on one breast
    - Cannot guarantee sensation will be preserved
    - If patient wants sensation preserved do not operate
    - Not correctable
  - Increased sensitivity 6-9 weeks postop normal
  - Pneumothorax (rare)
    - Thoracic surgery consult
    - Chest tube may or may not be needed
  - Hematoma (0.5-2%)
    - Treatment: Return to OR and drain
      - Untreated hematoma may result in: Scarring and contracture
  - Infection <1%
    - Treatment
      - Early infection
        - Implant may be salvaged with antibiotics alone
        - Immediate replacement with new implant after aggressive washout
          - Likelihood of salvage 70%
      - If antibiotics fail:
        - Washout pocket
        - Send cultures
        - Remove implant
  - Asymmetry and implant malposition
    - Re-operate to correct if deformity is amenable to correction
    - Implant visibility
    - Rippling
    - Synmastia
    - Perforation
    - Implant extrusion
    - Double bubble deformity
      - Type B-implant significantly lower than IMF below breast mound
      - Type A- implant above breast mound
      - Your management algorithm?
    - Deformation during pectoralis muscle contraction
    - Re-operation rates
      - Saline 13% at 3 years
      - Silicone 21% at 3 years

- - - o Interference with cancer surveillance (Eklund views vs. MRI)
  - Capsulectomy Indications
    - o Baker III and IV
    - o Calcified or thick capsule
    - o Ruptured silicone implant
    - o Silicone granulomas
    - o Infection around implant
    - o Previous implant that needs to be changed to larger volume
    - o New plane needed
    - o More difficult hemostasis
    - o Reduces recurrence of contracture
    - o Controlled scoring through capsule, concentric, radial

6. Demonstrate ability to structure alternative plan

   - Cancer surveillance
     - o Standard mammogram with additional Ecklund view
   - Management of different breast shapes and sizes
   - Familiarity with various access incisions
   - Indications and familiarity with saline and silicone implants
   - Patient doesn't agree with your surgical plan

Chapter Four

Mastopexy

4
Mastopexy

1. Identify General Problem /Diagnosis/Planning
   (Describe photo, working diagnosis, key problems, evaluates patient)

   - Ptosis Classification (Regnault)
     - Grade I- NAC at IMF, above lower contour of gland
     - Grade II- NAC below IMF, above lower gland contour
     - Grade III- NAC points downward, at lower contour of gland
     - Pseudoptosis- Gland hangs below IMF
   - Hx:
     - Prior surgery
     - Family Hx of breast cancer
       - Preop mammogram if risk factors > 35 yo
       - If + family history and age <35 screening US
   - PE:
     - Note:
       - Breast shape
       - Tissue laxity
       - Symmetry
       - Parenchymal distribution
       - Nipple position
     - What are patient goals?
       - Patient must be willing to accept scars
     - Note asymmetries preop
     - Breast exam
       - Check for lumps and masses
       - Examine axilla for lymphadenopathy
       - Measurements
       - Breast width
       - Breast height
       - Intermammary distance
       - Nipple to suprasternal notch
       - Nipple to inframammary fold (N:IMF)
     - Adequacy of skin envelope

- o Plans for more pregnancies +/- future breast feeding?
  - If yes, may be better to defer surgery
  - Pregnancy found to be a key factor of ptosis, NOT breastfeeding
- o Depending on age of the patient mention basic medical history
  - DM
  - HTN
  - Smoker
  - Steroid use
  - Anticoagulants
  - Birth control, risk for DVT
  - Other

2. Consider reasonable goals in diagnosis and management *(Management and treatment, surgical indications, operative procedures and anesthesia)*

- INDICATION
  - o Breast Ptosis
  - o Goals
    - Reshape breast by tightening skin envelope with or without adding volume to breast
    - Raise NAC
    - Decrease skin envelope
    - Achieve symmetry
    - Improve breast shape
    - Maintain or increase volume
  - o May require augmentation
    - Especially if loss of upper pole volume
  - o Factors
    - Involution
    - Aging/gravity
    - Weight loss or weight gain
    - Multiple pregnancies
  - o Minimize scars if possible
  - o Individualize plan for each patient
    - Determine need for augmentation
      - Implant vs. flap
    - Breast shaping

- Sutures
- Local flaps
- Muscle slings
- Internal mesh support
  - Mark while sitting:
    - NAC measured from:
      - Sternal notch
    - Mid-clavicular area
    - Submammary fold
    - Midline
    - Current IMF
    - Planned nipple position
  - Nipple position
    - Use IMF as guide
    - Mark breast meridian
    - Palpate fold and mark approximately 20cm +/- 3cm from suprasternal notch
  - Excision pattern
  - Post op antibiotics 3 days
  - Vigorous exercise resumed 2-4 weeks

3. Select appropriate options in diagnosis and management

   - Present your proposed operative plan.
     - IF augmentation and mastopexy performed:
       - Safe answer:
       - Ideal stage in two surgeries
     - If pushed to do in one surgery:
     - AUGMENTATION FIRST THEN MASTOPEXY TO AVOID SKIN SHORTAGE AFTER MASTOPEXY PEFORMED.
   - MINOR PTOSIS
     - Breast augmentation alone
     - May correct mild ptosis
     - Downgrades ptosis
     - One stage
     - Periareolar approach if minor ptosis <3cm of nipple movement needed
       - Concentrically or eccentrically marked
       - Scar at border of areola

- Nipple marker 38-42mm size for NAC
- Tends to flatten breast shape
- MODERATE PTOSIS
    - Vertical excision
        - Determine nipple position
    - Distance from center of nipple position to new NAC border sets width of excision
    - Vertical limbs end 1-2 cm above IMF
    - Tightening lower poles redistributes fullness superiorly
    - Improves shape and projection
- SEVERE PTOSIS
    - Inverted-T Wise pattern excision pattern
    - Shorter horizontal component
    - Superiomedial pedicle used here vs. inferior pedicle in reduction surgery
- SIMULTANEOUS IMPLANT AND MASTOPEXY
    - Breast augmentation through planned mastopexy incisions
    - Tailor tack and adjust incisions prior to completion of mastopexy
- IMPLANT SELECTION SEE BREAST AUG CHAPTER
- Use periareolar purse string which enhances tightening, minimizes scarring in all types of mastopexy
    - Nonabsorbable Gortex

4. Understand risks and benefits of various approaches

- Consider one vs. two stages in simultaneous augmentation and mastopexy
- Consider indications for different types of mastopexy
- What is your surgical goal?

5. Address complications and unexpected problems adequately

- Hematoma
- Infection
- Paresthesia
- Anesthesia
- Nipple areola necrosis
- Capsular contracture
- Errors in nipple placement

- Revision for asymmetry
- Recurrent ptosis
- Wide scars
- Skin necrosis
- What is your management plan/algorithm for common complications?

6. Demonstrate ability to structure alternative plan

    - Inadequate correction of ptosis
    - Overcorrection with high nipple
    - Abnormal implant position
    - Double bubble deformities
    - Patient does not agree with suggested plan of operation
    - Reasonable alternative choices?

Chapter Five

Gynecomastia

5
Gynecomastia

1. Identify General Problem/Diagnosis/Planning
   (Describe photo, working diagnosis, key problems, evaluate patient)

   - Gynecomastia vs. Pseudogynecomastia
     - Describe photo, comment on:
       Excess skin and ptosis (Will skin excision be needed? Your best guess)
       - Quantify and classify amount of skin excess and ptosis
       - Multiple classification systems, use one and be familiar with it
       - Amount of fatty tissue
       - Suction-assisted lipectomy (SAL) or Ultrasound assisted lipectomy (UAL) vs. direct excision or combination of techniques
       - Amount of glandular tissue (UAL vs. direct excision)
       - Size of nipple areolar complex (NAC)
         - (reduce nipple or transpose? size >2.7cm is abnormal)
       - Grade of gynecomastia (I-III)
     - >2cm enlargement of nipple
     - Bilateral vs. Unilateral
     - Risk of malignancy (not increased)
   - History and PE to delineate etiology
     - Age of patient (infantile, adolescent, old age)
     - Most cases asymptomatic but can have associated pain
     - Is it stable? Persistent 1 year or longer?
     - Testicular masses
     - Breast examination
     - Grade of Gynecomastia (Simon Classification)
       - Grade 1: Small enlargement, no skin excess
       - Grade 2a: Moderate enlargement, no skin excess

- Grade 2b: Moderate enlargement with extra skin
- Grade 3: Marked enlargement with extra skin
  - Asymmetric enlargement
  - Discrete lesion
  - Tenderness
  - Check for lymphadenopathy
  - Clinical signs of feminization
  - Clinical signs of endocrine disorders
- CAUSES OF GYNECOMASTIA
  - Sporadic cases
  - Increased estrogen
  - Decreased testosterone
  - Infectious
  - Neoplastic local or distant
  - Systemic disease (liver dysfunction, others)
  - Drugs (marijuana use, H2 Blockers, other)
- INDICATIONS FOR INTERVENTION
  - Functional problems
  - Limitation of ability to exercise
  - Pain
  - Suspicion of malignancy
  - Psychosocial adjustment
    - Primary reason in pediatric cases
  - Rule out (R/O) coexisting medical conditions
    - Testicular tumors increased
    - Liver disease
    - Renal failure
    - Endocrine disorders (in 12% of teens)
    - Medication use or drug use
      - Marijuana
      - Heroine
      - Cimetidine (H2 Blockers)
      - Digoxin
      - Theophylline
      - Tricyclic antidepressants
  - Preop work up
    - R/O testicular mass
    - Consider Endocrine and nutrition consults
    - Labs
      - Endocrine work up

- LFT's
- Estradiol
- LH
- FSH
- Beta HCG
- Consider urine studies
  - Teens allow one to two years for regression prior to surgery
    - Most cases are sporadic but endocrine work-up should be done pre-op
  - Note any breast asymmetry preoperatively, likely to be persistent postoperatively (eg. nipple position, breast size)

2. Consider reasonable goals in diagnosis and management *(Management and treatment, surgical indications, operative procedures and anesthesia)*

   - Management Based On Etiology
     - Sporadic
     - Drugs
     - Endocrine
     - Tumor
   - Medical treatment if medical cause found:
     - Testosterone replacement- testicular failure
     - Tamoxifen- for non-operative candidates who are older men
     - Danazol androgen- may reduce pain
     - Clomiphene anti-estrogen agent in teens
     - Treat testicular tumor if present
   - Surgical options based on clinical presentation: Must address:
     - Excess skin
     - Ptosis
     - Amount of glandular vs. fibrous tissue
     - Size of nipples
   - Options:
     - SAL
     - UAL
     - Direct excision
     - Skin reduction techniques
     - +/- NAC reduction, reposition or free nipple grafting
     - Combination of techniques
   - What are your personal indications for each of these options?

- Surgical Techniques
    - Direct excision no skin resection
    - Circumareolar excision
    - Dounut mastopexy
    - Wise pattern skin excision (avoid)
    - Inframammary fold excision/mastectomy with nipple free graft
- Detail how you perform each operation? (5 Main Steps)
- Goals of surgery
    - Minimize scarring
    - Improve shape and contour
    - Match patient goals
    - Alleviate symptoms if present
- Male nipple- How do you position the nipple?
    - Suggestion
        - Ideal nipple size 2.8cm (Same size as a quarter (2.5cm) + marking (0.3cm))
        - Nipple plane located at 0.33 distance of sternal notch to pubis
        - Inter-nipple distance 0.23 x chest circumference
        - Nipple position lateral to breast meridian

3. Select appropriate options in diagnosis and management

- Present your proposed operative plan based on patient pathology and available surgical options.
- Specify your choice of operation and operative plan.
- Justify your choice.
- Discuss your expectations and anticipated outcome.
    - Easy vs. difficult case
    - Risk of residual skin
    - Chances of needed a revision
- Periop and postop management.
    - Postop care
        - Drains?
            - Remove when <30ml/day general guideline
        - Pressure Garment 6wks
        - Activity restriction 6wks
        - Periop antibiotics yes or no? (your choice, justify)

- Avoiding complications
  - Preserve 1.5cm button of tissue in circumareolar excision
  - Thick skin flaps in periareolar excision
  - Periareloar excision no more than 2-3cm skin excision from areola
  - Permanent 2-0 suture around areola (Nylon, Gortex, other)
  - Drains +/- Compression garments minimum 2 weeks
  - Pressure garments/silicone sheeting/scar massage
  - Thrombin/Fibrin glue?
- Safety Measures
- In UAL:
  - Wet cloths
    - Cannula sheath
    - Prevent burn injury
  - Control tip of cannula with nondominant hand
    - Avoid intraabdominal perforation
  - Sequential Compression Device initiated prior to anesthesia induction
    - Prevent DVT

4. Understand risks and benefits of various approaches

   - What are the potential risk benefits of different procedures?
   - May require revision if inadequate result. When would you time revision?
   - Skin shrinkage post-op generally anticipated except in bariatric cases
   - Marked enlargement generally warrants skin excision
   - Avoid overresection of breast tissue- saucer deformity can result

5. Address complications and unexpected problems adequately

   - Asymmetry- requires revision
   - Inadequate volume reduction
   - Overcorrection- saucer deformity
   - Post-op irregularity common

- Recurrence
- Hematoma may require drainage
    - Most common complication 5-15% of cases
- Seroma
- Infection- periop antibiotics only
- Drains for wide resections
- Nipple areolar complex (NAC) necrosis 2-3%
    - How would you manage this?
- Nipple numbness- uncorrectable if permanent
- Hypopigmentation
- What is your management plan for various complications?

6. Demonstrate ability to structure alternative plan

- Medical therapy
- Revision plans (SAL, UAL only vs. additional skin excision)
- Management of skin necrosis
- Nipple position asymmetry
- Multiple surgical options
- Timing of re-operation

Chapter Six

Poland Syndrome

6
Poland Syndrome

1. Identify General Problem/Diagnosis/Planning
   (Describe photo, working diagnosis, key problems, evaluates patient)

   - Describe chest asymmetry in detail, what do you see?
   - Hx:
   - Determine etiology
     o Based on presentation what is most likely?
     o Surgery iatrogenic from breast lesion intervention
       - Neonatal chest tube
       - Any surgery during infancy or childhood?
     o Congenital (intravascular accident in utero)
   - When was deformity noted?
     o Frequently not noted at birth
   - Functional limitations?
   - Occupation/avocations
     o May contraindicate latissimus use for reconstruction
     o Athletes
   - Medical hx
   - Family Hx breast disease
   - Smoker?
   - Psychosocial concerns- self-esteem peer interaction
   - Most young women with chest wall asymmetry DO NOT have Poland syndrome
   - PE
   - Classification of Poland Syndrome
     o Class I- Chest asymmetry from:
       - Hypoplastic breast
       - Small elevated nipple
       - Hypoplastic pectoralis major
       - Normal thoracic skeleton
     o Class II- Chest asymmetry from:
       - Hypoplastic breast
       - Hypoplastic/absent nipple
       - Absent sternal head pectoralis major
       - Minor thoracic skeleton abnormalities
     o Class III- Chest asymmetry from:

- - - Hypoplastic breast
    - Hypoplastic/absent nipple
    - Absent sternal head pectoralis major
    - Marked thoracic skeleton abnormalities
  - Identify and describe specific chest wall asymmetries
  - Hand anomalies?
    - Brachydactyly
    - Syndactyly
    - Both?
  - Breast exam
    - Underdevelopment on one side, hallmark of Poland
    - Third phase of breast development at puberty from hormonal influences
    - Check:
    - Breast volume
    - Position of IMF
    - Asymmetry in position and volume of NAC
    - Note discrepancies with opposite breast
    - Usually hypoplastic but nipple and/or areolar complex is formed
  - If bilateral look for other causes: R/O
    - Amastia
    - Athelia
    - Tuberous breast
    - Polymastia
    - Polythelia
  - Chest wall exam
    - Absence of pectoralis major muscle
    - Absence or hypoplasia
      - Pectoralis minor
      - Serratus
      - Infraspinatus
      - Supraspinatous
      - External oblique
      - **Latissimus dorsi- test for presence**
    - Skin quality
    - Hypoplastic
    - Absence of subcutaneous fat
    - Thoracic skeleton
      - Sternal deformity
      - Winged scapula (Sprengel deformity)
      - Absence of anterolateral ribs?

- o Vascular anomalies? Esp. thoracodorsal, IMA
    - Extremity
        - o Shortening of the limb
        - o Brachysyndactyly
        - o Symphalangism with syndactyly
        - o Hypoplasia or absence of middle phalanges
    - About Poland Sequence
    - Poland incidence 1:30K
        - o Sporadic
        - o Generally unilateral
        - o More common on the right
        - o Ratio Right:Left 2:1
    - Poland sequence
        - o Congenital hypoplasia of subclavian artery
        - o More proximal occlusion more severe deformity
    - Associated anomalies
        - o Moebius CN VI and VII 1 in 500K
            - Especially in left sided Poland
        - o Leukemia
            - Non-Hodgkin's lymphoma
    - Presents in teen years unless distal extremity involvement present and diagnosed in infancy
    - Elaborate patient concerns
        - o What are the patient's goals?
    - Preop patient education is critical
    - Perfect symmetry not possible
    - Additional work-up
    - IS PREOP MAMMOGRAM NEEDED?
        - o Generally NOT indicated
        - o Dense breast parenchyma in young patients
        - o Poor study for evaluating breast in young patients.
        - o American cancer society now recommends baseline mammogram at age 50, up from age 40.
        - o Over 40 and family history of breast cancer get baseline mammogram
        - o Not necessary in young pt (20's) and no FHx
    - GET SCREENING MAMMOGRAM IF AGE 35 or OLDER AND PLANING TO OPERATE ON BREAST.
        - o Consider screening ultrasound in patients under 35 with strong family history of breast cancer.
        - o Mammogram is **not** indicated in patients under 35.
    - Other Imaging

- o Chest x-ray important to check presence of absence of ribs.
- o CT scan or MRI considered in severe deformity
  - Delineates abnormal chest wall anatomy
  - May be helpful in planning reconstruction or designing implant
  - Consider preop angiogram for thoracodorsal vessel
- o Consultations: Genetics

2. Consider reasonable goals in diagnosis and management *(Management and treatment, surgical indications, operative procedures and anesthesia)*

    - INDICATIONS
      - o Cosmesis/breast aesthetics
      - o Psychosocial issues
    - TIMING
      - o May be postponed until after breast maturity, if possible
        - Improves ability to achieve symmetry
      - o Earlier correction if major psychosocial reasons
      - o Tissue expansion beginning in childhood through puberty to keep pace with developing breast with definitive treatment after completion of breast development
    - CHEST WALL IS FOUNDATION FOR RECONSTRUCTION
      - o Severe defects
        - Customized chest wall implants
        - Autogenous rib grafts
        - Marlex or prolene mesh
        - Sternal wedge osteotomy
      - o Brachysyndactyly
        - May benefit from widening first web space
        - Syndactyly reconstruction in infancy as indicated

3. Select appropriate options in diagnosis and management

    - Multiple treatment options:
    - Female patients

- Tissue Expander (TE) and/or implants
    - TE advantage in developing patients to mirror growth of opposite side
    - TE useful if significant skin shortage present
- Latissimus dorsi muscle flap/implant most popular technique
    - Pedicled
    - Free latissimus from opposite side
- TRAM may be needed if:
    - Hypoplastic skin
    - Muscle coverage poor for implant
    - Thoracodorsal vessels will not support latissimus
- Alternative flap: superior or inferior artery gluteal artery flap
- Male patients
    - Latissimus dorsi muscle flap and/or customized implant
        - Pedicled latissimus
        - Free latissimus from opposite side (especially in male patients)
        - No consensus on best technique
        - Benefit of muscle flap no additional surgery needed
        - Try to recreate axillary fold in males
    - Prepare to discuss main steps of latissimus reconstruction or customized implant placement.
    - Be prepared to describe your surgical approach and postop management short-term and long-term.

4. Understand risks and benefits of various approaches

- Understand benefits and risks of each approach in the male or female patient
    - Tissue expanders and or implant only
    - Latissimus reconstruction with or without implant
    - TRAM flap
- Discuss your approach to the timing of surgical intervention based on patient age and circumstances.
- What is your tissue expansion protocol? Your preferred implant for tissue expansion?
- Management of implants (See Breast Augmentation chapter)

5. Address complications and unexpected problems adequately

    - More common in cases of severe thoracic wall deformity treated with implants
    - Infection
    - Infected implant
    - Hematoma
    - Seroma in latissimus reconstruction
    - Asymmetry- guaranteed, educate
        - Revise if amenable
    - Implant capsular contracture
    - Partial or total flap loss
    - Re-explore compromised flap
        - Debride
        - Allow healing
        - Revise
    - Donor site morbidity
        - Specific to site
    - Long thoracic nerve injury (C5-C7)- serratus innervation- winged scapula (Sprengel deformity)
    - Ventral hernia or abdominal bulge in TRAM
    - Interference with cancer surveillance
        - Baseline mammogram after healing in patients older than 35
    - Hypertrophic scar or keloid formation
    - How do you manage these complications?
    - What is your timeframe for intervention?
    - Do you try to salvage infected implants?

6. Demonstrate ability to structure alternative plan

    - Family does not agree with your suggested operative approach
    - Failed latissimus or implant
    - Contracture of implant
    - Insurance will not approve surgery
    - Family wants money back, they are not satisfied with the result
    - Significant residual postop asymmetry
    - At what age do you start reconstruction?

Chapter Seven

Tuberous Breast Deformity

7
Tuberous Breast Deformity

1. Identify General Problem/ Diagnosis/Planning
   (Describe photo, working diagnosis, key problems, evaluates patient)

   - Describe deformity:
     - Typical tuberous breast deformity
       - Narrow constricted base of breast
       - Large areola
       - Parenchyma seems to herniate into areola
       - Elevated IMF
   - Accurate diagnosis important, critical in management
   - Hx:
     - Prior surgery/trauma should be absent
       - Iatrogenic trauma
       - Neonatal chest tube
     - Age of patient
     - When was deformity noted? Often late teens early 20's
     - Psychosocial issues
       - Will not change in locker room
       - Teasing or bullying from peers
       - Self-image issues
       - Other
     - Emotional impact
     - Medical conditions
     - Past surgery for syndactyly
       - Consider Poland rather than tuberous breast
     - Concomitant Moebius can be seen with Poland
   - PE
     - Key findings generally limited to breasts themselves
     - Shape of breast
       - Tuberous breast
         - Narrow, typically associated with inferior and medial parenchymal deficiency
     - NAC
       - Typically widened diameter from herniation

- o IMF
  - ▪ Usually high, more lateral
- o NAC to IMF distance shortened
- o Unilateral or bilateral
  - ▪ Tuberous breast typically bilateral
  - ▪ Symmetric constriction
- o Ptosis
- o Chest wall findings
  - ▪ May indicate alternative diagnosis i.e. Poland Syndrome or other
  - ▪ Absence sternal head of pectoralis major
  - ▪ Absence of other chest wall muscles
- o Additional findings
  - ▪ No associated musculoskeletal abnormalities
  - ▪ Presence of musculoskeletal abnormalities suggests alternative diagnosis i.e. Poland Syndrome or other condition

▪ Main Components of Tuberous Breast Deformity
- o Elevated IMF
- o Breast parenchyma constriction
- o Enlarged NAC with breast herniation
- o Hypoplastic skin envelope

▪ Classification of Tuberous Breast Deformity
- o Type 1: Inferior medial hypoplasia
- o Type 2: Inferior medial and lateral hypoplasia
- o Type 3: As above with subareolar skin shortage in circumferential plane
- o Type 4: Severely constricted base

▪ Consider and R/O other congenital breast conditions
- o Amastia- absence of breast w/ or w/o NAC
- o Athelia- absence of NAC alone
- o Polymastia
- o Polythelia

▪ WORK-UP
- o Pre-op mammogram in older patients >35 and planning surgery on breast
- o Mammogram age 50 current American Cancer Society recommendation
- o Consultation consider psychological evaluation if significant emotional trauma.

▪ Condition has an enormous emotional impact
▪ Etiology unknown

- o Error in breast development or result of limited growth of investing fascia

2. Consider reasonable goals in diagnosis and management *(Management and treatment, surgical indications, operative procedures and anesthesia)*

    - INDICATIONS
        - o Restore breast symmetry
        - o Alleviate psychosocial impact of condition
        - o Improve self-esteem
    - Strategy based on presentation of deformity
        - o Moderate-severe with paucity of overlying skin
            - May require two-stage approach
                - Primary tissue expansion followed by secondary augmentation
    - TIMING
        - o Ideally when breast growth is complete
    - Goals of surgery
        - o Expand breast circumference
        - o Expand skin envelope in lower pole
        - o Release constriction at the breast-areola junction
        - o Lower IMF
        - o Increase breast volume when appropriate
        - o Reduce areola size and correct herniation
        - o Correct nipple location and breast ptosis

3. Select appropriate options in diagnosis and management

    - Present your proposed operative plan based on presented deformity. Individualize treatment plan.
    - MANAGEMENT PRINCIPLES
    - Simple augmentation (subglandular)
        - o Many patients have hypoplastic breast
        - o Augmentation with implant helps achieve symmetry
        - o Smooth, round silicone gel-filled subglandular
        - o Textured or anatomically shaped okay
        - o Saline implants may be used
    - Skin approach
        - o Periareolar or Inframammary
    - Circumareolar mastopexy

- - -
      - o Typical tuberous breast NAC 7-8cm
      - o New NAC 3-4 cm
        - ▪ Cuff of dermis 2-3cm left around new NAC
    - ▪ Radial parenchymal incision release
      - o Performed on deeper aspect of gland
      - o Addresses constricting ring at base of breast
    - ▪ Internal glandular flaps
      - o Used to compensate for lack of parenchyma in hypoplastic areas
    - ▪ Lowering of IMF
    - ▪ **Enlargement of lower pole skin envelope is needed if significant skin shortage is present!**
      - o 1st stage of 2-stage approach via tissue expansion
    - ▪ In unilateral cases consider augmentation prior to mastopexy

4. Understand risks and benefits of various approaches

    - ▪ Have understanding of the approach to tuberous breast deformity.
    - ▪ What are the deformities present and how do you correct them?
    - ▪ When do you stage the correction?
    - ▪ Be able to individualize treatment on case-by-case basis by identifying abnormalities present.
    - ▪ What is your tissue expansion protocol? Your preferred implant?

5. Address complications and unexpected problems adequately

    - ▪ Most complications related to postop appearance of the breast.
    - ▪ More than slight asymmetry is concerning (some asymmetry is expected)
    - ▪ Augmentation alone can result in double bubble deformity
    - ▪ Subpectoralis placement can cause double IMF if implant large and ptosis of glandular tissue is small
    - ▪ May require further expansion for correction (two-stage approach)
    - ▪ Infection-may require removal of implant
    - ▪ Hematoma
    - ▪ Contracture of implant capsule

- Interference with cancer surveillance
- Be able to manage implant and mastopexy related complications.

6. Demonstrate ability to structure alternative plan

    - Base plan on presented deformity
    - Staging with tissue expansion followed by final reconstruction a safe approach for complex cases.
    - Be able to manage post-op double bubble deformity in tuberous breast reconstruction.
    - Timing of reconstruction
    - Temporizing measures till completion of breast growth options?

Section Two
Breast Reconstruction

Chapter Eight

Breast Reconstruction Overview

———

8
Breast Reconstruction Overview

1. Identify General Problem
   - Describe photo
   - Give working diagnosis
   - Note key problems
   - Evaluate patient
   - Note pertinent positives and negatives in history
     - Medical history
     - Radiation
     - Chemotherapy
     - Status of cancer and other breast (nodes)
     - Family history
     - Indications for prophylactic mastectomy
     - BRCA status and management
   - Note previous surgery that may affect available reconstructive options
     - Previous lymph node dissection- scarred axilla
   - Patient's desires and goals
   - Classify defect
     - What is present?
     - What is missing?
     - Volume needed
     - Compare to normal breast
   - Long term and short term breast cancer management issues
     - Chemo
     - Radiation

2. Consider reasonable goals in diagnosis and management

   - Management and treatment
   - Surgical indications
   - Operative procedures and anesthesia
   - Your surgical goals
   - Plan to give symmetry (match other breast)
     - Need for reduction or augmentation of unaffected breast

3. Select appropriate options in diagnosis and management

- Your surgical plan and why?
- Do you stage your reconstruction?
  - What are the stages and timing between?
- How will you prevent complications?
- Your post-op management
- Your nipple reconstruction?
- Cancer surveillance plan
- How is procedure performed?
- Key steps of surgery
- Markings and relevant anatomy

4. Understand risks and benefits of various approaches

   - Note benefits, risks of various approaches
   - Anticipated effect of previous radiation or planned post-op radiation,
   - How will you deal with this?

5. Address complications and unexpected problems adequately

   - Anticipate and manage common complications
     - Skin necrosis
     - Implant exposure
     - Infection
     - Asymmetry
     - Wound complications
     - Flap failure
     - Ischemic flap
     - Wound problems with chemo/radiation pending
     - Radiated field

6. Demonstrate ability to structure alternative plan

   - Your plan if reconstruction fails
     - Why did reconstruction fail? Alternatives
   - Plan if complication occurs during chemo-radiation period
   - Patient refuses nipple reconstruction
   - Wants prophylactic mastectomy but not indicated?
   - Insurance denies coverage for procedures

Chapter Nine

Breast Reconstruction
———

9
Breast Reconstruction

1. Identify General Problem/Diagnosis/Planning
   (Describe photo, give working diagnosis, key problems, evaluates patient)

   - Describe deformity, defect or shape of breasts presented in photo in detail.
   - Detail your working diagnosis, key problems and potential operative challenges.
   - Follow with thorough but concise and pertinent history (hx) and physical exam (PE) to determine reconstructive (recon) options.
   - Hx:
     - Overall health of patient?
     - Patient age
     - Timing of initial surgery
     - Based on plan for immediate reconstruction vs. delayed reconstruction note pertinent history needed for reconstruction plan.
     - For delayed case:
       - Prior adjuvant therapy
       - Especially Radiation/Chemotherapy
       - Prior lymphadenectomy?
       - How long ago was radiation completed?
         - Guideline: Wait 6 months prior to initiation of recon
     - Manage patient expectations:
       - Usually match contralateral breast
         - If excessively large or ptotic as per patient
         - New goal for size selected by patient.
       - Plan for symmetry procedures
         - Reduction mammoplasty
         - Mastopexy
         - Augmentation
         - Combination?
     - What is the oncologic status of uninvolved breast?

- Mammogram prior to intervention
    - Surgical history?
        - Prior abdominal procedures
        - Pelvic surgery
        - Thorocotomy
        - May affect choice of flap in autologous recon
    - Medical conditions
        - Older patient with multiple medical problems
            - Less invasive procedure may be more appropriate
                - Eg. Tissue expander rather than free-flap
        - Diabetes mellitus
        - Scleroderma
        - Lupus
        - Cardiac or vascular disease
        - Smoking
        - May increase risk of complications
    - SMOKER
        - Increased risk
            - Flap loss
            - Skin complications
            - Free flap may have better vascularity than pedicled flap in a smoker.
    - Medications
        - Herceptin- need cardiac clearance prior to sx
        - Tamoxifen- stop minimum 2 weeks prior to surgery avoid venous thromboembolism
- PE
    - BMI> 30 relative contraindication to TRAM
    - Very obese large enough expander may not be available
    - Mastectomy must include NAC, previous biopsy scars
        - Conservative approach
        - Be familiar with indications for skin-sparing mastectomies
    - Focus on contralateral breast
        - Dimensions

- Ptosis
- Need for symmetry procedure
- Examine possible donor sites
  - Adequacy of tissue volume
  - Presence of scars
- Breast exam
  - Residual or recurrent disease
    - Palpate
      - Skin flaps
      - Suture line
      - Axilla
  - Skin of treated breast, radiation changes?- autologous recon best
  - RADIATION EFFECTS
    - Induration
    - Less pliability
    - More healing complications
- Abdominal exam
  - Adequate tissue for recon?
  - Check for
    - Diastasis of rectus abdominis muscle
    - Palpable hernia
      - Avoid bowel injury
    - Old scars from previous surgery?
- Functional latissimus dorsi
  - Radiation unlikely to affect pedicle
  - If prior axillary dissection can affect this
  - If not functioning uninjured during axillary dissection
  - TEST- press inwards with hands on hips

- PATHOLOGY
  - Most cancers from ductal elements
  - Ductal Carcinoma In Situ (DCIS)- confined to basement membrane
  - Infiltrating ductal carcinoma- 75% of breast cancer cases
    - (variants medullary- favorable, tubular- excellent prognosis, mucinous or colloid- favorable)
  - Lobular Carcinoma In Situ (LCIS)
    - Marker for breast ca

- - Increased risk for cancer in either breast
  - Invasive lobular ca 5-10%
- Work-up
  - Recent mammogram of contralateral breast within 1 year of planned surgery
  - Doppler to check blood supply to abdominal wall if prior surgery
  - Multidisciplinary management of breast cancer
    - Oncologist
    - Breast surgeon
    - Plastic surgeon
    - Radiation oncologist
    - Pathologist
    - Psychologist
  - Discuss completion of reconstruction may require 2-3 surgeries.
- IS RADIATION PLANNED? MAJOR IMPACT ON TIMING OF BREAST RECONSTRUCTION
  - Reconstruction associated with high level of quality of life and patient satisfaction
    - Most effective means for restoring psychological well-being
  - Multidisciplinary approach
  - Mandated coverage by insurance companies
    - 1998 Women's Health and Cancer Rights Act (Clinton)
  - Patient satisfaction immediate vs. delayed recon equivalent
  - Timing
    - Immediate okay in stage I or II disease
      - Major complication rate
        - 46% Implants
          - Infection 35%
          - Capsular contracture 16%
        - 31% TRAM pedicle
        - 46% Free TRAM
    - Delayed preferred in stage III or IV or post radiation therapy
      - Significantly lower complication rate
  - Radiation

- - - Decreases local recurrence by 2/3 regardless of chemo
    - Indicated for all locally advanced cases
    - Tumor >4cm
    - 4 or more positive LN
    - Diffuse calcification in DCIS
    - TE/implant complication rate 50%
    - Increased risk
      - Autogenous flap loss
      - Fat necrosis
      - Contour deformity
      - Volume loss
    - Worse outcomes aesthetically
    - Must have FRANK discussion with patients about risks of radiation
  - Chemotherapy
    - Reduces mortality in node positive and negative patients
    - Tumor >1cm
    - Weight gain during chemo
    - Based on # of positive nodes
    - Wait until blood counts normalized, fatigue resolved before recon
  - Genetic testing
    - 1/3 of patients have family hx of cancer
  - Cancer Surveillance
    - Recon does not impair
    - No increase in local failure
    - Annual oncology exam
    - Autogenous flaps annual mammography of recon
  - Reconstruction does not delay cancer treatment or increase morbidity
  - Most frequent site of recurrence
    - Remaining chest wall skin
  - Delayed Recon not sooner than 6 months from mastectomy allow maturation of scars
  - Some argue immediate results are better than delayed
    - No scar to overcome
    - Early filling of defect mimics borders of natural breast

2. Consider reasonable goals in diagnosis and management *(Management and treatment, surgical indications, operative procedures and anesthesia)*

- GOAL OF RECON: Symmetry in clothing
- GOALS OF BREAST RECON
    - One-stage procedure
    - Restore deficient skin
    - Replace contour of absent pec major
    - Restore lost breast volume
    - Replace NAC
    - Match remaining breast in symmetric, pleasing way
    - Autologous recon preferred in setting of radiation
    - If radiation planned opt for delayed reconstruction if possible:
        - Recon delayed with autologous tissue
        - Minimum 6 months
    - Plan timing of symmetry procedures:
        - Can be same time contralatateral reconstruction.
        - Can be after contralateral reconstruction
    - Implant selection:
        - Based on dimensions of contralateral breast
        - Width and approximate volume
    - Surgical options:
        - Tissue expanders and implants
        - Autologous tissue
        - Combined approach- implant with autologous tissue
    - Considerations
        - Skin required for wound closure?
            - Flap required
            - Thin skin replace by flap
        - Quality of mastectomy flap
            - Poor quality- NO IMPLANT
            - Non-irradiated flap
        - Size and shape contralateral breast
            - Symmetry procedure (reduction, mastopexy, aug?)

- INDICATIONS AND CONTRAINDICATIONS
  - Stage III and IV disease or need for adjuvant radiation therapy relative contraindication to immediate recon
  - Autogenous better in radiation
  - Delayed recon wait 2-3 months post chemo, minimum 6-8 weeks
  - Post radiation as long as 6 months post radiation
  - Contraindications- COPD, CAD, severe asthma, fragile diabetes, extreme obesity
  - Relative contra- hypercoagulable state, rheumatologic disorders, smoking

3. Select appropriate options in diagnosis and management

- Implant recon
- Single stage (Used to be rare, becoming more popular)
  - Provide breast mound of acceptable shape and volume
  - Candidates:
    - Small to moderate sized breast
    - Placement beneath pectoralis- complete submuscular
    - +/- alloderm sutured to inferior edge of muscle and chest wall
    - Requires ample skin and soft tissue coverage in mastectomy flaps
- Two Stage: Expander then implant, more reliable than single
  - Most common form of breast recon in U.S.
  - Obese patients less satisfied
  - Implant saline or silicone based on contralateral breast dimensions
  - Anatomic expanders preferentially expand lower pole facilitating breast ptosis
  - Delayed recon reduces complications
  - Chemotherapy does not increase risk of complications if timed appropriately.
    - Standard or adjustable prosthesis
  - Best suited to adequate skin envelope, small, non-ptotic breast
  - Small breasted women with minimal skin deficiency

- Always submuscular or subpec with alloderm- reduces risk of exposure
- Compared to autologous recon
  - Breast mound
    - More round, less ptotic
    - Symmetry inferior to autologous recon
- Advances in breast recon
  - Anatomic implants
  - Alloderm
  - Skin sparing mastectomy resection:
    - Breast tissue
    - NAC
    - Previous biopsy scar
      - Ideal for small to moderate breast size
      - Large breast will need skin excision
  - At mastectomy TE placed submuscular
    - Partially filled
    - At 1-2 week intervals expander is injected 50-100ml per week
    - Over 4-6 months
    - Allows safe stretching of skin envelope
    - Over expansion is critical
    - Precise placement and accentuation IMF with suture placement
    - Create ptosis
    - Routine circumferential capsulectomy at time of exchange
- Advantages
  - Smaller operative procedure
  - Faster recovery
  - Better in bilateral recon
  - Adjacent tissue similar color, texture, sensation
  - No donor site morbidity
- Disadvantage
  - Frequent office visits for percutaneous expansion

- Mild discomfort with expansion
- Capsular contracture
- Device failure
- Infection
- Exposure
- Implant migration
        - Use of alloderm is an advancement of the technique
            - Indications for implant recon
                - Most mastectomy patients
                - Most have favorable results
                - Moderate breast volume 500g or less
                - Mild to moderate ptosis
                - Large or markedly ptotic breast will need matching procedure
            - Contraindications for implant recon
                - ABSENCE of skin envelope to cover implant
                - Will need ipsilateral latissimus or other soft tissue coverage
            - Relative contraindications
                - Smoking
                - Obesity
                - Previous chest wall radiation
                - Postmastecomy radiotherapy (increased infection, exposure, extrusion, capsular contracture)
                    - Some say absolute contraindication
                    - Some say timing and radiation dose dependent
- OPERATIVE APPROACH FOR IMPLANT RECON
    - Periop antibiotics
    - Arms at sides/hands padded and tucked
    - Re-prep entire field
    - Hemostasis mastectomy flaps
    - Complete, submuscular pocket
        - Do not elevate pec minor
        - Elevate serratus and anterior rectus sheath
    - Expander chosen based on base dimensions and volume capability
        - Textured anatomic preferred

- - Close muscle pocket with 2-0 vicryl
  - Drains
  - Tailor mastectomy flaps
  - Skin closure
  - Intraop expansion to tissue tolerance
    - Up to 50% expander volume
  - Markings
    - Midline over sternum
    - Medial limits of expander pocket marked 2-3cm lateral to midline
    - Lateral limits in line with anterior axillary fold
    - Inferior limit 2cm below native inframammary fold
- POSTOP
  - Remove drains when output <30ml in 24 hours
  - Absence of problems begin expansion in 10-14 days
    - Weekly or bi-weekly 60-100ml/session
    - Final volume 20-30% > than planned implant volume or 20% > than recommended volume of expander
    - OVEREXPAND!
  - Exchange procedure
  - Minimum 4-6 weeks following last expansion
  - AND/OR 4-6 weeks following postop chemotx
  - Prep both breasts in op field
  - Excise mastectomy incision
  - Elevate mastectomy flaps
  - Access pocket and remove expander
  - Circumferential capsulectomy, full release of skin muscle envelope
  - Upright position
    - Recreate IMF, 0-0 silk sutures
    - Precise repositioning of fold
    - Sizers, select prosthesis
  - Return to supine
  - Irrigate pocket & hemostasis
  - Re-prep, glove change
  - Place implant
  - Close muscle running absorbable
  - Double layer skin closure

- Key Points
  - Anatomic expander
  - Overexpansion
  - Circumferential capsulectomy
  - Precise re-positioning of IMF
- AlloDerm
  - 20-30 minutes reconstitution
  - Elevate pectoralis only
    - Leaving serratus and rectus down
  - AlloDerm placed over inferior and lateral portions of expander pocket
  - Shiny side facing vascularized mastectomy flaps
  - Suture laterally to serratus
  - Place implant and close lateral pocket AlloDerm to Pec
  - Close
  - Exchange
    - AlloDerm incorporated into mastectomy flaps
    - Revision of the pocket
    - Standard technique
    - NAC as in TRAM
    - Skate flap
    - Areolar tattooing
    - Skin Graft
    - Combination
    - At time of exchange or 2 months later
- AUTOGENOUS RECONSTRUCTION
  - Like tissue
  - Potential for return of sensation
  - Better contour
  - Pedicled transverse rectus abdominis myocutaneous (TRAM)- most common
    - Abd skin and fat transferred to chest based on superior epigastric system
    - Beware
      - Previous abdominal surgery
      - Smoking and DM relative contraindication
    - Delay procedure- division of inferior epigastrics prior to recon
      - May decrease complications

- 14% decrease in trunk function
- ANATOMY
    - Rectus originates from pubic symph inserts on 5th, 6th and 7th rib cartilage
    - Flexes vertebral column
    - Motor lower 6-7 segmental intercostals
    - Dual blood supply
    - Skin island 4 zones
    - Zone over muscle most reliable
    - Zone furthest from muscle discarded (can keep in free flap)
    - Advantage
        - No implant
        - Abdominal wall contouring- abdominal lipectomy
        - Potential good long-term results
    - Reinforce donor site closure with mesh
- CONTRAINDICATIONS
    - Smoking
    - Obesity
    - COPD
    - Previous abdominal surgery
    - DM
- TRAM OPERATION
    - Markings
    - Made preop in standing position
    - Skin island follow natural creases
        - Just above umbilicus and at suprapubic region
    - Elevate skin superior to TRAM island
    - Expose upper rectus muscles
    - Maintain skin bridge between abdominal dissection and mastectomy defect
        - Leave support for IMF
        - But make large enough to pass skin island
    - Can pedicle one or two muscles
    - All attachments except to skin island separated
    - Can take whole muscle or preserve lateral or medial segments
        - High-risk patients
            - Bipedicle
            - Supercharge

- Delay procedure- 1 week prior to surgery
  - Ligate inferior epigastrics
- Reinforce defect with on-lay and or in-lay mesh
- Transfer flap closure abd defect as in abdominoplasty
  - May also plicate abd wall if indicated
- In sitting position inset, tailor trim TRAM flap
- FREE TRAM OPERATION
  - Uses inferior epigastric system
  - Microvascular anastomosis
    - Internal mammary artery (preferred) (IMA) or thoracodorsal vessels
  - Advantage
    - Dominant blood supply- minimized fat necrosis
    - Better option for smokers
    - Easier inset
  - Disadvantage
    - Risk of thrombosis and total flap loss
    - <5% failure rate, some lit <1% failure rate

  - ONLY ABSOLUTE INDICATION
    - Previous upper abdominal surgery
  - ONLY CONTRAINDICATION
    - Previous lower abdominal surgery
- Muscle sparing free TRAM or DIEP (deep inferior epigastric perforator)
- FREE TRAM OPERATION
  - Differences from pedicle TRAM
  - Same initial approach
  - Muscle splitting dissection to identify and expose inferior epigastric vessels
  - Opposite side of flap is elevated to first row of medial perforators
  - Fascia split here
  - Muscle splitting dissection
  - Repair fascial defect with mesh
  - Upright for inset
  - Loupe magnification or microscope for vessel anastomosis
  - Anastomosis 8-0 or 9-0 nylon sutures

- Thoracodorsal vessels
    - Exposed during axillary dissection
    - Thoracodorsal a. and v. dissected free
    - Flap secured temporarily anastomosis performed
    - Flap inset
- IMA
    - Avoids axilla in delayed case
    - Allows more medial placement of flap in immediate recon
    - Preferred if mastectomy alone performed or sentinel node only performed
    - Separate fibers of pec overlying 3rd costal cartilages
    - Perichondrium incised, separated off cartilage
    - Costal cartilage removed with rongeur
    - Perichondrium on deep side incised and IMA exposed
    - Larger on right than left
    - Temporarily secure flap end-to-end anastomosis
    - Post op flap checks Q1 hour first 24/then Q2 hours 48 hours/then Q4 24 hours. Monitor in ICU first 24-48 hours.
    - Dextran +/-
    - Sequential compression device (SCD) started before induction then postop till ambulating.
- What is your protocol?
- Abdominal perforator flaps
    - No muscle sacrifice
    - Deep inferior epigastric artery perforator flap (DIEP)
    - Rectus abd muscle is split to allow dissection of perforator
    - Disadvantage less perfusion
    - Perforator from inferior epigastrics
    - Superficial inferior epigastric perforator flap (SIEP)
    - Perforators arise from common femorals
    - 20-30% of the time large enough for use
    - No involvement of rectus abdominis muscle
    - Not available in all patients
    - Contraindicated in large breast recon, planned postop RT
- Main advantage
    - No effect on abdominal wall
    - No hernias, bulging, weakness

- o Usually not clinically significant in muscle sparing free TRAM for the average patient
- OPERATION
  - o Identify perforator with doppler
  - o Loupe magnification
  - o Atraumatic technique
  - o SIEP identified during dissection of lower incision
  - o Medial to iliac crest
  - o Just above or below Scarpa's fascia
- LATISSIMUS RECONSTRUCTION WITH OR WITHOUT IMPLANT
  - o See below for full description
  - o Generally considered a second-line option but can be used as a first choice.
- NIPPLE RECONSTRUCTION
  - o Can be performed with second procedure or deferred as a third procedure
  - o Local or general anesthesia
  - o Method depends on:
  - o Size
  - o Color of opposite nipple and areola
  - o Type of breast mound
  - o Patient and surgeon preference
  - o Composite graft from opposite nipple
    - If adequate size
    - Harvested from lower half or tip
    - Graft sutured to central portion of de-epithelialized areola site
    - Generally good take
  - o Local flap
    - Skate flap most common
    - Linear configuration
    - Central base with large wings on each side
    - Wings elevated at level of deep dermis
    - Deep fat harvested at central portion
    - Can augment with cartilage from ear
  - o Areola
    - Skin graft
    - Intradermal tattooing

4. Understand risks and benefits of various approaches

- Consider risks benefits of implant vs. autogenous reconstruction
- Consider difference between different autogenous options
- Consider need for symmetry procedures and best way to proceed
- What will you do for a bilateral reconstruction case?

5. Address complications and unexpected problems adequately

    - Complications
    - Specific to type of reconstruction
    - Mastectomy flap necrosis- common unrelated to recon type
        o Can result in expander extrusion or exposure
        o Careful evaluation of mastectomy skin flaps and debridement as appropriate
        o Minimizes this problem
        o Do you have any preventative measures?
    - Hematoma
    - Seroma
    - Fat necrosis
        o Manage expectantly
        o May require return to OR
    - Infection
        o May require device removal
        o IV antibiotics and close observation in early cases
    - Expander malfunction
        o Deflation, malposition, malfunction of port
    - Capsular contracture and replacement of implant
    - Abdominal wall complications
        o Minimize tension at closure
        o Flap slough
        o Abdominal wall weakness
        o Hernia formation
    - Preserve rectus muscles as perforator flaps, minimizes hernia formation
    - Expander Complications
    - Skin flap necrosis
    - Hematoma
    - Seroma
    - Infection
    - Implant exposure/extrusion

- In rare cases implant may be salvaged
- If no signs of infection
  - Irrigate and exchange
- Signs of infection
  - Remove
  - Treat infection
  - Wait 3-6 months following explantation for delayed reconstruction
- Rippling
  - Changing from saline to silicone may help

- How do you manage various simple complications?
  - Seroma
  - Hematoma
  - Flap necrosis
  - Compromised flap
  - Wound dehiscence

6. Demonstrate ability to structure alternative plan

- If TRAM not available
- Gluteus flap
  - Two main flaps
    - Superior gluteal artery perforator (SGAP)
    - Inferior gluteal artery perforator (IGAP)
  - If inadequate abdominal tissue
  - OR
  - Secondary contralateral recon
  - Limited skin paddle width
  - OPERATION
  - Flap harvest decubitus or prone position
  - Inferior gluteal flap 4-5cm inferior to superior gluteal vessels
- Latissimus dorsi (lat)
  - Alone or with implant
  - Most commonly with implant
  - High seroma rate
    - Any preventative measures?
    - How do you manage Seroma?
  - Requires lateral position for harvest
  - Flap muscle with skin paddle
  - Excellent choice for foreign body coverage

- Excellent choice for partial mastectomy recon
- Excellent choice for chest wall reconstruction alone
- Ideal candidate
  - Thin, fit, can undergo longer operation
  - Obese patients encourage to lose weight first
- Low complication rates
- Rapid rehab
- Can be used as a miniflap for small or large volume deficits
- ANATOMY
  - Pedicle in axilla allows transposition to anterior chest
- INDICATIONS
  - Breast and chest wall recon
  - Head and neck coverage
  - Sternal recon
  - Recon abd wall
  - Functional restoration arm and shoulder
  - Coverage lower extremities
  - Good choice in recon post radiation
- Other Indications
  - Thin body habitus
  - Previous abdominal operations
  - Preferred dorsal donor site
  - Prior chest wall radiation
  - Failed implant or TRAM
  - Desire future pregnancy (Poland's patients)
  - Irradiated wound or require postop radiation
- CONTRAINDICATIONS
  - Posterior thoracotomy
  - Large breasts and implants not desired
  - Requiring latissimus for muscle activity (tennis player, mountain climber)
  - Severe CAD, COPD
  - Need for minimum operative time
- Relative contraindication
  - Smoking
  - Obesity
- Unlikely radiation to axilla will affect latissimus dorsi flap
- Frequently used with implant to fill volume deficit
- Operative approach

- Markings
  - Marked with patient sitting or standing
  - Arms relaxed at patients sides
  - Dimensions 30cm x 15cm
  - Width of skin island 10cm
  - Superior posterior skin island most commonly used
  - Scar masked under bra strap
  - Alternative oblique skin flap
  - Skin flap situated over muscle
  - Superior margin tip of scapula
  - Inferior margin posterior iliac crest
  - Skin island ends 8-10cm superior to this line
  - Anterolateral border flap best visualized at the posterior axillary line
    - Hands on hips contract lat to palpate posterior medial border
  - Mark IMF's of both breast pre-op!
- Positioning
  - Lateral decubitus position for flap harvest
  - Prep and drape ipsilateral arm to allow shoulder manipulation
  - Bean bag for support
  - Axillary roll to prevent nerve injury from compression
  - Abduction of ipsilateral arm limited to 90 degrees to prevent brachial plexus injury
  - Reposition and reprep for flap inset
  - Implant based on opposite breast
- Incision
  - Muscle elevated via skin island incisions
  - If no skin harvested
    - Incision placed at posterior axilla and extends 5-20cm depending on desire to minimize scar
  - Elevation of subcutaneous tissue extends over border of planned muscle flap
  - Extended latissimus flap can increase tissue volume
- Raising the flap
  - Superior medial fibers divided at scapula
  - Lat is separated from serratus anterior

- - - Fibers of origin separated from vertebral column, paraspinous muscle fascia, lumbosacral fascia
      - Hemostasis from minor vascular pedicles
      - Identify thoracodorsal a. and v. located near insertion
      - Separate lat from teres major
      - Can separate from insertion into humerus to increase arc of rotation
    - Transposition
    - Tunnel made from back to chest wall defect
    - Close donor site
    - Drains 2 weeks minimum
    - Reposition
    - Shape and tailor breast and closure
    - Can use implant as a spacer and replace later if needed
    - Implant can be place below pec or under latissimus flap
    - May require denervation, can do at primary operation
    - Complications
      - Hematoma
      - Seroma common
      - Flap loss
      - Brachial plexus injury from poor positioning
      - Hypertrophic scars at donor site
  - TREATMENT OF ASYMMETRY IN BREAST CANCER PATIENTS
    - Manage pt expectations pre-op
    - Asymmetry somewhat natural state
    - Breast recon cannot duplicate natural breast
    - Unilat recon always asymmetry with native opposite breast

    - Liposuction useful in volume excess and contour asymmetry
    - IMF defining architectural structure in revisional surgery
    - Capsule is surgeon's friend in revision
    - Fat transfer useful in small peripheral contour deformities

- Revision may salvage a significantly suboptimal recon- improves aesthetic outcome
- Asymmetry may not be amenable to complete correction
- INDICATIONS
  - Evaluate
  - Volume
    - Excess
    - Deficiency
  - Volume distribution or shape
  - IMF discrepancies
  - NAC appearance
  - Skin envelope asymmetry
  - Contour abnormalities
  - Minor or major flap loss
- CRITICAL ANATOMIC FEATURES
  - Supra-sternal notch to nipple distance
  - Breast base width
  - Nipple to IMF distance
  - General shape including lateral contour
- OPERATIVE APPROACH
- VOLUME EXCESS
  - Liposuction/Lipo-contouring- wet technique
- VOLUME INSUFFICIENCY
  - Additional volume via implant
    - First step correct base width dimension
  - Fat transfer not used for large volume deficiency
- SKIN ENVELOPE
  - In unilateral delayed, may be able to measure directly
  - Immediate- skin needed equal to skin excision
  - If excess then resection
    - Volume reduction and re-shaping of breast
  - IMF asymmetries
  - IMF is a condensation of connective tissue which emanates from superficial fascial system of anterior trunk at 6th intercostals
    - Definition varies from tight to loose

- If asymmetry noted preop
  - Then correct at initial surgery
  - It can be incrementally lowered
    - Done by incrementally sitting pt up to 90 degrees
    - Releasing scar tissue to achieve lowering
  - Use 2-0 Prolene to fix the SFS to muscle fascia
  - IMF can be raised
    - Raising the fold can increase upper pole fullness
    - In implant and autologous flap
    - Flap
    - Elevate inferior most portion from flap and fold under Implant
    - Interrupted capsulorraphy sutures or strip resection
      - 2-0 prolene sutures
    - Plan suture position by simulating effect of suture placement with fingers
- CONTOUR DEFORMITIES
  - Secondary to scar release or resect
  - Small defects dermis fat grafts may be used
    - Harvest site- adj scars, or groin
    - Deep dermis
  - Adipose advancement
  - Autologous fat grafts
  - 70% or grafts take

Section Three
Trunk Reconstruction

Chapter Ten

Trunk Reconstruction Overview

10
Trunk Reconstruction Overview

1. Identify General Problem

   - Describe photo
   - Give working diagnosis
   - Note key problems
   - Evaluate patient
   - Diagnosis/Planning
   - Specify what is missing in the defect
     - What is classification/grade/stage of wound?
   - Relevant medical history
     - Non-smoker
     - DM
     - CAD
     - HTN
     - Steroids
     - Cancer
   - Pertinent positives and negatives in history
   - Nutritional status and work-up
     - (Pre-albumin, anemia)
   - Previous surgeries
   - Relevant medications especially anticoagulants
   - Need for further work-up or consultations?
     - Imaging studies
     - Lab work
     - Orthopedics
     - General surgery
     - Other surgical subspecialist

2. Consider reasonable goals in diagnosis and management

   - Management and treatment
   - Surgical indications
   - Operative procedures and anesthesia
   - What are your options?
   - What type of coverage do you need?

- Skin
- Muscle
- Bone
- Fascia
- All of the above?
        - Why is surgery indicated?
        - When should surgery be undertaken?
        - Level of urgency

3. Select appropriate options in diagnosis and management

    - Choose your operative approach and why?
    - Anticipate outcome and potential complications.
    - Preventative measures?
    - Your post-op management
    - How is procedure performed?
    - Key steps of procedure
    - Markings and relevant anatomy

4. Understand risks and benefits of various approaches

    - Note risks, benefits of various approaches- upsides and downsides.
    - How well does each accomplish the clinical goal?

5. Address complications and unexpected problems adequately

    - Manage partial or complete flap loss
    - Wound complications
    - Infection
    - Recurrence
    - Contracture
    - Need for revision
    - Pneumothorax
    - Bowel injury

6. Demonstrate ability to structure alternative plan

    - Why did reconstruction fail?
    - Life boat or back up plan if initial approach is not available

Chapter Eleven

Abdominal Wall Reconstruction

11
Abdominal Wall Reconstruction

1. Identify General Problem Diagnosis/Planning
   (Describe photo, give working diagnosis, key problems, evaluates patient)

   - Describe photo and give your working diagnosis
     - Describe defect and mention what is missing *(skin/fascia/muscle)*
       - What is exposed? Internal organs, mesh?
   - History (Hx):
     - Elicit nature of injury, give your clinical impression
     - Previous attempts at reconstruction
     - Areas of compromised skin from old scars
     - Size of defect: <5cm or > 5cm
     - Infection of mesh, mesh placement?
     - Radiation?
       - Less viable tissue local flaps not as reliable
     - Enterocutaneous fistula
     - Hernia history?
     - Comorbidities (DM, BMI, COPD, smoking)
     - Loss of domain
       - Chronic herniation in extra-abdominal sac
       - Will abdominal space be adequate for reduction?
     - Length of time
   - Physical Exam
     - Examine patient while supine and legs bent
     - Define borders of defect
     - Examine intra-abdominal content
     - Note old scars
     - Wounds, wound edges intact?
     - Graft adherence to bowel
     - Unrecognized masses
   - Determine safety of further intervention
   - Pre-op work up:
     - Imaging
       - CT scan

- Evaluate intra-abdominal contents and hernia
      - Fistulograms
    - Labs
      - CBC
      - CHEM 7
      - Albumin
      - Prealbumin
      - PT/PTT
      - LFT's
    - Medical control of comorbidities
    - Nutritional optimization
    - Consultations
      - GI
      - General Surgery
        - Fascial exposure and lysis of adhesions
      - Nutrition

2. Consider reasonable goals in diagnosis and management

   - Surgical goals
     - Repair of muscle, fascia, skin and subcutaneous tissue
     - Avoid bowel incarceration
       - Risk of strangulation in hernias (never 0%)
     - Restore function of abdominal wall
       - Barrier protection of viscera
       - Posture
       - Flexion, rotation of trunk
       - Ventilation
       - Cough
       - Emesis
       - Defecation
       - Micturition
       - Childbirth

3. Select appropriate options in diagnosis and management
   - Medically and nutritionally optimize patient
     - Smoking cessation
     - Increase pre-albumin pre-op
   - General surgery consultation

- o Fascial exposure
- o Lysis of adhesions
- Bowel management
  - o Pre-op bowel prep
    - Magnesium sulfate
    - Other
- Surgical goal
  - o Tension free closure
- Indication for reconstruction
  - o Myofascial defects of abdominal wall
  - o Immediate reconstruction after trauma or oncologic resection
- Surgical options
  - o Closure by secondary intention and skin graft
  - o Tissue expansion with inherent risks
    - Placed through vertical incision in posterior leaf of internal oblique muscle between int. obl. and transversalis muscle
  - o <5cm defect: mesh repair acceptable
  - o >5cm: components separation +/- alloderm or mesh onlay, underlay or bridge in hernias with excess tension at fascial closure
  - o Components separation preferred option in most cases
  - o Synthetics contraindicated in infected or potentially contaminated procedures
- About Components Separation
  - o Release external oblique 1cm lateral to rectus
  - o Separate to midaxillary line from internal oblique (avascular plane)
  - o Rectus and anterior sheath can be separated from posterior sheath (extra 2cm mobility)
  - o Flap
    - Rectus with internal oblique and transversalis fascia
      - Moves medially
  - o Each side of abdominal wall moves:
    - 5cm at epigastrium (10cm total)
    - 10cm at waist (20cm total)
    - 3cm at suprapubic region (6cm total)
  - o Internal oblique- inferolateral oriented fibers
  - o External oblique- inferomedial oriented fibers

- Other surgical options, dependent on location of wound:
    - Anterolateral thigh flap
    - Tensor fascia lata
    - Rectus abdominis
    - Latissimus dorsi
    - Free flaps
- Skin defect only
    - Lateral undermining and closure
    - Skin graft over fascial closure
    - Fasciocutaneous or musculocutaneous flap
- Fascial defect options
    - Primary closure
    - Mesh Repair
    - Components separation
    - Bridging material soft polyprolene vs. acellular human dermis
- Make a plan and select your surgical approach based on presented clinical scenario.

4. Understand risks and benefits of various approaches
    - Mesh
        - Primary risks- infection, dehiscence, recurrence
        - Primary benefit- availability
    - Components separation
        - Dehiscence: 22%
        - Autologous reconstruction, resistant to infection
    - Muscle flaps
        - Donor site morbidity
        - Eventual atrophy from non-use
        - Fascial flaps better than pure muscle flaps
    - If possible await resolution of active infection or inflammation prior to reconstruction
        - Antibiotic therapy
        - Remove infected mesh
        - Drain pockets of fluid or abscess
    - General Considerations
        - Stability of patient
        - Reconstructive options may be limited
        - Wound contamination
    - In case of failed prosthetic or simple flap closure:
        - Do not reattempt same repair

- - - Must use components separation or other major flap closure
    - Infection or excess tension frequent cause of failure
  - Postop Management
    - Drains: long-term
    - Closed suction: minimum 1 week
    - Early ambulation
      - DVT prophylaxis- what is your protocol?

5. Address complications and unexpected problems adequately

   - Dehiscence
   - Wound infection
   - Postop ileus
   - Bowel injury
   - Skin necrosis/wound healing problems
   - Enterocutaneous fistula management
   - Delay closure if ostomies present
   - Abdominal compartment syndrome management
   - Give your rationale as to why the complication occurred

6. Demonstrate ability to structure alternative plan

   - Stabilize acute problems
   - Alternatives if primary operation fails
   - In case of ostomies, close with component separation at time of ostomy closure
     - May require mesh vs. acellular human dermis for closure

Chapter Twelve

Chest Wall Reconstruction

12
Chest Wall Reconstruction

1. Identify General Problem/Diagnosis/Planning
   (Describe photo, give working diagnosis, key problems, evaluates patient)

   - Describe defect
     - Note what is missing, exposed organs
     - Anticipate coverage needs based on potential surgical defect
     - Give working diagnosis
     - Note key problems
   - History
     - Sternal wound
       - Usually post-op complication following median sternotomy
         - Dehiscence or infection (1-3% incidence)
         - Usually early post-op
       - Etiology
         - Mechanical problem in closure
         - Ischemic injury
         - Severe COPD
         - Diabetes
         - Infection
     - Risk factors
       - DM
       - Obesity
       - Nutritional status
       - Ischemia
       - Immunocompromised
       - Smoking
     - Comorbid considerations
       - Can patient tolerate big surgery?
         - Hemodynamically stable
         - Pressors in use?
     - Anticoagulants in use?
       - Must coordinate with cardiology, ICU, cardiac surgeon

- Switch to heparin if on Coumadin
- Surgical Hx:
    - Is internal mammary artery (IMA) intact?
        - Affects use of pectoralis
        - Avoid turnover flap if IMA used for bypass
        - Avoid use of rectus on that side
    - Other procedures?
        - May affect flaps available for use
        - Previous abdominal surgery
            - Affects rectus, possibly omentum
        - Previous thoracotomy
            - Do not use latissimus on that side
- Categorize wound
    - Acute: first two weeks post-op
    - Subacute: between 2-4 weeks post-op
    - Chronic: over 4 weeks post-op
- Acute wound
    - May require early, emergent intervention if fresh coronary artery grafts are exposed
- Subacute and chronic wound
    - May tolerate period of wound preparation and medical optimization prior to reconstruction
- Flap closure of sternal wound is preferred option
- Flap closure decreases mortality (5-15%) compared to local wound care alone (50%)

- Physical Exam
    - What does wound look like?
    - Infection present, drainage?
    - Note any surgical scars
    - Size of wound
    - What is exposed?
    - Radiation damage
    - Tumor present?
    - Thin body habitus (omentum may not be available)
    - Don't forget to palpate wounds
    - Check for mobility of sternum
- Work-up
    - **Culture and sensitivities** most important
    - Chest x-ray
    - Medical and nutritional evaluation

- Lab work (CBC, Pre-albumin, Lytes, LFT's, PT/PTT) prior to any surgery
- Consultations
    - ID
    - Cardiology
    - CT surgery
    - Other as medically indicated
- Oncologic Chest Wall Defects
    - Need immediate coverage!!
    - Isolated chest wall lesion
        - Establish diagnosis
        - Determine extent of disease
            - Physical examination
            - Imaging as indicated
            - Plan resection and reconstruction
            - Consider post-op therapy
                - Chemotherapy
                - Radiation
    - Consider prior radiation or surgery
    - Consults
        - Thoracic surgery
        - Oncology

2. Consider reasonable goals in diagnosis and management *(Management and treatment, surgical indications, operative procedures and anesthesia)*

    - Medically optimize
        - Cardiac workup
            - EKG's, check arrhythmias, coronary circulation
        - Chest x-ray
            - Pleural fluid or collection
        - CT scan not needed in acute wounds
            - Useful in chronic wounds to evaluate extent of disease
    - Treatment based on type of infection
        - Pairolero (Three types of sternal wound):
            - Type I (Subacute)
                - Early separation with or without sternal instability
                - Within days or weeks of surgery

- Treatment:
    - Debridement
    - Removal foreign materials
    - Closure over closed suction
- Type II (Acute)
    - Fulminant mediastinitis within first weeks after sternotomy
        - Frank cellulitis and purulent drainage
    - Tx:
        - Wide debridement
        - Dressings
        - Serial debridement
        - Secondary flap closure
- Type III (Chronic):
    - Chronically infected >4 weeks, sinus tracts that drain into sternum several weeks to months after procedure
    - Tx:
        - Wound exploration
        - Wide debridement
        - Aggressive wound care
        - Secondary flap closure
- Conservative therapy
    - Debridement/drainage/extended wound care only
        - For patients in poor medical condition that cannot tolerate an extensive procedure
- Drainage
    - Evacuate infectious material
    - May be emergent at bedside
    - Ideally performed in OR
    - Gross purulent fluid: immediate drainage needed
- Complete sternal debridement necessary first step!
    - Exposed hardware or bone in OR
    - Done in conjunction with cardiac surgeon
    - Serial debridement until ready for closure in OR
- Wound closure
    - Flap choice based on
        - Size of wound
        - Amount of contamination
            - Omentum ideal for:

- - -
        - - Severely contaminated wounds
          - Implant salvage e.g. aortic grafts
      - Available donor sites
    - Oncologic wound with prior radiation
      - Radiation can cause new tumors
        - Basal cell
        - Squamous cell
        - Osteosarcoma
        - Fibrosarcoma
        - Lymphangiosarcoma
        - Other
      - Tx:
        - Wide excision of all devitalized tissue
        - Reconstruct with muscle or myocutaneous flaps
        - Skeletal defects <5cm do not require reconstruction
        - Skeletal stabilization needed in:
          - Chest wall resection >5cm
          - Resection of more than 4-5 ribs
          - Chest flail may occur without stabilization
            - Paradoxical respiratory motion and abnormal ventilation
            - Reconstruction avoids chest flail, preserves respiratory function
    - Options for skeletal reconstruction
      - Autogenous bone grafts
        - Ribs
        - Iliac crest
        - Fibula
        - Graft must be opposed to large surface area of trabecular bone for osteoinduction to occur
      - Autogenous fascia lata graft
        - Semi-rigid skeletal substitute
      - Prosthetic materials (many advantages)
        - Conform to shape easily

- Materials (Gore-Tex, Teflon, Marlex, vicryl mesh) promote incorporation
- Marlex mesh with methyl methacrylate sandwich
  - Good option- adaptable, durable, biologically inert, radiographically translucent

3. Select appropriate options in diagnosis and management

- Plan for closure when all nonviable tissue and foreign material (wires) have been removed
- Irrigation with pulsed antibiotic solution
- Minimize dead space
- Interim dressings until closure
  - Wet to dry antibiotic dressing in gross purulence
  - Negative pressure therapy for cleaner wounds
- Support chest stability
  - Velcro binders and "coughing pillows"
- Surgical procedure
  - Begin once wound clean 48 hours or more after cleansing areas of frank pus
    - Exception: omental flap can be done earlier
  - Cover exposed bone and myocardium with healthy vascularized tissue
  - Minimize dead space
    - Use prolonged aggressive post-op wound suction (drains on wall suction at 100mmHg)
    - Facilitates flap adhesion and obliterates dead space
  - Airtight/watertight wound closure
- Flap options
  - Pectoralis muscle
    - Most commonly used flap
    - Unilateral or bilateral
    - Blood supply
      - IMA for turnover flap
        - Generally not an option as IMA frequently used for bypass

- - -
    - - -
        - Contralateral turnover frequently limited reach
        - Some institutions still use turnovers routinely and split the muscle to enhance coverage
    - Thoracoacromial artery for medial advancement flap
        - Steps:
            - Release from sternum, clavicle
            - Islandize flap, release insertion on humerus
  - Rectus abdominis
    - Unilateral or bilateral
    - Blood supply: superior epigastric (IMA must be intact)
    - More morbid harvest using abdominal flaps
  - Latissimus dorsi
    - Secondary or tertiary choice because harvest requires lateral decubitus or prone position
    - Blood supply: thoracodorsal pedicle
  - Omentum
    - Third choice if no muscle flaps available
    - Rescue flap in cases of severe infection
    - Important consideration in diabetic patients
        - Decreases incidence of second operation in diabetics
    - Steps:
        - Preserve gastroepiploic vessels
        - Separate from attachments to transverse colon
    - Disadvantages
        - Residual small abdominal wall hernia
        - Suture omentum to fascial edges to decrease need for re-operation
  - Free flap if other options not available
    - Anterior lateral thigh flap
  - Skin usually available for closure

- o Non-operative therapy can be done with extended VAC therapy with eventual granulation tissue and split thickness skin graft
  - ▪ Option for unstable patients that cannot tolerate a big procedure
  - ▪ More morbid
- ▪ Oncologic Chest Wall Defects
  - o Describe what is missing, anticipated defect
  - o Aggressive wide debridement for irradiated areas
  - o Select flap for coverage
  - o Consider the need for chest wall stabilization if ribs are resected
  - o Reconstructive options are above-mentioned flaps as well as:
    - ▪ Trapezius flap
      - • Type II dominant vessel transverse cervical artery and vein
      - • Spinal accessory nerve
      - • Covers superior aspect of posterior chest wall
    - ▪ Parascapular flap
      - • Pedicle circumflex scapular artery
      - • Covers shoulder, axilla, lateral chest wall
    - ▪ Serratus Anterior flap
      - • Intrathoracic cavity defects
      - • Cannot use entire muscle (may cause winging of scapula)
    - ▪ External Oblique flap
      - • Covers anterior chest wall defects
    - ▪ Free flaps
  - o Choose coverage based on size of defect, exposed underlying structures and available donor sites.
  - o **Don't forget thoracic surgery/oncology consultation!**

4. Understand risks and benefits of various approaches

   - ▪ Select flap based on size of defect, available muscle flaps considering prior surgeries
   - ▪ Consider timing of surgery
   - ▪ Pectoralis - first choice flap; note status of IMA

- Rectus - increased morbidity from abdominal flap harvest
- Omentum- residual abdominal wall hernia
- Consider indications for plate and screw fixation of sternum
  - Sterile dehiscence with minimal contamination
- Immediate coverage scenarios
  - Exposed bypass grafts
  - Oncologic resection with exposed viscera

5. Address complications and unexpected problems adequately

- Potential complications
  - Hematoma/bleeding
    - Infrequent, frequently secondary to anticoagulants
    - Manage anticoagulation in conjunction with cardiac team
    - +/- Drainage: when will you go back to OR?
  - Seroma
    - Manage/prevent via wall suction up to 5 days to minimize dead space and promote flap adherence
  - Avoid injury to heart or grafts during debridement
    - Debridement with cardiac surgeon present or available
  - Infection
    - Prevention best course
    - Usually secondary to inadequate debridement
      - Debride all exposed cartilage as completely as possible
    - Intense pre-op wound care
    - Incision, drainage, adequate debridement
    - VAC therapy
    - Use cultures to target proper antibiotics
    - Antibiotic irrigation: minimum 3L
    - In event of reinfection:
      - Reopen and debride
      - Allow healing by secondary intention
      - VAC therapy
      - Second flap rarely needed unless frank flap necrosis

- - Omentum good salvage flap option
  - Wound breakdown
    - Work-up cause
      - Infection vs. ischemia
    - Appropriate post-op antibiotics in conjunction with ID recommendations

6. Demonstrate ability to structure alternative plan

   - If patient too unstable for wound closure, consider prolonged therapy with VAC
   - Optimize medical status
   - What will you do for flap failure?

Chapter Thirteen

Pressure Sores

13
Pressure Sores

1. Identify General Problem/Diagnosis/Planning
   (Describe photo, give working diagnosis, key problems, evaluates patient)

   - Describe the defect
     - Note stage of pressure sore
     - Size of wound
     - What tissue is missing?
     - What is exposed?
     - Chronicity of wound
   - History
     - What pertinent medical information do you want to know?
     - Investigate underlying cause
       - Noncompliance
       - Social circumstances
       - Pressure from wheelchair, other
       - Attempted pressure relief measures
       - Acute illness
         - ICU admission with intubation/deep sedation
       - Immobility and etiology of immobility
       - Other
     - Co-morbidities
       - DM
       - PVD
       - CAD
       - Stroke
       - Acute neurologic disease
       - Orthopedic injury (femoral head fracture)
       - Smoking
       - Spina bifida
       - Other
   - Primary Factors Causing Pressure Sores
     - Unrelieved pressure
     - Shear
     - Frictional forces

- o Force >32mmHg impairs perfusion
  - Sitting position generates 100mmHg
- Risk Factors
  - o Braden Scale based on:
    - Skin Moisture
    - Activity
    - Mobility
    - Friction and shear
    - Nutrition
  - o Elderly with femoral neck fracture
  - o Quadriplegic/Paraplegic
  - o Neurologically impaired
  - o Chronically hospitalized or facility residents
  - o Altered level of consciousness
  - o Malnutrition
  - o Anemia
  - o Altered sensation
  - o Immobility
  - o Ischemia and sepsis (ICU patients)
  - o Infection
  - o Small vessel occlusive disease
- Physical status
  - o Ambulatory (better outcomes)
  - o Wheelchair bound
  - o Bed bound
- Location of wound
  - o Ischial
    - Wheelchair bound, able to sit
  - o Sacrum, heels, occiput
    - Bed bound
- Physical Exam
  - o Extent of Ulcer
    - Stage
      - I - erythema, non-blistering
      - II - blisters, partial skin loss
      - III - subsequent full thickness skin loss, not to fascia
      - IV - fascia, muscle, bone, joint
    - Size of wound
    - Exposed tissue
    - Previous operations/scars
      - Check for available donor sites

- General work-up
- R/O Osteomyelitis
  - MRI
  - Bone Culture/Biopsy
- R/O associated infection (warmth, erythema, tenderness, edema)
  - Wound infection
  - Untreated UTI in catheterized patients
  - Pneumonia in quadriplegics/paraplegics
- Incontinence
  - Rectal
    - Consider diverting ostomy in extreme cases
      - Ostomy generally not needed, morbid procedure
  - Urinary
    - Must address prior to surgery
- Spasm
  - Treat prior to wound closure
  - Potentially increases tension
  - PT to prevent contracture; if this fails, tenotomies may be needed
- Nutrition work-up
  - Oral intake
  - Minimum
    - Check for anemia (CBC)
    - Check pre-albumin levels/albumin levels
      - Low pre-albumin may be associated with zinc deficiency; normalize prior to surgery
- Work-up in all chronic wounds
  - Labs
    - CBC
      - WBC with differential
      - Hb/Hct (check for anemia)
    - Iron
    - Transferrin levels
    - Glucose + Hgb A1C
    - Albumin >3.0 ideal
    - Pre-albumin (16-35 normal range)
    - ESR
    - C-reactive protein
    - Cultures, bone biopsy ideal

- Consider core needle bone biopsy
    - Imaging (as indicated)
        - Plain x-rays
        - MRI (97% sensitivity, 89% specificity for osteomyelitis)
- Evaluate and note options for closure and initial plan based on:
    - Medical status
    - Previous surgery
    - Current state of wound
    - Previous operation records are important

2. Consider reasonable goals in diagnosis and management *(Management and treatment, surgical indications, operative procedures and anesthesia)*

- Prevention
    - General
        - Maintain good medical/nutritional status
        - Routine pressure relief measures
        - Avoid frictional forces
        - Control incontinence and spasm
    - Ischial Ulcers
        - Cushion Status
        - Cushion change
            - Gel
            - Foam
            - Air
            - Water
        - Wheel-chair bound, seated patient should routinely lift and shift weight for 10 seconds every 10 minutes.
    - Sacral Ulcers
        - Mattress, bedding
            - 4" of foam minimum
        - Alternating air cell
        - Low air loss bed
        - Clinitron (periop use, too heavy for home therapy)
- Nutrition management
    - Optimize nutrition prior to surgery
        - Prevents wound complications

- o Consider enteral feeds vs TPN
  - Enteral feeds ideal
  - 25-35 calories/kg non-protein
  - 1.5-3.0 gm/kg protein
- o Correct vitamin deficiencies
  - Vit C
    - Affects collagen synthesis
  - Vit A
    - Supplementation reverses steroid effects
    - Deficiency impairs wound healing, increases risk of infection
  - Zinc
    - Deficiency inhibits epithelialization and fibroblast activity
- Chronicity of wound dictates initial management
  - o New wound
    - Trial of non-operative management
      - Wound care
      - Pressure relief measures
      - Medical optimization
      - Monitor wound response
  - o Chronic
    - More recalcitrant to non-operative management
    - More likely to require operative management
    - Small wounds: may debride then attempt trial of local wound care
- If osteomyelitis (osteo) present
  - o IV antibiotics to downstage wound
  - o Delay flap closure 6 weeks conservative approach
  - o Can do immediate biopsy and closure at time of debridement if wound seems clean enough
    - Treat osteo after surgery if bone culture is positive

- Initial wound care and management
  - o Topical antibiotics/enzymatic debridement
    - Silvadene
    - Collagenase/polysporin powder
    - Sulfamylon

- o Topical acetic acid or Dakin's solution
- o VAC therapy
- o Optimize nutrition
- o Pressure relief measures, control spasm
- o Control infection
- o Control friction/shear
- o Debridement
  - Surgical and mechanical to decrease bacterial load
- o Complete medical evaluation
- Decide on surgical intervention and timing based on:
  - o Medical status
  - o Status of wound
  - o Response to wound care
  - o Generally, not an emergent problem
- If non-operative treatment is working, continue until closure or until wound healing is no longer progressing
- If non-operative therapy fails, consider surgery
  - o Always monitor response to non-operative therapy first unless wound is obviously too large for closure by non-operative measures
- Continue non-operative therapy for poor surgical candidates
  - o Avoidance of unrelieved pressure
  - o Control of infection
  - o Control of incontinence
  - o Improve nutrition
  - o Goal is to stabilize wound
- Goals of management
  - o Best treatment is prevention
    - Prevent progression
      - Pressure relief (foam, air-mattress, cushion changes, etc.)
      - Turning at regular intervals
    - Correct and optimize medical co-morbidities
      - DM
      - Infection
      - Other
    - Spasm therapy
      - Medical therapy
        - o Diazepam
        - o Baclofen
        - o Dantrolene

- Surgical therapy
  - Peripheral nerve blocks
  - Epidural stimulators
  - Baclofen pump
  - Neurosurgical ablation
  - Cordotomy/rhizotomy
  - Amputation
    - DVT Prophylaxis
    - Operative treatment only after failure of non-operative options
    - Stage III or IV ulcers generally require surgical treatment
    - May consider no intervention (non-operative treatment only) in:
      - Post-traumatic paraplegic males aged 20-30
        - Poor compliance
          - 80% recurrence in 10.9 months
      - Stroke in elderly patients
        - 69% recurrence
  - Contraindications to surgical reconstruction
    - Terminally or critically ill unable to undergo general anesthesia
    - Sepsis
    - Wound bacterial load $>10^5$ cfu/gm tissue beta hemolytic strep
    - Albumin <2.0
    - Preop vital capacity <1500 ml
    - Failure to control spasticity
    - Noncompliance with previous rehab protocols, multiple recurrences
    - Insufficient social support system for post-op care
    - Most contraindications can be addressed directly and allow for surgical intervention

3. Select appropriate options in diagnosis and management

- Choose appropriate operation based on:
  - Wound status
  - Previous surgery
  - Available donor sites
- Surgical Principles

- o Complete excision of ulcer bursa and heterotopic calcification
  - Wetting solution for hemostasis
  - Methylene blue to mark area for excision
  - Indurated tissue tends to leave dead space
- o Ostectomy of all devitalized/infected bone
  - Debride to hard, healthy, bleeding bone
- o Minimize ischial excision
  - Increased risk contralateral ulcer
  - Bilateral ischiectomy: increased risk urethral fistula
  - 38% recurrence in total ischiectomy
    - i.e. contralateral ulcer
- o Bone culture for antibiotic coverage
- o Meticulous hemostasis
- o Avoid radical ostectomy in all cases
- o Eliminate dead space with flaps
- o Never do primary closure (always fails)
  - Tension free closure critical
- o Avoid incisions on weight bearing surfaces
- o Anticipate next flap i.e. secondary flap use
  - Use large flap of simplest design that allows re-rotation
  - REMEMBER 80% recurrence
- o Skin graft acceptable for superficial ulcer
  - 30% success rate
  - Plan for flap if it fails
- o Only undermine what is needed for closure
- o **Modify all predisposing factors prior to surgery!**
- Ischial Ulcers
  - o Most common ulcer in paraplegic patients
  - o Operative approach
    - Jack-knife flexed position
      - Best way to access size of ulcer
    - Adequate padding of pressure points for pressure sore prevention during surgery
    - Sequential compression devices
  - o Options
    - Fasciocutaneous flaps
      - Axial blood supply
      - Durable
      - Minimal functional deformity

- Important in ambulatory patients
- Can be re-rotated
- Disadvantage
    - Minimal bulk for large ulcers
- Flaps
    - Posterior thigh flap
    - Gluteal fasciocutaneous flap
    - Anterolateral thigh fasciocutaneous island flap
- Musculocutaneous flaps
  - Excellent blood supply and bulk
  - Can be re-rotated
  - Disadvantages
    - Atrophic in older patients and spinal cord patients
    - Functional impairment in ambulatory patients
  - Flaps
    - Superiorly based gluteal musculocutaneous flap
      - Gluteus maximus NOT expendable in ambulatory patients
      - Can be split
    - Posterior thigh musculocutaneous advancement flap
      - Hamstrings includes biceps femoris/semimembranosus/semitendinosus
      - Can be used as a V-Y advancement flap
    - Tensor fascia lata (TFL)
      - Occasionally used for ischial pressure sores
      - Thin padding
- Sacral Ulcers
  - Operative approach

- Prone positioning
- Adequate padding for pressure prevention
- Sequential compression devices
        - Options
            - Gluteal V-Y Advancement
            - Gluteal rotation advancement fasciocutaneous or muscle flap
                - Superiorly or inferiorly based
            - Lumbosacral (fasciocutaneous)
                - Requires back grafting of donor site
    - Trochanteric Pressure Sores
        - Etiology: pressure in lateral decubitus position
        - Options
            - Tensor fascia lata (TFL) flap
                - Highly reliable
                - Perforators from TFL muscle
                - Pivot point 8cm below anterior superior iliac spin (ASIS)
                - Sensation L1, L2, L3, lateral femoral cutaneous nerve
                - Can reach ischial and sacral ulcers
                - Problem: Distal tip of flap not well padded
                - Probably best for trochanteric ulcers or as adjunct flap in large sacral or ischial ulcer
            - Rectus femoris muscle
                - Can interfere with extension of leg at the knee
            - TFL + vastus lateralis
            - Girdlestone procedure
                - Closure with proximal femurectomy and vastus lateralis
                - Consider consultation with Ortho with operative assistance
                - Femurectomy reduces pressure in trochanteric region
    - Extreme recurrent cases or multiple prior surgeries
        - Carefully consider:
            - Total thigh flap
            - Amputation

- Hemipelvectomy
- Hemicorpectomy
- Hip disarticulation
            - All highly morbid surgical options
            - Must have an ideal patient or life threatening clinical situation
        - Post-op management
            - Inpatient for initial peri-op period, minimum 2 weeks
            - Clinitron bed
                - Ordered pre-surgery
                - Confirmed and waiting in PACU prior to starting case
                - Transfer into clinitron immediately from OR table
            - Maintain flat supine position 2 weeks
            - IV antibiotics 3-6 weeks based on culture results
            - Seat mapping for customized cushion for wheelchair
            - Start sitting protocol at 6 weeks
            - Drains minimum of two weeks
            - Occlusive dressing for 1 week, then keep wounds clean and dry
                - Wash wounds twice a day after removal of dressing
            - Staple removal starts at week 2
            - Continued control of incontinence
            - Nutritional repletion

4. Understand risks and benefits of various approaches

    - Risk-benefit ratio of surgery based on acute and chronic medical issues
    - Optimize patient for surgery
        - Identify etiology of pressure sore
        - Nutrition
        - Post-op management plan
        - Pre- and post-op operative plan
        - Social support
    - Is patient a good candidate for surgery?
    - Fasciocutaneous flap vs. musculocutaneous flap
    - Management of ambulatory vs. non-ambulatory patient
    - Attend to preventative measures for recurrence

- Medical
- Surgical
- Social

5. Address complications and unexpected problems adequately

- Complications
    - Autonomic dysreflexia
        - Can happen with bedside debridement or with surgery under general anesthesia (avoid by using local)
        - Cause
            - Overstimulation
            - Noxious stimuli
        - Symptoms
            - Paroxysmal hypertension
            - Throbbing headache
            - Profuse sweating
            - Flushing of skin
            - Bradycardia
        - Treatment
            - Antihypertensives
            - Remove stimuli
    - Hematoma - evacuate or drain if large
    - Seroma - evacuate or drain if large
    - Persistent wound infection
        - Decrease risk of infection by staging debridement and flap closure
            - Debride first
            - VAC therapy followed by flap at separate operation
        - Inadequate debridement: potential cause of infection
        - Missed osteo
    - Flap necrosis management
    - Recurrence most common complication (as high as 80%)
        - Underlying medical problems still exist
        - Noncompliance with post-op care
        - Must be able to identify and modify predisposing factors prior to embarking on surgical closure (if not, NO SURGERY)

- Get control of wound (reconsider timing for repeat surgery)
    - Not emergent to reclose wound
- Avoid radical ostectomy
    - Increased risk of bleeding, hematoma
    - May cause skeletal instability
    - Redistribution of pressure points, especially in ischial pressure sores (Contralateral side increased pressure)

6. Demonstrate ability to structure alternative plan

- What if planned flap not available?
- Back-up plan for flap failure
- Recurrent infection
- Patient persistently non-compliant, but wants repeat surgery
- Recurrent pressure sore

Chapter Fourteen

Abdominal Compartment Syndrome

14
Abdominal Compartment Syndrome

1. Identify General Problem/Diagnosis/Planning
   (Describe photo, give working diagnosis, key problems, evaluates patient)

   - Abdominal compartment syndrome is a risk of:
     - Components separation
     - Closure and reduction of abdominal contents into a smaller volume space
     - May be secondary to bowel injury or general bowel edema post-op abdominal wall closure
   - Hx:
     - Recent abdominal surgery or abdominal trauma
   - Pertinent PE findings:
     - Abdominal distention
     - Tight abdomen
     - Hypotension
     - Tachycardia
     - Oliguria
     - Increased peak inspiratory pressure (in vented patient)
     - Decreased urine output
   - Clinical sign: Poor response to fluid resuscitation
   - Work-up:
     - Check bladder pressure with a-line or CVP line via Christmas tree in foley
       - Pressure > 20-25mmHG diagnostic

2. Consider reasonable goals in diagnosis and management
   (Management and treatment, surgical indications, operative procedures and anesthesia)

   - Treatment goal: relieve excess abdominal pressure
     - Can progress to multi-system organ failure untreated
   - Treatment: open the abdomen in OR!
   - Resuscitate in ICU

- Temporize abdominal wound

3. Select appropriate options in diagnosis and management

    - Treatment: open the abdomen!
    - Temporize abdominal wound
    - VAC followed by skin graft
    - Delay re-repair
    - Evaluate and consider reasons abdominal compartment syndrome occurred prior to reclosing abdomen.

4. Understand risks and benefits of various approaches

    - If not treated, ongoing hemodynamic instability will ensue with possible multisystem organ failure
    - What are the risks benefits of immediate attempts at reclosure vs. delayed reclosure after reopening the abdomen?

5. Address complications and unexpected problems adequately

    - Manage open abdomen until stable
        - What is your management plan?
    - Manage concurrently with ICU, General Surgery teams

6. Demonstrate ability to structure alternative plan

    - Operative plan for future closure depends on etiology of compartment syndrome
        - If secondary to decreased intraabdominal volume, then consider mesh in combination with component separation for repair
        - If secondary to bowel injury or bowel edema, reattempt repair without mesh may be acceptable
    - Consider tissue expansion of abdominal wall to accommodate volume in case of loss of domain
    - Can temporize wound with skin graft
    - Timing of reoperation minimum 6-12 months post recovery

Chapter Fifteen

Bariatric Reconstruction

15
Bariatric Reconstruction

1. Identify General Problem/Diagnosis/Planning
   (Describe photo, give working diagnosis, key problems, evaluates patient)

   - Describe what you see
     - All visible deformities and areas to address
     - Evaluate: Face, breast, trunk, arms, thighs
     - Note key problems present for reconstruction
   - Hx:
     - Specify what you want to know regarding the overall health status of the patient
     - Determine if patient a candidate for major surgery?
     - What previous surgeries did the patient undergo?
       - Any abdominal operations?
     - Previous bariatric procedures?
       - Restrictive vs. Malabsorptive Procedures
       - Lap Band
       - Roux-en-Y Gastric Bypass
       - Biliopancreatic diversion-duodenal switch
     - How long ago was surgery?
       - Ideal surgical candidate for bariatric reconstruction
         - 1 year past surgical date **and** stable weight for 6 months
         - Maximized weight loss
         - Stable weight for 2-3 months minimum prior to surgery
       - Ideally stable weight for:
         - 18 months after roux-en-y gastric bypass
         - 24 months after gastric band or duodenal switch
     - Nausea, emesis sign of dumping syndrome
     - Other pertinent medical history
       - DM, HTN, Sleep Apnea
       - Prior surgeries, history of pregnancies
       - DVT

- Increased risk
- Consider IVC filter preop
- Smokers
  - 46% complication rate vs. 14% in non-smokers
- Physical Exam:
  - BMI >35: More weight loss prior to surgery
    - Except for disabling pannus
  - Evaluate key areas
    - Abdomen/Posterior trunk
      - Shape of torso
      - Double panniculus
        - Excess laxity above and below level of umbilicus
      - Hernias or fascial defects
    - Size and shape of mons pubis
    - Breast
    - Arm
    - Thigh
    - Neck
  - Note:
    - Skin laxity
    - Remaining adiposity
    - Rolls and folds
    - Skin tone
    - Skin Integrity (rashes, folliculitis, infections, lymphedema)
    - Scars (appearance HTS or keloid)
    - Abdominal wall structure
    - Panniculus grade
      - 1-barely covers pubic hairline
      - 2- covers entire mons
      - 3- covers upper thigh
      - 4- covers mid-thigh
      - 5- covers knee or beyond
- What work-up is necessary prior to surgical intervention?
- Work-up
  - Check current nutritional status
    - Hypoproteinemia
    - Hypocalcemia
    - Prolonged bleeding time

- ▪ Anemia frequent
  - • Check coags/Hb/Hct
  - • Hct of 20 not uncommon
- o Noncompliant patients are poor surgical candidates
- o Nutritional Supplements
  - ▪ Iron
  - ▪ Calcium
  - ▪ Vitamin A, D, E, K
    - • Vitamin K deficiency causes coagulopathy
- o Pre-op Labs
  - ▪ CBC
  - ▪ Lytes
  - ▪ LFT's
  - ▪ Coags- PT/PTT
  - ▪ Protein (albumin, pre-albumin)
  - ▪ Iron studies (transferrin, TIBC, increases ferritin)
- o Imaging
  - ▪ Consider pre-op CT scan Abd/pelvis to evaluate abdominal wall
    - • Especially in the case of large pannus
    - • Substantial abdominal wall defect may be present but not detectable on PE
  - ▪ Lymphoscintigraphy
    - • Prior to thigh lift if lower extremity swelling present
    - • R/O lymphatic or venous outflow obstruction
    - • Surgery may cause lymphedema
- o Consult with primary medical doctor and bariatric surgeon
  - ▪ May consult bariatric surgeon for hernia repair
  - ▪ Consider repair options if asked to perform yourself
- o Other preop consultations based on lab work and chronic medical comorbidities
  - ▪ Hematology- anemia, h/o DVT, clotting disorder

- Cardiology for high-risk patients
- Endocrinologist for DM management, thyroid issues, polycystic ovary disease
- Pulmonary- if on-going sleep apnea
- Psychiatry- screen for likelihood of post-op compliance
- Nutrition

2. Consider reasonable goals in diagnosis and management *(Management and treatment, surgical indications, operative procedures and anesthesia)*

- Contraindications to intervention
    - Only absolute contraindication to surgery:
        - Systemic disease that precludes safe general anesthesia
- Relative contraindications:
    - Smoking
        - Stop smoking 1 month prior to surgery to decrease risk of complications
        - Check urine nicotine level day of surgery
            - Cancel if positive
    - Active intertrigo
    - BMI >35
    - Coagulopathy
    - Collagen diseases
    - COPD
    - CAD
    - Renal failure
    - Suspicion patient will not be compliant with post-op management
- Manage patient expectations
    - Scarring
    - Waistline unlikely to be slender
    - Asymmetries will be present
        - Point them out to patient pre-op
    - Potential complications
        - DVT-PE-Death!
        - Seroma
        - Wound dehiscence
        - Bleeding
        - This is big time surgery!

- Admit to hospital for initial postop period
- Always get preop consent for blood transfusion
- Set up social support/family groups
- Umbilicus management
  - May have long stalk
  - In cases of long stalk, amputation and delayed umbilicoplasty may be necessary
- Abdomen management
  - Pannus
  - Abdominal wall defects
  - Old scars
  - Abdominoplasty
  - Panniculectomy
  - Lower Body Lift
  - Adjunct: liposuction flank and lower back
- Breast
  - Ptosis secondary to volume loss
  - Mastopexy +/- Augmentation
  - Gynecomastia surgery
- Arms
  - Candidate for brachioplasty?
- Thigh
  - Ptosis
  - Thigh lift
- Liposuction
  - Adjuvant therapy
- Most procedures will be done under general anesthesia

3. Select appropriate options in diagnosis and management

- Torso management
  - Frequently addressed first
  - Severe panniculitis
    - Panniculectomy only
- In Cases of >100lb weight loss
  - Lower body lift
    - Addresses: buttocks, lateral thighs and anterior trunk
  - Abdominoplasty (extended)
  - Fleur-de-lis Abdominoplasty (T-shape abdominoplasty)

- Consider in patients with midline scar
- Adjunct: liposuction flank and lower back
- Surgical Techniques
- Abdominal contouring
    - Aesthetic and functional
    - Aesthetics based on:
        - Adequate undermining
        - Abdominal wall plication
        - Umbilical transposition
- High-risk patients
    - Panniculectomy ONLY if indicated for function
        - No plication
        - Umbilicus sacrificed
        - 2 Drains
        - Skin closure 2-0 prolene, vertical mattress
- Giant Pannus Management
    - Suspend by technique of choice, options:
        - Suspend from ceiling bars
        - Hydraulic lift with Steinman pins
        - Traction bars
    - Benefits of suspension
        - Better exposure
        - Allows venous drainage
        - Facilitates ventilation
- Variation in Abdominoplasty
    - Some patients may require vertical incision to eliminate horizontal excess
    - Consider especially in patients with old midline incision
    - Downside:
        - Increased risk of postop complications (skin necrosis)
        - Limiting undermining may decrease complication risk
        - May avoid liposuction in these cases
- Monsplasty
    - Important adjunct to abdominoplasty in more cosmetic cases
    - Give appropriate attention to mons correction
    - Key points:
        - Lower margin incision

- 6cm above anterior vulvar commissure
- Just above pubic symphysis
- May require higher marking
            - Suspend tissues to abdominal fascia
              - Heavy suture (2-0 or 0 braided nylon)
            - Reduce thickness of mons by direct defatting
              - Lipo not preferred for defatting here
        - Potential benefits of monsplasty:
            - Improved sexual function
            - Does not impair sexual function
        - May temporarily change angle of urinary stream
    - Lower body lift
        - In massive weight loss patients
        - Correction of abdominoplasty alone may not be adequate
        - Lower body lift
            - Belt lipectomy
            - Circumferential torsoplasty
        - Goal:
            - Circumferential correction of laxity
              - Buttocks, lateral thigh, abdomen
            - Elimination of rolls and festoons
            - Ted Lockwood the innovator
        - Operative positioning options:
            - Two position procedure
              - Prone
              - Supine
            - Three position procedure
              - Lateral decubitus x2 (Left then right)
              - Supine
        - May not have specific landmarks
        - Try to keep resection low
        - Abdominal wall plication and vertical abdominal skin resection helps waist definition
        - Plan to preserve some adipose tissue to shape buttock region
    - Markings for lower body lift

- - -
      - Start supine, with upward stretch on lower abdominal tissues
      - Mark midline 6cm above anterior vulvar commissure
      - Mark should be above pubic symphysis on stretch
        - If not move mark superiorly until 1 or 2cm above symphysis
      - In Standing Position
        - Facing away from surgeon
        - Select superior anchor line
        - Keep low to minimize tension
      - Extend from mid-axillary line to midline
        - Make vertical reference marks every 6cm
        - Use **Pinch Test** to check margins of resection
          - Roll inferior tissue under anchor line
          - Mark lateral margin of resection
    - Lower body lift: operative details
      - Prone 1st
      - Foley
      - Warming blankets (bair hugger)
      - Padding for pressure
      - **HIGH RISK FOR PE, DVT**
        - Sequential Compression Devices
          - Start prior to induction
          - Pre- and/or Post-op lovenox
      - Chloroprep
      - Tumescent solution with epi along planned incisions
      - Areas for gluteal preservation
        - De-epithelialize with versajet or knife
      - Inferior flaps mobilized
      - Secure to muscle fascia
      - Plicate dermis
      - Contour skin for closure
      - Drains
      - **Turn supine**
      - Lower incision first
      - Standard abdominoplasty technique
    - Breast: Female Patients
      - Goal: Address breast deflation and distortion
      - Problems:

- Loss of volume
            - Loss of elasticity
            - Asymmetry
            - Medialization of nipples
            - Laxity of lateral chest wall and rolls to back
        - Many options:
            - Individualize management
        - Wise pattern mastopexy
            - Goal:
                - Remove excess skin of deflated breasts
        - AVOID simultaneous augmentation and mastopexy
            - If done, best sequence ("safest"):
                - Augmentation followed by mastopexy
        - Recommendation
            - Mastopexy first stage
            - Augmentation second stage
        - Consider dermal suspension techniques
        - Dermal suspension and total parenchymal reshaping
            - Goal:
                - Create internal brassiere; gives long lasting shape
        - Modified Wise pattern
            - Auto-augmentation with excess tissue from lateral chest wall
            - Area for skin excision is de-epithelialized
            - Lateral wing of wise-pattern augments breast
            - Nipple position moved laterally
            - Dermis is incised and sutured to pectoralis fascia with 0-braided permanent suture
- Breast: Male Patients
    - General Clinical Presentation:
        - Grade III Gynecomastia with excess skin
        - Pseudogynecomastia after massive weight loss
    - Breast management:
        - Individualize treatment
        - Most bariatric patients require skin excision
            - Elliptical mastectomy and nipple repositioning

- Review Gynecomastia Chapter 3
  - Nipple Management:
    - Skin excision with free nipple graft or elliptical excision with nipple preserved on thin broad based pedicle
    - How do you position the male nipple?
      - Male nipple position
      - 1/3 the distance from sternum to pubis
      - Inter-nipple distance 0.23 x Chest circumference
      - Nipple should lie lateral to mid-clavicular line
      - Approximately 2.5 cm above the IMF
    - Ideal nipple size 2.8cm
      - U.S. quarter (2.5cm) as sizer
      - 2.5cm marking from marking pen gives additional 3mm if you cut on the outside of the line
- Arms
  - Goal: Correct arm, axillary region, and chest wall together
  - General Problem:
    - Excess skin- "bat wings"
    - Folds on flank
  - Options:
  - Liposuction alone
    - Generally not helpful in bariatric patients
  - Brachioplasty
    - Marking
      - Sitting or standing with arms bent
        - 90 degrees at elbow
        - 90 degrees abduction at shoulder
      - Mark bicipital groove
      - Avoid crossing the elbow for distal extent of resection
      - Proximal extent of resection ends at dome of the axilla

- May extend inferiorly at 90 degrees onto chest wall
- Length of incision determined by skin laxity
- IV placement
  - Foot ideal
  - Okay if distal to elbow
- Procedure
  - Incision placed along bicipital groove- L-shape
  - Longitudinal elliptical pattern with extension into axillary region
  - Step-by-Step excision
    - Allows concomitant closure with resection
    - Decreases risk of inability to close arm
  - Do not discard excised skin until complete closure in case short of skin on closure
  - Z-plasty may be added in axilla if additional skin excision needed, risk of tissue breakdown
  - Keep dissection above brachial fascia
- Important anatomy
  - Medial antebrachial cutaneous nerve
    - Emerges from inner aspect of mid-humerus from subfascial plane
    - Lies superficial and inferior around the elbow
    - Associated with basilic vein
- Liposuction
  - Useful adjunct for thinning posterior aspect before excision
  - Risk of edema making closure more difficult
  - If skin elasticity is good:
    - Lipo alone is okay; not usually an option for massive weight loss population

- o Brachioplasty incisions have tendency for hypertrophic scar (HTS) formation
  - Manage patient expectations
    - State "expect red thick scar for 12-18 months until final scar maturation"
  - Scar management initiated early
    - Scar massage
    - Silicone
    - Pressure garment
    - Steroids
    - Laser therapy
  - Minimum 12-18 months before considering surgical scar revision
- Thighs
  - o Problem: Excess skin and fat
  - o Treatment: Thigh lift
    - Impacts medial thighs
    - Decreases leg circumference
    - No effect on lateral thigh
      - Lower body lift affects lateral thigh
    - Usually performed after lower body lift as second stage
  - o Medial thighs
    - Address 3 months after abdominoplasty
    - Liposuction + crescent shaped skin excision superiorly within the groin
  - o Thigh Lift
    - Ideal table position
      - Start prone in jack-knife position
      - Finish with patient supine
    - Attempt to preserve the lymphatics
    - Minimize dissection over femoral triangle
    - Keep plane of dissection above saphenous vein
    - Preserve saphenous vein and overlying fat
    - Superficial fascial suspension system important to close
      - Minimizes widening of scars
      - Suture to firm tissue above Cooper's ligament

- Suture superficial fascial suspension system to Colle's Fascia
- Periosteum of ischium
- Very uncomfortable in immediate post-op period
  - Best not to combine thigh lift with other procedures
    - Review Ted Lockwood papers
  - AVOID longitudinal scar on inner thigh
    - Never used unless absolutely necessary
    - Increased recovery time
    - Increased pain
    - Increased risk of lymphedema if too much vascularity removed or damaged
    - If used, restrict incision above the knee, not below!
    - Incision goes from groin to knee
    - Sometimes requires T incision in groin
- Vertical thigh lifts
  - Better results if lower body lift performed first
  - Some patients will require vertical thigh lift
  - Medial thigh excision will undercorrect most massive weight loss patients
- Marking for thigh lift
  - Patient supine in frog leg position
  - Mark 4cm lateral to mons mark
  - Groin crease to gluteal fold
  - Estimate vertical skin resection by:
    - Pinch test
    - Anchor line drawn on each leg
  - Check symmetry

4. Understand risks and benefits of various approaches

- Consider general risks and benefits of different approaches to each anatomic area
- Consider sequence of reconstruction

- Limit undermining in abdominoplasty to costal margin to decrease risk of complications from decreased blood supply
- Brachioplasty risks
    - Long scars, hypertrophic scars
    - Residual excess skin
    - Compartment syndrome from tight closure
    - Medial antebrachial nerve or intercostals nerve injury
- Use superficial fascial system in all closures to decrease widening of scars

5. Address complications and unexpected problems adequately

- Post-op Management: Lower Body Lift
    - Drains
    - Beach Chair position 10 days
- Post-op Management: Thigh Lift
    - Drains
    - Leg elevation
    - Compressive hose 2-4 weeks
    - Anticipate leg swelling 2-6 weeks post-op
- Post-op Management: Brachioplasty
    - Drains
    - No heavy lifting 2 weeks
    - Active ROM to start 2 weeks post-op
- Complications
    - Seroma in 1/3 of cases
        - Frequent problem
        - Progressive tension sutures decrease the risk
        - Increased risk in prolonged OR time
        - Use drains in these cases to manage and decrease risk
        - Treatment:
            - Serial aspiration
            - Reinsertion of drain (technique of choice)
            - Sclerosing agents
            - V.A.C. Therapy
        - Prevention
            - Compression garments
            - Quilting techniques
            - Fibrin glue?

- Hematoma
  - Increased risk in bariatric patients
  - Post-op hematomas may be difficult to diagnose
  - Clinical sign:
    - Increased heart rate in absence of hypertension
  - May require CT scan for work-up to make diagnosis
  - Labs- CBC, PT, PTT
  - Gold standard- clinical exam to determine need for return to OR
- Unfavorable scars
  - Especially after brachioplasty
  - HTS, management:
    - Scar massage
    - Silicone sheets
    - Steroids
    - Pressure garments
- Lymphedema
  - Primarily post-thigh lift surgery
  - Secondary to lymphatic interruption
  - Prevent by preserving lymphatic drainage at primary surgery
- Wound dehiscence
  - Frequent problem
  - Secondary to:
    - Overly aggressive excision
    - Smoking
    - DM
    - Fat has poor blood supply
  - Prevention:
    - Avoid excessive undermining
    - Only undermine necessary areas
  - Treatment:
    - Local wound care
    - Topical antibiotics
    - Enzymatic debridement
    - V.A.C. therapy

6. Demonstrate ability to structure alternative plan

    - Consider operative timing based on patient's weight and timing post bariatric surgery
    - Consider patient's goals: are they realistic?
    - How will you stage surgeries and how much will you do at any one sitting?
    - Management of dog-ears and excess folds
    - What if patient does not agree with management plans?

Chapter Sixteen

Abdominoplasty & Liposculpture

———

16
Abdominoplasty & Liposculpture

1. Identify General Problem/Diagnosis/Planning
   (Describe photo, give working diagnosis, key problems, evaluates patient)

   - Describe given photo
     - Note areas of excess skin and subcutaneous tissue and/or laxity
     - Where are the major problem areas?
     - Extent of affected areas?
     - Is it limited to anterior abdominal wall and abdominal wall musculoaponeurotic laxity?
   - History
     - Any weight fluctuations?
     - History of pregnancy
     - Diet and exercise regimen
     - Previous abdominal surgery and/or hernia
     - Smoking
   - Physical Exam
     - BMI kg/m2
     - Three main components of evaluation:
       - Skin
         - Skin quality
         - Scars
         - Stretch marks (where will they end up)
         - Laxity
       - Subcutaneous fat
         - Thickness of fat
         - Is abdomen protruding?
           - Poor candidate
         - Thick panniculus may require thinning of flap (bariatric patients, massive weight loss)
           - Lipo and limited undermining

- Abdominal wall laxity
  - May contribute to protruding abdomen
  - Addressed by abdominal wall plication
  - Diver's test
    - Flex at waist
    - Supine on table lift head and back off table while palpating abdomen
- Check abdominal contour rib cage to mons
- Check mons
  - Ptosis
  - Excess fat
  - Special attention in high BMI patients
- Check waist, hips, and flank for localized fat deposits
- Previous abdominal scars
  - McBurney or lower abdominal scars little effect
    - Resected in panniculus
  - Lower abdominal transverse scars okay
  - Subcostal incision
    - Contraindication to abdominoplasty
    - High risk of skin necrosis
  - Midline scar
    - Acceptable
    - May limit flap advancement
    - Mild to moderate risk of skin necrosis
    - Revision of midline scar at second surgery safer
- Anatomy
  - Abdominal flap post abdominoplasty
    - Blood supply:
      - Lateral intercostals (interrupted by subcostal incision)
      - Old subcostal >3years may be safe with limited technique
      - Subcostal
      - Lumbar perforators

- High BMI superficial fat layer is thicker than deeper
- Vascular Zones
  - Zone I
    - Deep epigastric arcade
    - Central region xiphoid to pubis
    - Lateral edge of rectus to other lateral edge
    - Divided in abdominoplasty
  - Zone II
    - Lower abdomen one anterior superior iliac spine (ASIS) to the other
    - Superficial branches circumflex iliac and external pudendal vessels
  - Zone III
    - Critical zone to preserve
    - Blood supply to anterolateral abdominal wall above ASIS lateral to rectus sheath
    - Intercostals, subcostal, lumbar arteries
    - If disrupted during abdominoplasty, then skin necrosis!
  - Be able to draw vascular zones
- Sensation
  - 6-12th thoracic nerves and 1st lumbar nerve
  - Lateral femoral cutaneous nerve L2-L3 sensation to anterolateral thigh
    - Located 1-6cm medial to ASIS
    - Can be injured during abdominoplasty
    - Painful neuroma or paresthesia to anterolateral thigh
  - Iliohypogastirc and ilioinguinal nerve sensation to groin, symphysis pubis
    - Can be entrapped during plication
- Fascial attachments
  - Zones of adherence
    - Posteriorly midline over the spine
    - Anteriorly midline
      - Less defined zone of adherence over linea alba
    - Three horizontal zones of adherence
      - In inferior aspect of lower trunk
        - Prevents upward migration of abdominoplasty incision
      - Bilaterally at inguinal ligament

- o Above the mons pubis
  - Bilaterally between hip and lateral thigh
- Adipose tissue
  - o Two layers
    - Superficial
    - Deep
  - o Patterns
    - Androgenic- men abdomen and dorsal regions
    - Gynecoid- women thighs and ankles
- Ideal candidate
  - o Young, healthy, nonsmoker
  - o Weight within or slightly above normal range
- May have concomitant lipodystrophy of hips and lateral thighs
- Bariatric patients generally benefit more from circumferential truncal dermatolipectomy

2. Consider reasonable goals in diagnosis and management *(Management and treatment, surgical indications, operative procedures and anesthesia)*

- Abdominoplasty/Liposuction
  - o Manage patient expectations
  - o Psychologically stable
  - o Counsel risks and benefits
  - o Liposuction/abdominoplasty NOT an alternative to diet and exercise
- Goal of liposculpture
  - o Improve facial or body contour by removing localized fat deposits
- Indications
  - o Removal of fatty deposits with or without reinjection
  - o Areas that do not respond to diet or exercise
  - o Can be any anatomic area
    - Abdomen
    - Flank
    - Ankles
    - Thighs
    - Calves
    - Buttocks

- Back of arms
- Neck
    - Frequent adjuvant to other procedures without increased morbidity
        - Gynecomastia
        - Jaw and neck with facelift
    - Prior to:
        - Abdominoplasty (flanks)
        - Thigh lift
        - Brachioplasty
- Prep
    - Liposuction fluid injection
        - Determines amount of fat to be aspirated
        - Minimizes blood loss
        - Minimizes postop complications
    - Tumescent Solution
        - Saline 500ml
        - 1ml Epi (1:1,000,000) final concentration 1 in 500,000
        - 30ml 1% Lidocaine
    - Dry
        - No fluid injection
        - 20-45% blood loss in aspirate
    - Wet
        - 200-300ml infiltration
        - 4-30% blood loss in aspirate
    - Super-wet
        - Volume equal to volume anticipated for aspiration
        - 1% blood loss in aspirate
    - Tumescent
        - Volume 2-3 times amount anticipated for aspiration
        - Least blood loss
- Materials
    - Blunt tipped cannulas 2-4mm multiperforated
    - Complication rate related to cannula size
    - Smaller cannulas decrease trauma and blood loss
    - Syringe lipo best control over final volume of aspirated fat
        - Attach 20-35cm cannula to 60ml syringe
    - Antiseptic solution

- - - 15 blade for stab wounds for access
      - Closure 5-0 nylon or subdermal
      - Anesthesia local with sedation or general
  - Abdominoplasty
    - Indications
      - Skin and subcutaneous tissue excess and/or
      - Laxity limited to anterior abdomen and abdominal wall musculoaponeurotic laxity
    - Contraindications
      - Generalized obesity
      - Excessive intraabdominal content
      - Circumferential lower truncal excess
      - Smoking
      - Planned pregnancy in near future
        - Can affect results
      - Subcostal incision
        - Relative contraindication
    - Relative contraindications
      - DM
      - COPD
        - Abdominal wall plication contraindicated
      - CV disease
      - Thromboembolic events
    - Post-op care
      - Keep flexed in beach chair position
      - Walk same day of surgery (DVT prevention), bent at waist
      - Not allowed to straighten for 1 week

3. Select appropriate options in diagnosis and management

   - Suction-assisted liposuction
     - For fat excess only, no skin excess, and anticipate good post-op skin retraction
     - Power-assisted liposuction
       - Reduces fatigue and trauma
       - Device makes mechanized movement
     - Ultrasonic assisted liposuction
       - Transmits vibrations, ruptures fat
     - Vibrating cannulas
     - Technique

- Bimanual technique
  - Control and monitor position of cannula tip
  - Avoid perforation
- Pre-tunneling
- Cross radial tunneling
- Use multiple incisions with small cannulas
- Feathering
- Avoid suctioning too superficial (i.e. too close to skin)
  - Contour or skin deformity may occur
- DVT Prevention
  - Compressive stocking
  - Compressive devices for lower limbs
  - Low-molecular-weight heparin
- Abdominoplasty Options
- High lateral tension abdominoplasty
  - Maximum tension is created laterally
  - Improved contour and appearance of anterior thighs
  - Zone I
    - Always interrupted in abdominoplasty
  - Key to evaluate previous abdominal scars
  - Scar patterns focus on accommodating clothing patterns
  - Try to avoid dog-ears while balancing scar width
  - Abdominal wall plication important
  - Can increase intra-abdominal pressure
  - Problem in pts with COPD
  - Appropriately position mons
- Mini-abdominoplasty
  - Abdominal laxity restricted to infraumbilical region
  - Minimal laxity
  - Infraumbilical diastases
  - Diver's test
  - Good skin elasticity
- Abdominoplasty: Operative Approach
  - Landmarks and Anatomy
    - Umbilicus normally sits midline at level of iliac crests
      - Sometimes 2.5cm superior to crests

- Narrowest aspect of waist 2.5 cm cephalad to iliac crests
- Ideally, distance from umbilicus to anterior vulvar commissure is 18-21 cm
- Pubic hairline
- 5-7 cm cephalad to anterior vulvar commissure
- Large umbilical hernias or previous transection of umbilicus puts umbilicus at risk

o Markings
- French Bikini pattern
  - Scar at natural junction between abdominal and thigh units
- Mark 1-2 days before surgery
- Balance scar length with dog-ears
- Inferior line longer than superior
- Lower BMI: less dog-ear issues
- Mark midline
- For ptotic mons, mark line 7cm above top of anterior vulvar commissure or penis

o Steps
- Supine position
- Intermittent compression devices
- Peri-op antibiotics
- IV sedation or general
- Foley if long procedure planned (>4 hrs.)
- Incise around umbilicus first
  - Leave fat on umbo, periumbilical dissection
  - Retraction sutures at 6 and 12 o'clock
- Inferior mark incised
- Elevate flap at level of muscle fascia
  - Around umbilicus
  - Up to xiphoid to costal margins
- Leave subscarpal fat in femoral region
- Avoid extensive liposuction to flaps
  - May devascularize tissue
- If lipo used, limit elevation on either side of midline
- Flex at waist

- Examine abd wall laxity
- Vertical elliptical plication marked
- Two-layer vertical plication
  - First layer
    - Interrupted permanent braided
  - Second layer
    - Permanent monofilament running
- Flap advanced
- Tailored and skin closed with drains
- Scarpas and skin closed
- Consider indwelling pump for pain control
- Umbilicoplasty
  - Neoumbilicus: keep small, vertically oriented
  - Cone shaped
  - 1.5-2.0 cm vertical incision made overlying buried umbilicus
  - Three point fixation sutures placed
- Mini-abdominoplasty Approach
  - Abdominal flap raised to level of umbilicus
  - Flex
    - Examine laxity
    - Rectus muscle vertical plication
      - Umbilicus to pubis
  - Flap advanced excess tissue excised
  - Close
  - Drain
- Post-op Care
  - IV fluids, antibiotics 24 hours
  - Flex in beach chair position for 7 days
  - Diet as tolerated
  - Ambulate in flexed position 1 week
    - Then gradual stretching
  - Consider 23-hour stay
  - Abdominal binder or garment

4. Understand risks and benefits of various approaches

- Decide on operative plan based on physical findings and preop work-up

- o Individualize to patient needs
- o Consider lipo alone or combination of procedures
- o What are the risks?
- o Informed consent important
- o What is your anticipated outcome?

5. Address complications and unexpected problems adequately

- Liposuction
  - o Pulmonary embolism: most frequent cause of death
    - Etiology
      - Blood flow decrease in lower limbs, trauma, hypercoagulability
    - Work-up
      - ABG
      - CXR
      - Spiral CT scan
    - Tx:
      - Non-rebreather
      - Heparinization
  - o Fat Embolism
    - Difficult to avoid
    - Supportive care in ICU
  - o Abdominal perforation
    - Caution in patients with abdominal scars
  - o Lidocaine toxicity
    - Maximum dose 7mg/kg
    - Maximum subq dose 35mg.kg in super-wet technique
    - Serum level above 5microgram/ml
    - Super-wet technique
      - Deceased absorption
    - Lido absorption low in subq tissues
    - Diluted in large volume of fluid
    - Serum peak 6-8 hours post-op (while at home)
    - Symptoms and events
      - Agitation
      - Tinnitus
      - Seizure
      - Coma

- Cardiac arrest
- o Infection
  - Wound infection
    - Cellulitis
    - Abscess
  - Toxic shock
    - Initial signs non-specific
    - High temperature
    - Diarrhea
    - Vomiting
    - Hypotension
    - Cutaneous rash
    - Oliguria
    - Necrotizing fasciitis: Wide debridement
- o Prolonged edema and induration
- o Management of contour irregularities or skin problems from poor liposuction technique
- o Death: 1 in 5000
- o Limited liposuction to 5L reduces systemic complications
- Abdominoplasty
  - o Wound dehiscence
    - Technical error
    - Avoid by solid scarpas closure
    - Stay in flexed position 5-7 days even during sleep
  - o Hematoma
    - Meticulous hemostasis
    - Avoid bucking and coughing during extubation
    - Large evacuate
    - Small manage expectantly
  - o Wound infection
    - Increased with:
      - Obesity, DM, Smoking
    - Most common organisms:
      - Staph, Strep, Pseudomonas, E. Coli
    - Tx:
      - Antibiotics
      - Drainage of abscess

- Debridement and dressing changes
    - Toxic shock syndrome
        - Malaise
        - Very ill
        - Generalized discomfort
        - With or without fever
        - Tx:
            - Return to OR
            - Culture washout
            - ID consult
            - Staph coverage
    - Seroma
        - Drains
        - Aspiration initially
    - Tissue necrosis
        - Predisposing factors
            - Lipo in zone III
        - Debridement and dressing changes
        - Hyperbaric therapy
    - Contour irregularity
        - Inadequate plication
        - Lateral dog-ears
    - Scarring
    - Umbilical deformity
    - Paresthesia
    - DVT/PE
        - Prevention
            - Sequential compression garments
            - Early ambulation, day of surgery
            - Birth control pills stop one cycle prior to surgery
            - Chemoprophylaxis
            - High index of suspicion

6. Demonstrate ability to structure alternative plan

    - Indications for inverted "T" or fleur-de-lis
        - Increased risk of skin necrosis
    - Management of residual deformity
    - Management of abnormal scar and etiologies
    - What if patient is dissatisfied with result?

FACE

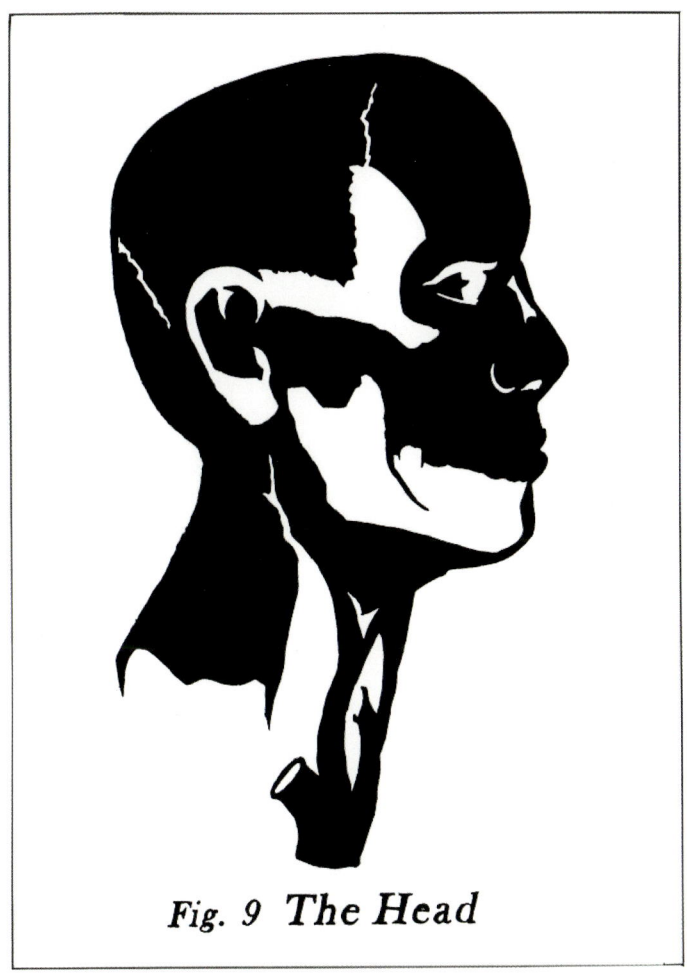

Fig. 9 The Head

Section Four
Facial Reconstruction

Chapter Seventeen

Facial Reconstruction Overview

17
Facial Reconstruction Overview

1. Identify General Problem

    - Describe photo
    - Give working diagnosis
    - Key problems
    - Evaluate patient
    - Diagnosis/Planning
    - Determine etiology of wound
        - Tumor, Trauma, Chronic wound, Infection
    - Be prepared to discuss reconstruction and management based on tumor type
        - Basal cell, Squamous cell, Melanoma, Merkel Cell
    - Classify problem
    - Describe what is missing and functional implications
    - Note anatomic location and all structures involved
    - Detail your physical exam including:
        - Palpation of lesion
        - Mobile vs. fixed
        - Oral examination
    - Give your clinical impression
    - Relevant medical history
        - Smoking, DM, CAD, HTN, Steroids
    - Pertinent positives and negatives in history
        - Drug abuse- cocaine
    - Previous surgeries
    - Relevant medications especially anticoagulants

    - Need for additional work-up and or consultants?
        - Imaging studies
        - Tear duct drainage
    - Oncology staging?

2. Consider reasonable goals in diagnosis and management

    - Management and treatment
    - Surgical indications
    - Operative procedures and anesthesia

- What is your surgical goal and why?
- Cancer management including lymph nodes

3. Select appropriate options in diagnosis and management

    - Your choice of surgical management and why?
    - Post-op management plan
    - Cancer management short-term and long-term
    - How is procedure performed?
    - Key steps of surgery
    - Details of procedure (main 5 steps)
    - Markings and relevant anatomy

4. Understand risks and benefits of various approaches

    - Be prepared to discuss the risks and benefits of various approaches
    - Functional advantages or disadvantages of different approaches
    - Consider:
        - Risk of microstomia
        - Ectropion
        - General scarring
        - Ability to eat
        - Effect on vision

5. Address complications and unexpected problems adequately

    - Hematoma
    - Flap loss
    - Recurrence
    - Bad scar
    - Bulky flap
    - Patient refuses treatment
    - Noncompliant patient
    - Patient belligerent with office staff

6. Demonstrate ability to structure alternative plan

    - Lifeboat or back-up plan if flap fails
    - Surgical plan for cancer recurrence

Chapter Eighteen

Scalp and Calvarial Reconstruction

18
Scalp and Calvarial Reconstruction

1. Identify General Problem/Diagnosis/Planning
   (Describe photo, working diagnosis, key problems, evaluates patient)

   - Take time to describe photo
     - Note what is missing, what is exposed
       - Hair
       - Layers of scalp
       - Bone
       - Brain
     - Note extent of wound, size of defect
       - This will influence choice of coverage
       - Use reconstructive ladder
     - Note key problems due to injury
       - Brain exposure- urgent coverage needed
       - Bone exposure- risk of osteomyelitis
       - Alopecia
   - History
     - Details of wound
       - Traumatic
       - Iatrogenic- tumor resection
     - Age of patient
     - Duration of wound
     - Loss of consciousness
     - Fall from height
     - Chronicity
       - In chronic wound
         - What is the duration?
         - Are the wounds stable?
     - Concurrent medical problems
       - PVD
       - Cardiac disease
       - DM
       - Smoker
     - Etiology of wound

- Electrical injury
  - Progressive tissue necrosis
  - Resembles crush injury
  - May require multiple debridements prior to definitive closure
  - Extent of injury depends on
    - Type of current
    - Duration of contact
    - Voltage
    - Low <1000 volts
      - Behaves like thermal burn
      - Household injury
    - High >1000 volts
      - Deep tissue destruction
      - Power line, industrial injury
- Traumatic scalp avulsion
  - Consider replant
- Burn injury
  - Acute vs. chronic
- Tumor
  - Plan for resection and reconstruction
  - Radiation exposure?
    - Decreased skin vascularity
    - Increased necrosis
- Pressure ulcer
- Congenital defect
  - Cutis aplasia

- Physical Exam
  - Trauma cases
    - ATLS Protocol/Full exam
    - Neuro status GCS
    - May influence timing of intervention
  - Other injuries
    - Head trauma
    - Thoracic trauma
    - Abdominal trauma
    - Extremities
    - Previous surgeries
  - Scalp avulsion

- Are vessels available for replant?
  - Minimum 2 arteries, 2 veins
  - The more veins the better
  - Post-op congestion a problem
- Acute wounds
- Chronic wounds
  - Are wounds stable?
- Electrical injury
  - Entry and exit wound?
  - Ocular exam in all patients
    - Late cataracts may occur 6 months or more after injury
  - EKG for arrhythmias in high voltage injuries
  - Abdominal exam for tenderness
  - Check extremities for:
    - Long bone fractures
    - Distal perfusion
    - Compartment syndrome
- Tumor
  - Is lesion mobile or fixed?
  - Check for lymphadenopathy
  - Is bone involved?
    - i.e. will craniectomy be needed?
    - Be prepared for brain exposure

- Work-up
  - Trauma
    - ATLS Protocol
    - Imaging
      - C-spine
      - Chest and pelvis
      - Head CT
      - As per current trauma protocol
  - Electrical injury
    - EKG
    - Labs
      - CBC
      - Lytes, K+
      - ABG, check for acidosis
      - Urine myoglobin
  - Tumor
    - Incisional or excisional biopsy for diagnosis

- Determine extent of disease
- Pre-op imaging
  - CT scan or MRI
  - Bone involvement?
- Staging
  - Metastasis?
  - Burn injury
    - Photos
    - Lund/Browder evaluation for burn injury
      - Estimate size of burn
        - Dictates resuscitation
        - i.e. Parkland or No Parkland
  - Other
    - Imaging studies as indicated
    - Pre-op blood work
    - Type and screen
  - Consultants
    - Neurosurgery
    - Trauma evaluation
    - Ophthalmology
    - ENT
    - Oncology

2. Consider reasonable goals in diagnosis and management *(Management and treatment, surgical indications, operative procedures and anesthesia)*

    - Electrical injury management
      - Management of compartment syndrome
        - Fasciotomy
          - In lower extremity
            - Anterior compartment
            - Lateral compartment
            - Superficial compartment
            - Deep posterior compartment
          - In upper extremity
            - Flexor compartment
            - Extensor compartment
            - Mobile wad
          - Be able to draw and describe
    - Burn injury management
      - Fluid resuscitation (Parkland)

- o Keep urine output
  - ▪ 0.5-1.0 ml/kg/hour minimum (adults)
  - ▪ 1.5ml/kg/hour (children)
- o Circumferential burn
  - ▪ Escharotomy if constricting
  - ▪ Decompress median and ulnar nerves
- o Tetanus
- o Topicals
  - ▪ Silvadene
  - ▪ Sulfamylon (mafenide acetate)
  - ▪ Collagenase and Polysporin
- o Early debridement
  - ▪ Decreases necrotic burden of tissue
- ▪ Reconstructive goals
  - o Soft tissue coverage for bone exposure
    - ▪ Early coverage for bone exposure avoids full thickness calvarial desiccation and bone loss
    - ▪ Can use VAC to temporize wound till definitive coverage
  - o Rigid protection for brain exposure
    - ▪ Exception in elderly patients
    - ▪ Acceptable not to reconstruct calvarium in the elderly
    - ▪ If rigid protection not able to be immediately provided, helmet for protection until definitive coverage
- ▪ Options and Indications
  - o STSG over pericranium (acute wounds) or granulating wound bed
    - ▪ Burring outer table + VAC may stimulate granulation tissue
      - • Burring may not be possible in infants and young children- thin vault
  - o Local and Regional Flaps
    - ▪ Indicated for limited defects
    - ▪ Pericranial flap + STSG if pericranium available
      - • Always elevate large pericranial flap
    - ▪ Temporoparietal fascia flap
      - • Blood supply superficial temporal artery

- An extension of the galea
  - Temporoparietal-occipital flap (Juri flap)
    - Can be used for frontal or frontoparietal defects
    - Width 4cm length up to 32cm!
  - Orticochea flap
    - For defects up to 30%
    - Elevate to deep galea
    - Incise galea to allow for additional stretch
    - Blood supply
      - Anterior pedicle- ophthalmic vessels
      - Lateral pedicle- superficial temporal artery
      - Posterior pedicle- medial and lateral occipital vessels
  - Fasciocutaneous Flaps
    - Rotation flap
      - Make large
      - Back graft residual defect if necessary
    - Rhomboid flaps
    - Other
  - Pedicled flaps
    - Latissimus dorsi
    - Trapezius
    - Pectoralis major
      - Limited reach in head and neck
- Free flaps
  - Indications
    - Large defects
    - Electrical injuries
  - Latissimus
    - Work horse flap
    - Ideal for large complex wounds
  - Omentum
    - For large complex wounds
  - Radial forearm
  - Anterior Lateral Thigh

- Recipient vessels
  - Superficial temporal artery can be used but is small and difficult to expose
  - If long pedicle available external carotid branches better
- Tissue Expander
  - Not for acute wounds
  - Two-stage elective reconstruction to correct large areas of alopecia
  - Place in subgaleal plane
  - For defects up to 50% of scalp
  - > than 50% hair starts to thin notably
- The Avulsed Scalp
  - Consider immediate replant if:
    - Minimal trauma to scalp itself
    - Short ischemia time <24 hours
  - Can survive on single artery and vein but the more the better chances of survival
    - Scalp has extensive collateralization
    - Superficial temporal artery and vein most common recipient
    - Can consider vein graft to branches of external carotid artery
  - Hair will grow if replant is successful
- Calvarial Recon Options
  - Full thickness skull defect
    - Autogenous bone
      - Cranial bone graft
      - Rib grafts
    - Alloplastic implant
      - Titanium mesh
        - Coverage with scalp or flap
      - Acrylic implant
      - Methylmethacrylate

3. Select appropriate options in diagnosis and management

- Choose intervention based on:
  - Size of defect
  - Amount of contamination

- o Chronicity of wound
- o Available donor sites
- Surgical goals
  - o Soft tissue coverage
  - o Calvarial reconstruction
  - o Protection of the brain
  - o Correction of scalp alopecia
- In cases of scalp alopecia
  - o Hair transplant?
  - o Small defects (<5cm) may be amenable to serial excision or local flap based on pliability of skin
  - o Pliability decreases with age
  - o Newborn extreme pliability vs. Eldery minimal pliability
  - o Larger defects (>5cm) will need tissue expansion
    - Expansion probably more reliable in most cases
- In elderly patients who may not tolerate long procedure:
  - o May consider soft tissue coverage without immediate calvarial reconstruction
  - o May delay recon or use helmet for protection

4. Understand risks and benefits of various approaches

- Based on size of defect must determine feasibility of various treatment options
- What are the upsides/downsides of different options?
- Autogenous vs. alloplastic reconstruction
- Risk of residual alopecia
- Growth considerations in pediatric patients?

5. Address complications and unexpected problems adequately

- Manage:
  - o Skin graft failure
  - o Local flap problems
  - o Free flap failing or failed
  - o Tissue expander complications
  - o Osteomyelitis
  - o Extensive alopecia
- Complications of Electrical Burn
  - o Arrhythmias

- o   Renal failure from myoglobin
- o   GI bleed
- o   Stress ulcers- antacid prophylaxis
- o   Flap loss
- o   Alopecia

6. Demonstrate ability to structure alternative plan

   - Exposed brain needs urgent coverage
   - Exposed bone need eventual definitive coverage
   - Back-up plan for failed flap or other initial intervention
   - FOREHEAD CONSIDERATIONS
     - o   May present as area for reconstruction electively for giant congenital nevus reconstruction or acutely after trauma or tumor resection.
     - o   Can be combined with scalp and/or facial defect.
     - o   Approach based on:
       - Etiology of anticipated defect
       - Size of defect
       - What is missing
       - Consider need for calvarial reconstruction
     - o   Note the goals of your reconstruction
       - Some cases may be temporization of wound with plan for definitive reconstruction at a later time
       - In the case of exposed brain immediate recon is needed to prevent life threatening complications
       - In the case of congenital nevi plan to optimize aesthetics and minimize functional impact. Tissue expansion frequently used in these cases.
       - Respect anatomic boundaries as much as possible
         - Hairline
         - Eyebrows
           - o   What are the options for eyebrow reconstruction?
           - o   How should hair transplants be oriented?

- What is your preferred modality of eyebrow reconstruction?
- Reconstructive Options
  - Healing by secondary intention
    - As in forehead flap for nasal reconstruction
  - Skin grafting
    - Ideal donor sites?
  - Local flaps
    - What are your favored local flaps in this region?
  - Pericranial flap with skin graft
  - Integra with skin graft
  - Tissue expansion
  - Free flaps to cover calvarial reconstruction and/or defects
  - Most complications related to local problems or modality of reconstruction.
- Be prepared to manage:
  - Common tissue expander related complications
    - Exposure
    - Infection
    - Devise malfunction
  - Microsurgical related problems
  - Skin graft or local flap related issues

Chapter Nineteen

Upper Eyelid Reconstruction

19
Upper Eyelid Reconstruction

1. Identify General Problem/Diagnosis/Planning
   (Describe photo, working diagnosis, key problems, evaluates patient)

   - Describe the photo.
     o What is missing?
       - Skin
       - Muscle
       - Septum
       - Tarsal plate
       - Conjunctiva
       - Lacrimal ducts/punctum
     o Note all details of the defect
       - Partial thickness vs. full-thickness
       - Amount of tissue loss
         • Partial <50% vs. Near Total or Total
         • Affects reconstructive choice
     o Note anatomic structures involved
       - Especially note if upper or lower lacrimal ducts are involved
       - Beware of medial lesions- management more complex
   - Determine etiology of defect, your presumptive working diagnosis
     o Congenital
     o Traumatic
     o Iatrogenic
     o Malignancy (Tumor)
     o Other
   - History
     o Useful to determine etiology of lesion
     o Increased risk of melanoma or non-melanoma skin cancer
       - Age >60
       - Fair skin
       - Chronic repeated sun exposure
       - History of radiation

- Length of time lesion has been present
  - Chronic lesion- likely malignant in adult
- Traumatic injury
- Previous surgery
- Painful eye
  - May indicate corneal exposure, keratopathy
- Watery eye
  - May indicate duct obstruction
- Visual symptoms
  - Indicates more extensive involvement
    - Pre-op CT scan
- Ensure patient is suitable for surgery
  - Concomitant medical conditions
    - Controlled HTN, DM, Smoker
  - Medications: NSAID, Anticoagulants
- In congenital cases
  - Are there other medical conditions?
    - Cardiac
    - Renal

- Physical Exam
  - In significant upper lid defects
    - Is Bell's phenomena intact/present?
    - Protects eye from corneal exposure during sleep
  - Middle third defects
    - High risk for corneal exposure
  - If lesion is present
    - Where is it located?
    - What is your estimated resection size?
    - Tumors generally require full-thickness excision
    - Fixed vs. mobile
    - Ulcerated/bleeding indicates cancer
  - Colobomas
  - Is vision intact?
    - Ophthalmology exam important
  - Best guess which lamellae are involved?
    - Anterior- skin/orbicularis
    - Middle- septum, tarsus
    - Posterior- tarsus (support) and conjunctiva
  - Other areas involved in defect especially in trauma cases

- Lymphadenopathy?
  - Parotid/cervical lymph node chains
- Don't forget to palpate lesion
- What are the key problems?
  - Avoidance of corneal exposure
  - Patency of lacrimal ducts
- Work-up
  - Consultants
    - Ophthalmology
      - Check if vision intact
      - R/O other problems pre-op
      - For congenital cases
    - Oncology
      - Evaluation for adjuvant treatment
- Tumor cases
  - Biopsy to determine etiology of lesion
  - Consider if imaging needed to determine extent of disease
  - Staging of malignant lesions
    - Consider need to r/o visceral metastasis:
      - Chest x-ray
      - CT scan head and neck/abd/pelvis
      - MRI
      - PET scan
- Skin cancer types
  - Basal Cell Carcinoma
    - Most common
    - Localized
    - Nodular
    - Sclerosing type
    - Recurrent
      - More aggressive
      - High recurrence rate after repeat excision
      - Candidate for Moh's resection
    - Generally no distant metastasis in basal cell carcinoma can be locally invasive
  - Squamous Cell Carcinoma
    - Less common (2-10% of eyelid tumors)
    - Tendency to spread to orbit, cranium or bone
    - Increased tendency for metastasis

- Risk factors
  - Sun exposure
  - Radiation
  - Chronic wound
  - Chronic exposure
  - Actinic keratosis
  - Bowen's disease
- Melanoma
  - Rare in eyelids (<1% of eyelid tumors)
  - Superficial spreading
  - Nodular
  - Lentigo maligna
  - Poor prognostic signs
    - Bleeding
    - Ulceration
  - Evaluate lymph nodes
  - Sentinel node biopsy
- Only 10% of upper lid lesions are malignant
- Congenital Cases
  - Ophthalmology
  - Genetics evaluation
  - Echocardiogram
  - Renal US
- Must know etiology of lesion/defect prior to reconstruction
- Benign lesions can be less aggressive with margins, better prognosis

2. Consider reasonable goals in diagnosis and management *(Management and treatment, surgical indications, operative procedures and anesthesia)*

- Determine etiology of lesion
- Skin cancer
  - Be able to manage:
    - Basal cell carcinoma, Squamous cell carcinoma, Melanoma
    - Review staging for above
  - Biopsy: Permanent vs. Frozen
    - Permanent better than frozen section for definitive diagnosis

- If frozen done in OR, better to temporize defect and do definitive reconstruction after permanent section complete.
- Moh's resection
  - Adequately evaluates margins and pathology during resection
  - Beneficial in areas of skin conservation like the eyelid
  - Not appropriate for melanoma at this time
  - Acceptable to reconstruct immediately based on Moh's resection in BCC and SCC
- Prior to surgery be sure cornea managed properly
  o Prevent or treat keratopathy
  o Ocular lubricant and ointments
  o Eye shield
  o Taping
  o Temporary tarsorrhaphy
- What will be involved in the reconstruction?
  o Anterior lamella (skin, orbicularis)
  o Middle lamella (septum, tarsus)
  o Posterior lamella (tarsus, conjunctiva)
- Anticipated involvement or excision
  o Small defect <1/3 of eyelid
    - Primary repair
  o >1/3: additional maneuvers will be needed
  o Large defects
    - Lid-switch- advancement transfers lashes
    - Lid-sharing flaps from lower lid
- Surgical goals
  o Restore form and function
  o Upper lid function
    - Primary function protect cornea
  o Avoid lagophthalmos with reconstruction
  o Smooth mucous membrane on inner lid
    - No suture knots to avoid irritation of conjunctiva and cornea
- Surgical Indications
  o Primary
    - Protection of cornea
    - Preservation of vision

- Secondary
  - Restore aesthetics
- Surgical options
  - Skin only/small or partial thickness defects
    - Skin graft
      - Potential donor sites
        - Contralateral upper eyelid
        - Retroauricular
        - Supraclavicular
        - Scalp
    - Local flap
      - Eyelid
      - Temporal skin
      - Glabella
    - Flaps of adjacent eyelid ideal
      - Maneuvers to increase laxity of flap
        - Release upper limb of lateral canthal tendon
        - Z-plasty can give further release
  - If orbicularis in intact:
    - FTSG is okay decreases contracture
      - 1st choice lax skin from opposite upper lid via bleph incision
      - 2nd choice postauricular or preauricular skin
    - Primary closure of donor site may require undermining
  - Extensive defects (multilayered reconstruction)
    - Posterior lamella and middle lamella
      - Composite graft
        - Nasal mucosa and septal cartilage
        - Replaces conjunctiva (inner lamella) and tarsus (middle lamella)
      - Hard palate mucosa
        - Lubricated and rigid
        - Replaces conjunctiva (inner lamella) and tarsus (middle lamella)
    - Anterior lamella

- Requires vascularized flap from lower lid
- Donor defect may require FTSG from opposite eyelid or ear
- Lower eyelid sharing
  - Tarsoconjunctival flap- caudal border of tarsus is transferred
    - Cover with FTSG
    - Divide in 7-10 days
  - Lid Switch Flap
    - Divide/insertion: 7-10 days
    - Flap is narrower than defect so donor site can be closed primarily
  - Lower limb of lateral canthus can be divided
  - Advancement flap from temporal area can close donor site

3. Select appropriate options in diagnosis and management

   - Algorithm
     - Reconstructive choice determined by defect
       - Partial thickness vs. full thickness
       - Size <1/3, >1/3, total
       - Involved structures
     - Must choose what you think is the best option based on scenario
       - Skin graft
       - Direct closure
       - Local flaps
     - Upper lid excisions
       - Shield pattern decreases risk of notching
       - Skin graft (contralateral lid best if available)
     - Cross Lid Flaps
       - Medial pedicle more reliable
   - What is your postop management and follow-up?
   - Be prepared to mark/draw flaps.

4. Understand risks and benefits of various approaches

- Demonstrate understanding of the risks and benefits of various approaches
- Understand morbidity of donor sites
- Advantage of various techniques based on defect
- What is the most appropriate approach and why?
- What is predicted outcome? Anticipated future problems?

5. Address complications and unexpected problems adequately

- Complications primarily related to delay in treatment with inadequate protection
- Post-op bleed
    - Retrobulbar hematoma
        - Dx: Excessive edema, Periorbital pain
        - Tx:
            - Open incision in OR
            - Control bleeders
            - Mannitol
            - Steroids
- Infection- uncommon
- Lagophthalmos- inability to close eyelid
    - Initial Tx:
        - Lubrication and massage
    - Persistent problem:
        - Scar release and replacement with more adequate tissue for reconstruction
- Corneal injury
    - Dx:
        - Pain in cornea
        - Woods lamp
        - Fluorescein dye
        - Ophthalmology consultation if unsure of etiology or not resolving with treatment
    - Tx:
        - Topical antibiotics
        - Observation

6. Demonstrate ability to structure alternative plan

- Have plan of intervention for postop complications
- Other options if initial flap fails
- Management changes based on skin cancer type and stage?

Chapter Twenty

Lower Eyelid Reconstruction

20
Lower Eyelid Reconstruction

1. Identify General Problem/Diagnosis/Planning
   (Describe photo, working diagnosis, key problems, evaluates patient)

   - Describe the photo. What is missing?
     o Note all details of the defect
       - Partial thickness vs. full-thickness
       - Partial <50% vs. Near Total or Total
       - Affects reconstructive choice
     o Note anatomic structures involved
       - Beware of medial lesions
       - Are upper or lower lacrimal ducts potentially involved?
   - Give your presumptive working diagnosis
   - Determine etiology of defect
     o Congenital
     o Traumatic
     o Iatrogenic
     o Malignancy (Tumor)
   - Establish diagnosis
     o Directed history:
       - Length of time lesion has been present
       - Any changes in lesion?
         • Size, Ulceration, Bleeding
       - Chronic wound?
         • Consider: Marjolin's ulcer, squamous cell carcinoma
       - Signs of malignancy
         • Rapid growth, Ulceration, Bleeding
   - Hx
     o Not critical, useful to determine etiology of lesion
     o Risk factors for melanoma or non-melanoma skin cancer
       - Age >60
       - Fair skin
       - Chronic repeated sun exposure
       - History of radiation

- Painful eye- may indicate corneal exposure, keratopathy
- Watery eye- may indicate duct obstruction
- Visual symptoms present
  - Indicates more extensive involvement
  - Pre-op CT scan to evaluate
- Ensure patient is suitable for surgery
  - Medical conditions
    - Controlled HTN, DM, Smoker
  - Medications
    - NSAID's, Anticoagulants, Steroids
- Length of time lesion has been present
  - Chronic lesion- likely malignant in adults
- In congenital cases
  - Are there other medical conditions?
  - Cardiac/Renal/Other
- Traumatic injury
- Previous surgery

- PE
  - Palpate lid and turn down to exam completely
  - Evaluate fixed vs. mobile lesion
  - Ulcerated vs. bleeding may indicate cancer
  - If lesion is present
    - Where is it located?
    - What is your estimated resection size?
    - Tumors generally require full-thickness excision
  - Is vision intact?
    - Ophthalmology exam important
  - Best guess which lamellae are involved?
    - Anterior- skin/orbicularis
    - Middle- septum
    - Posterior- tarsus (support) and conjunctiva
  - Other areas involved in defect especially in trauma cases
  - Palpate for lymphadenopathy?
    - Parotid/cervical lymph node chains
  - What are the key problems?
    - Avoidance of corneal exposure
    - Patency of lacrimal ducts
    - Potential for ectropion
- Work-up

- Tumor cases
  - Biopsy to determine etiology of lesion
  - Pathologic diagnosis- most important step
    - Incisional biopsy
    - Excisional biopsy
      - Small lesions if they can be closed primarily
  - Consider if imaging needed to determine extent of disease
    - Eg. Extensive or fixed lesions
- Staging of malignant lesions
  - Consider need for:
    - Chest x-ray
    - CT scan head and neck/abd/pelvis r/o visceral metastasis
    - MRI
    - PET scan
    - Oncology consultation
  - Lower lid/medial canthus increased incidence of malignant lesions
- Skin cancer types
  - Basal Cell Carcinoma
    - Most common
    - Localized
    - Nodular
    - Sclerosing type
    - Recurrent
      - More aggressive
      - High recurrence rate after repeat excision
      - Candidate for Moh's resection
    - Generally no distant metastasis in basal cell carcinoma can be locally invasive
  - Squamous Cell Carcinoma
    - Less common (2-10% of eyelid tumors)
    - Tendency to spread to orbit, cranium, bone
    - Increased tendency for metastasis
    - Risk factors
      - Sun exposure
      - Radiation
      - Chronic wound

- Chronic exposure
- Actinic keratosis
- Bowen's disease
    - Melanoma
        - Rare in eyelids (<1% of eyelid tumors)
        - Superficial spreading
        - Nodular
        - Lentigo maligna
            - Poor prognostic Signs: Bleeding, Ulceration
        - Evaluate lymph nodes
    - Sentinel node biopsy
- Congenital cases
    - Coloboma: Manage as an eyelid defect
    - Ophthalmology consultation
    - Genetics evaluation
    - Echocardiogram
    - Renal US
- Must know etiology of lesion/defect prior to reconstruction
    - Benign lesions can be less aggressive with margins, better prognosis

2. Consider reasonable goals in diagnosis and management *(Management and treatment, surgical indications, operative procedures and anesthesia)*

- Multidisciplinary approach in eyelid tumors
    - Pathologist
    - Oncologist
    - Radiation/Oncology
    - Ophthalmology
    - ENT
    - Tumor board for complicated cases
- Prior to recon
    - Ensure negative margins
        - Moh's: Permanent sections safer than frozen for definitive margins
    - Tumor recurrence in eyelid catastrophic
- Surgical goal
    - Closure of defect
    - Stable lid margin
    - Support eyelid in opposition with globe

- If eyelid margin is involved
  - Defect requires
    - Full thickness excision and primary closure at minimum
    - Shield excision preserves vertical height of eyelid
      - Modified pentagram
- Superficial partial thickness defects
  - Defects less than 4mm
    - Close by primary approximation if enough adjacent eyelid skin is available
    - Vertical closure preferred
      - Prevents ectropion which is more likely with horizontal closure
      - Preserves vertical height
  - Primary closure is generally feasible in defects up to 25-30% of horizontal dimension
    - Sometimes larger defects in elderly patients
  - Lateral canthotomy adjunct to primary closure
    - Allows medial advancement of lid
    - Additional 1-2mm
    - Lining provided
  - If persistent gap after lateral canthotomy
    - Undermine cheek
  - If still not approximated (Cheek flap)
    - Subcutaneous back-cut end of lateral cheek incision
    - 4-5cm lateral to canthal tendon
    - An incision from the lateral canthus is directed superiorly and laterally in an arch then downward toward the superior helix
    - This can close 75% defects
    - Cheek is mobilized as in Mustarde' flap
    - KEY TECHNICAL POINT:
      - Suture deep dermis of cheek flap to lateral orbital rim with periosteal sutures to Whitnall's Tubercle
      - Conjunctiva can usually be advanced for lining closure
  - When primary closure is not possible in superficial partial thickness defects
    - Partial thickness defects

- Skin graft
    - May heal with some stiffness
    - Stiffness may give some support
    - Full thickness graft is best
        - Least contracture
        - Good color match
- Donor site
    - 1st choice excess upper lid skin if available
    - 2nd choice postauricular area
        - Up to 5-6cm of full thickness skin available
        - Excellent color match
- Local flap
    - Bipedicled Tripier flap from upper eyelid
    - Fricke flap
    - Midline forehead flap
    - Superiorly based nasolabial flap
    - Cheek flap (described above)
    - Useful for near-total defects
- If needed perform posterior lamellar recon:
    - Hard palate mucosal graft
    - Septal cartilage-mucosal composite graft for support
    - Sagittal split of graft allows slight convex curvature

o Total or near total defect
- Large cheek flap + composite septal mucosa-cartilage graft for lining if conjunctiva insufficient
    - Estimate conjunctival defect with paper pattern (suture foil) in defect give idea of graft size needed
- Hard palate may be used in place of septal graft if not available
- May combine with glabellar flap
- Residual defect left to heal by 2nd intention

o Medial canthal area
- Small full thickness defect medial canthus and lower lid

- Use small medially based musculocutaneous supratarsal flap from upper lid and small cartilage graft
        - Small horizontal defect that cannot be closed primarily
            - Flap of skin and orbicularis from upper eyelid to cover small composite mucosal cartilage graft
            - Donor site closed primarily in supratarsal fold
        - Horizontal defects- entire lid width
            - Composite graft sutured beneath bipedicled skin and muscle flap from upper lid
        - If inferior lacrimal punctum, lacrimal canaliculus involved
            - Some cases may be able to mobilize and redirect medially
            - Intubate with 1mm silastic tube to maintain patency during healing
                - Minimum 4-6 mo
        - Other flap options
        - Hughes tarsoconjunctival flap
            - Turn down "book" flap of conjunctiva and tarsus from upper lid with full thickness skin graft
            - Requires that eye be closed several weeks to allow revascularization

3. Select appropriate options in diagnosis and management

    - Algorithm
        - Reconstructive choice determined by defect
            - Partial thickness vs. full thickness
            - Size <30%, 30-75%, >75%, total
            - Involved structures
        - Must choose what you think is the best option based on scenario
            - Skin graft, Direct closure, Local flaps
    - What is your postop management and follow-up?

- Be familiar with markings and main steps of commonly used flaps.

4. Understand risks and benefits of various approaches

    - Demonstrate understanding of the risks and benefits of various approaches
    - Morbidity of donor sites
    - Advantage of various techniques based on defect
    - What is the most appropriate approach and why?
    - What is your predicted outcome? Anticipated future problems?

5. Address complications and unexpected problems adequately

    - Ectropion
        - Decreased with the use of post-op temporary frost sutures or lateral tarsorrhaphy
        - Tx:
            - Scar massage 3-6 months
            - Persistent after 6 months
            - Re-op:
                - Lid shortening or soft tissue suspension procedure
    - Corneal injury
        - Tx: Ophthalmic antibiotic ointment 7-10 days Ophthalmology consultation
        - Prevention: Intraop Corneal Protector Shield
    - Entropion
        - Correct by excision of horizontal tangential "V" wedge of tarsus

6. Demonstrate ability to structure alternative plan

    - Have plan of intervention for postop complications
    - Other options if initial flap fails
    - Management plan changes based on skin cancer type and stage?
    - What if patient refuses treatment?
    - No insurance coverage
    - Consider other ethical scenarios

Chapter Twenty-One

Ectropion

21
Ectropion

1. Identify General Problem/ Diagnosis/Planning
   (Describe photo, give working diagnosis, key problems, evaluates patient)

   - Describe photo, give specific diagnosis
     o Ectropion
       - Implies outward eversion of the lower eyelid
       - Frequently secondary to increased laxity of tarsal support structures
     o Causes
       - Retraction of eyelid
       - True ectropion
     o Key problems:
       - Appearance
       - Epiphora
       - Irritation of globe and/or conjunctiva
       - Risk of keratopathy
   - Important to delineate etiology of problem
   - Several causes diagnose by history (hx):
   - History
     o Age of patient
       - Senile ectropion
         - Rare
         - Secondary to downward pull of malar structures (Theory: effect of gravity with aging)
     o Sun exposure
       - Alone should not cause retraction (if septum and conjunctiva unaffected)
     o History of trauma
       - Cicatricial ectropion
         - Following trauma or surgery (iatrogenic)
         - Cause
           o Excess resection of skin of anterior lamella

- - -
        - -
            - Scarring of septum in middle lamella
        - Higher risk in transcutaneous approach vs. transconjunctival approach in eyelid surgery
    - Time frame
        - Early (<6 months)
            - May respond to upper lid retraction or tarsorrhaphy
        - Chronic (>6 months)
            - May require surgical intervention
    - Excess tearing
        - Secondary to superior and/or inferior puncta being pulled away from globe
    - Antecedent history of nerve problems
        - Paralytic ectropion
            - Facial paralysis
                - Traumatic
                - Infection
                - Idiopathic (Bell's)
        - Spastic ectropion
            - In exophthalmos result of pull of orbicularis oculi m.
    - Congenital ectropion
        - Caused by deficiency in anterior lamella
        - Coloboma
    - Medical history
        - Smoker- may impair blood supply to skin flaps
    - Medications
        - Anticoagulants
        - NSAID's discontinue 7-10 days prior to surgery
- Physical Exam
    - Basic ophthalmologic exam
    - Malposition of lower lid noticeable by increase in lateral scleral show
    - Look for etiology of ectropion
        - Retraction of lower lid only
            - Tx: Canthal suspension
        - True ectropion- lid eversion
            - Tx: More complex

- Must identify involved structures:
  - Anterior lamella
  - Middle lamella
  - Posterior lamella
  - Combination
- Rounding of lateral canthus
  - Secondary to malposition of lateral canthal tendon
- Conjunctival exposure
  - Chronic exposure causes metaplastic change of epithelium to keratinized squamous epithelium causing persistent irritation
- Upward traction identifies which structures are insufficient
  - Tense lid lax skin
    - Suggests septal contracture of middle lamella
  - Tense skin
    - Suggests deficiency of skin of anterior lamella
- Lid Snap Back Test
  - Indicates tone of orbicularis muscle
  - Poor tone seen in senile ectropion and other disorders of the muscle
- Scars of external eyelid or within conjunctiva indicating previous surgery
- Palpate for bony step-offs
- Extraocular movement (EOM) intact all six visual axes
  - Medial
  - Lateral
  - Superior
  - Inferior
  - Down and out
  - Up and out
- Pupils equal and reactive
  - "Marcus Gunn" pupil
    - Paradoxical dilation of pupil rather than constriction with light stimulus
    - Indicates partial optic nerve injury
- Visual acuity
- Anterior chamber

- - - Check for hyphema, must be treated
 - - Facial nerve function
 - - - If abnormal may be related to ectropion
 - - Preop studies
 - - - Plain films to check any previously placed titanium plates for position, plates may require removal at time of surgery
 - - - CT scan optional

- Consultation
 - - MUST GET FORMAL OPHTHALMOLOGY CONSULTATION
 - - Ophthalmology exam
 - - - Dilation of pupils
 - - - Fundoscopic exam
 - - Tests for dry eyes prior to blepharoplasty
 - - - Schirmer test
 - - - - Filter paper, check moisture, low sensitivity
 - - - Lactoferrin level in tear fluid
 - - - - Decreased in dry eye diseases

2. Consider reasonable goals in diagnosis and management *(Management and treatment, surgical indications, operative procedures and anesthesia)*

- Treatment dictated by:
 - - Timing of inciting event
 - - Length of time problem has persisted
 - - Anatomic structures involved
- Must address:
 - - Patient expectations
 - - Anticipated results
 - - Potential problems
- Determine Lid Retraction vs. Ectropion
 - - Early lid retraction
 - - - Tape or sutures through lower lid and suspended to brow for 7-10 days
 - - Late lid retraction (but within 6 months)
 - - - May require division of scar tissue and resuspension of eyelid
 - - Exposure

- Through lateral canthotomy
- Exposes orbital rim and lateral canthus
  - Tarsal strip canthopexy
    - Strip of tissue developed
    - Conjunctival lining preserved
    - Tarsal strip attached to periosteum of lateral orbital rim and/or superior limb of lateral canthal tendon
    - Orbicularis also positioned and sutured to frontal process of zygoma
    - Postop Frost suture for additional support
  - Midface lift
    - May be appropriate especially in older patients
    - Resuspend malar structures into more youthful position
  - Kuhnt-Szymanowski Procedure
    - Triangular area of skin excised lateral to lateral canthus
    - Similar area excised from conjunctiva and lid margin
    - Medial extent of cut lower lid is sutured to lateral edge of upper lid at the canthus
    - Lower lid flap sutured to area of skin excised lateral to canthus
- Late lid retraction less common but more severe (> 6months)
  - Frequently require tissue placement in posterior lamella to fill space and compensate for secondary shortening of this layer
  - Posterior lamella spacer grafts
    - Hard palate mucosal graft
      - From one side of roof of mouth
      - Use Dingman mouth gag and epi
    - Ear cartilage
  - Recipient bed created after tarsal strip procedure
  - Width of graft determined by preop shortening
  - Recipient site may be left open
  - A second resuspension procedure may be required after complete healing
- Treatment of ectropion
  - Needs more than simple canthal suspension
  - Replacement of deficient skin from anterior lamella

- - - Full Thickness Skin Graft (FTSG)
    - Contralateral upper lid if sufficient or retroauricular sulcus
  - Defect is created 1-2mm below lash line
  - All scar excised
  - Subcutaneous dissection to orbital rim
  - Tie over bolster
- Middle or posterior lamellar shortening
  - Best addressed by addition of rigid mucosal graft
  - Horizontal defect is created just below the level of the lower eyelid tarsal plate

3. Select appropriate options in diagnosis and management

- Local with epinephrine
- Corneal shield
- Traction sutures for exposure
- Desmarre retractors
- Types of Ectropion
  - Involutional
  - Cicatricial
  - Paralytic
  - Mechanical
- Involutional
  - Senile ectropion
  - Laxity of supporting structures
  - Horizontal laxity
  - Degeneration or dehiscence of lower lid retractors
  - Tx:
    - Medial canthal plication, protect canaliculi
    - Attachment of lower lid retractors (rarely needed)
    - Correction of horizontal lid laxity (tarsal strip procedure)
- Cicatricial
  - Requires reconstruction of anterior lamella
  - FTSG vs. myocutaneous flaps vs. midface lift
  - Causes
    - Overly aggressive blepharoplasty
    - Actinic damage
    - Trauma
    - Laser resurfacing

- Malignancy
- Paralytic
  - Paralysis of orbicularis in facial nerve palsy
  - Many causes (overgenerous botox injections)
  - Problems
    - Exposure compounded by upper lid lagophthalmos
    - Interruption of lacrimal pump
    - Lacrimal gland dysfunction
    - Important to determine cause and anticipated return of function
    - If return of function anticipated:
      - Temporary measures:
        - Aggressive topical lubrication for corneal protection
        - Prevent keratinization
        - Taping of lateral aspect of lid
        - Tape shut when sleeping
        - Tarsorrhaphy if lesser measures failing
    - If return of function unlikely:
      - Horizontal shortening and tarsal strip
      - Suspension sling
      - Gold weight upper lid
      - Midface lift
- Mechanical
  - Mass effect pulling or pushing eyelid
  - Treat or excise mass
  - Usually readily recognized

4. Understand risks and benefits of various approaches
   - Understand risks and benefits of various treatment options based on duration and etiology of ectropion.
   - More about tarsal strips
     - Good for senile ectropion OR
     - As adjunct in management of other types of ectropion
     - Can tighten lid in lower lid blepharoplasty
   - Steps

- o Subciliary incision extended into crow's feet
  - Through skin and orbicularis muscle
  - Lateral canthotomy to expose inferior crus of lateral canthal ligament
- o Disinsert inferior crus of lateral canthus
  - Full release to allow upward mobility
- o Expose tarsal strip
  - Remove anterior skin and myocutaneous layer
- o Shorten strip to reduce horizontal laxity
- o Suture to inner periosteum of orbital rim
  - Higher than desired final position 5-0 suture
- o Excise redundant skin
- o Close skin
- Beware
  - o Medial punctual ectropion
    - Address with spindle procedure

5. Address complications and unexpected problems adequately

- Attempt to minimize further complications
- Complications
  - o Persistent deformity from inaccurate diagnosis and treatment
  - o Injury to globe
    - Avoid with corneal shield
    - Remove when positioning of lower lid in regard to limbus is needed to be assessed
  - o Skin graft failure
    - Poorly vascularized wound bed, shearing
    - Repeat graft
  - o Inferior oblique injury
    - Patient will c/o vertical dystopia
    - Trial period of observation prior to surgery
      - May resolve spontaneously
    - Corrective extraocular muscle surgery may be necessary
  - o Postop bleeding
    - Risk of retrobulbar hematoma
    - Avoid by aggressive management of:
      - Hypertension
      - Post-op pain

- Nausea control
- Careful hemostasis
  - Tx:
    - Release sutures
    - Lateral canthotomy
    - Mannitol
    - Acetazolamide- decreases intraocular pressure
    - Return to OR for wound exploration
    - Rare cases osteotomy of orbital wall may be needed for adequate decompression

6. Demonstrate ability to structure alternative plan

   - Know when to reassess and consider a different plan based on presented scenario.
     - Was there a missed diagnosis?
   - ENTROPION
     - Inward turning of eyelid margin
     - Clinical presentation
       - Corneal irritation, risk of corneal infection
       - Globe and conjunctival irritation
     - Etiology
       - Override of pretarsal orbicularis
       - Inwardly rotates eyelashes and secondary corneal irritation occurs
       - Increased eyelid laxity
       - Dehiscence of lower lid retractors cause this
     - Correction
       - Shortening lower lid
       - Repositioning lower lid
     - Options
     - Intermittent or mild cases
       - Quickert-Rathbun Sutures
       - Double-armed chromic passed from lower-lid palpebral conjunctiva 2mm below lower tarsal border and externalized 2-3mm below lower lid margin, 3mm apart
       - One suture placed medially one placed laterally (3-5 sutures)
       - Provides mechanical rotation of eyelid

- - Intent is scar produced by sutures results in permanent repositioning of eyelid
  - Unpredictable, poor long-term stability
- Mild to moderate eyelid laxity
  - Orbicularis strip
  - Subciliary skin only incision carried through mid-pupillary line
  - Starting 4mm below tarsal margin, 4mm strip of orbicularis is created laterally and extended inward to mid papillary line
  - Periosteum of inferolateral orbital rim is exposed with electrocautery dissection
  - Strip is then sutured with double armed 5-0 to periosteum of lateral orbital rim.
  - Results in outward turning of lid margin
  - Skin closed
  - Shorten via horizontal lid shortening technique if significant horizontal lid laxity present
  - Eyelid retractors may need to be directly visualized and sutured to tarsal plate

Chapter Twenty-Two

Nasal Reconstruction

22
Nasal Reconstruction

1. Identify General Problem/Diagnosis/Planning
   (Describe photo, working diagnosis, key problems, evaluates patient)

   - Spend time describing photo
     - Location of defect
     - What parts are missing?
       - Skin
       - Cartilage
       - Bone
       - Septum
       - Lining
       - Anatomic subunits of nose involved
     - Note skin type
     - Estimated size of defect
   - Establish a diagnosis
   - Determine etiology of defect
     - Your best guess based on clinical scenario
   - History
     - Useful to determine etiology of lesion
     - Increased risk of melanoma or non-melanoma skin cancer
       - Age >60
       - Fair skin
       - Chronic repeated sun exposure
       - History of radiation
     - Length of time lesion has been present
       - Chronic lesion- likely malignant in adults
     - Etiology of defect
       - Trauma
         - Acute
         - Distant
       - Malignancy
       - Post-surgical
       - Congenital
       - Other
     - Prior surgery

- Medical history
  - Hypertension
  - Smoker
  - Diabetes mellitus
  - Other
- Medications
  - Anticoagulants (aspirin, coumadin)
  - Steroids
  - Other

- Physical Exam
  - Location on nose and anatomic parts involved in defect
    - Skin (soft tissue coverage)
    - Cartilaginous or bony framework (support)
    - Internal mucosal lining (lining)
  - 9 anatomic subunits
    - Sidewall (2- Right, left)
    - Dorsum
    - Ala (2- Right, left)
    - Soft triangle (2- Right, left)
    - Tip
    - Columella
  - Skin types
    - Thick, glabrous
    - Thin, waxy
  - Assess facial scars
    - May interfere with reconstructive (recon) options
  - Laxity of surrounding skin
    - Elderly- generally more laxity in malar, glabellar and nasal skin
  - Palpate for lymphadenopathy
    - Parotid
    - Cervical regions
- Work up
  - In the case of tumors:
    - Most important to determine if benign vs. malignant, type of tumor influences management
  - Biopsy
    - Excisional if primary closure is possible
    - Incisional

- If diagnosis doubtful or in difficult area
- 2mm punch or knife incision
- Definitive recon after final pathology
- Local wound care until that point- your choice
  - Moh's surgery effective and reliable for:
    - Basal cell carcinoma
    - Squamous cell carcinoma
    - NOT for melanoma or Merkel cell
    - Moh's is generally very accurate and reconstruction can be based on Moh's pathology and defect
    - Moh's conserves tissue and adds in reconstruction
  - Permanent section is more reliable in demonstrating cell type than frozen section
  - Determine extent of disease
    - Focused PE
    - Imaging studies as indicated
      - CT scan
      - MRI
      - PET scan
    - Consider distant spread in the case of extensive disease
      - Check for metastasis
        - Lung/Brain/Liver
  - Pre-op Evaluation
    - Hypertension
    - CHF
    - Diabetes
    - Optimize medical status
      - Ideally controlled medical problems
    - Make plan if patient is on anticoagulants
  - Consultations
    - Oncology consultation in cancer cases
      - Evaluate need for chemotherapy or radiation

2. Consider reasonable goals in diagnosis and management *(Management and treatment, surgical indications, operative procedures and anesthesia)*

- Principles of Management
    - Skin/soft tissue coverage
    - Support
    - Lining
- Management by subunit principle
    - Not an absolute rule
    - Consider in defects with loss of >1/2 subunit
        - May require excision and reconstruction of entire subunit for optimal reconstruction
- **Skin Cancer Management Guidelines**
- Standard basal cell carcinoma (BCC)
    - 2mm margin
    - 5yr 90-95% cure rate
    - Other options
        - Radiation
        - Cryosurgery
        - Curette
- Recurrent or Morpheaform BCC
    - More aggressive resection needed
    - Good candidates for Moh's surgery
- Standard Squamous cell carcinoma (SCC)
    - 1cm margin
    - Large lesions may benefit from adjuvant radiation therapy
- Melanoma or Merkel Cell
    - Check histology depth to determine necessary surgical margin
        - Depth of lesion: Surgical Margin
            - <1mm: 1cm + sentinel node biopsy
            - 1mm: 1cm + sentinel node or lymphadenectomy
            - 1-2mm: 1-2cm margin
            - >2mm: 2cm margin
- Margins may be modified if strict adherence to surgical margin is too mutilating
    - e.g. Nasal sidewall lesion needing 2cm margin technically requires orbital enucleation
- In the case of large full thickness defects

- No role for non-surgical management EXCEPT
  - Unstable patients or unfit for surgery
  - Management
  - Partial or complete prosthesis
    - Requires negative surgical margin!
  - Silicone prosthesis
- Surgical steps
  - Negative margin by histology
    - Number 1 priority
  - Reconstruction of involved components
    - Skin
    - Support
    - Lining
  - Subunit approach
    - 9 anatomic subunits
    - Sidewall (2- Right, left)
    - Dorsum
    - Ala (2- Right, left)
    - Soft triangle (2- Right, left)
    - Tip
    - Columella
  - Adjuvant therapy in some cases
    - Radiation vs. Chemotherapy
    - Clinical trial
    - Merkel cell generally benefits from adjuvant radiation
- Perform definitive reconstruction when margin clear
  - Acceptable to perform immediate reconstruction after Moh's resection for BCC and SCC
- NASAL RECONSTRUCTION
  - All full thickness defects require
    - Skin coverage
    - Support
    - Lining
  - Nasal lining
    - Most difficult aspect of reconstruction
    - Options
      - Turn down flap of native skin on dorsum of nose
      - Unilateral or bilateral nasolabial turn in flaps

- Pedicled septal mucoperichondrial flaps
- Bipedicled mucosal flaps
- Extended forehead flap
- Prefabricated forehead flap with STSG on undersurface
  - Supporting framework
    - Options
      - Bone graft for dorsum and tip support
      - Can be done as a cantilever graft
        - Rib
        - Calvarium
        - Iliac crest
      - Cartilage graft for alar rim and columellar strut
        - Ear
        - Rib
  - Skin coverage
    - Use reconstructive ladder to consider choices available
    - Check size and shape of defect using foil template
    - Consider reconstruction entire subunit if > 50% is involved
      - More important in younger patients
        - Scars not as easily camouflaged

- OPTIONS
  - Healing by secondary intention
    - Good option for: Medial canthus, Sidewall defects
    - Sometimes good option for difficult areas
  - Primary closure if possible with minimal tension
  - Skin graft
    - Match area being replaced
    - Full-thickness or split-thickness
  - Donor site choices
    - Split thickness graft sites
      - Scalp- best color match
    - Full thickness graft sites

- - - Preauricular skin
      - Retro-auricular skin
      - Post-auricular skin
      - Supraclavicular skin
  - Local flaps
    - Be cognizant of arc of rotation
  - Dorsum and tip
    - Rotational flap from adjacent tissue
    - Banner flap
    - Limberg flap (rhomboid flap)
    - Variant Dufourmental flap
    - Bilobed flap
    - Dorsal advancement flap
      - Marchac
      - Reiger
      - Angelats
  - Alar rim
    - Kazanjian bipedicled flap
    - Z-plasty
    - Perialar transposition flap
  - Lateral dorsal advancement flap
  - Nasolabial flap
    - Axial pattern based superiorly or inferiorly
    - Blood supply:
    - Angular branch from anterior facial artery and branches from internal maxillary artery
    - Angular vein
    - Good option for lower nasal defects
    - Generally 2-3 mm of subcutaneous tissue on flap
    - Keep thicker in smokers or diabetics
  - Auricular composite graft for small defects of alar rim (1.5cm or less)
  - Columella
    - Nasolabial flap
    - Washio flap for pediatric cases
    - Composite graft from helical rim if <1cm in healthy patient
  - Large nasal tip or other defects >2.5cm
    - Paramedian forehead flap
      - Axial flap supratrochlear vessel

- Can prefabricate with cartilage and STSG lining
- Donor site
  - Mostly closed primarily
  - Distal aspect left to heal by secondary intention
  - 3-4 stage procedure
- Flap elevation:
  - Distal forehead flap keep thin, raised in subcutaneous plane
  - Proximal aspect submuscular plane to preserve vessels
- Scalping flap based on superficial temporal vessels if forehead flap not available
- Borrows tissue from behind the hairline
- Replaced after 3-4 weeks
- FTSG to donor site
- Washio flap
- Temprororetroauricular flap
  - Based on posterior branch or superficial temporal artery
  - Can fold on itself for lining
- Radial forearm free flap
  - Option for total nasal reconstruction

3. Select appropriate options in diagnosis and management

- For skin coverage choose best functional and aesthetic option
- A number of available options
  - Must choose best option based on:
    - Age and health of patient
    - Size and location of defect
    - Aesthetic goals
    - What is missing?
- Defects >2.5cm generally require paramedian fore head flap
- Smaller defects are amenable to local flaps
  - Most common:

- Bilobed flap
            - Dorsal nasal flap
            - Rhomboid flaps
        - Composite grafts
            - Useful in alar defects <1.5cm
            - Non-smokers best candidates
        - Skin grafts
            - Acceptable for small defects or in elderly patients that will not tolerate larger procedure- rare.
            - Generally poor color match and contour
            - Acceptable but not ideal
        - Reconstruction more difficult in younger patients, scarring more noticeable
        - Be familiar with how to draw, flap anatomy and main steps of your preferred procedures.

4. Understand risks and benefits of various approaches

    - Note risks benefits of each approach.
    - Always potential for scarring and distortion especially if larger lining defects are present.
    - Multiple stages and revisions may be necessary for optimal aesthetic result

5. Address complications and unexpected problems adequately

    - Avoid tension on flap minimizes risk of complications
    - Nasal collapse and contracture secondary to healing issues with lining common
        - Post-op stenting may help to prevent this
    - Bleeding rare
        - Evacuate any hematoma to prevent flap loss or graft loss
    - Infection- uncommon
    - Flap loss
        - Ischemia primary cause
        - Less frequently infection
        - Increased in smokers
    - Donor site complications
        - Abnormal scarring
    - How will you manage excessively bulky flaps, pin-cushioning or other reconstructive problems?

6. Demonstrate ability to structure alternative plan

    - Be prepared with lifeboat if initial flap fails
    - Have 2-3 ways to reconstruct defect based on reconstructive ladder taking into consideration clinical needs for soft tissue, framework and lining
    - If all else fails allow healing by secondary intention and plan for difficult re-op in the future.
    - What if patient refuses what you consider to be the best option?

Chapter Twenty-Three

Ear Reconstruction

23
Ear Reconstruction

1. Identify General Problem/Diagnosis/Planning
   (Describe photo, working diagnosis, key problems, evaluates patient)

   - Describe photo
     - Detail anatomic location of lesion
     - Size of defect
     - Note what is missing, specific anatomy involved
       - Skin only
       - Cartilage
     - Partial thickness vs. full thickness
     - In congenital lesions, classify deformity
       - Microtia (See microtia chapter)
       - Prominent ear deformity (See prominent ear chapter)
   - Discuss key problems of anticipated reconstruction
     - Aesthetic and reconstructive concerns
   - Give your working diagnosis based on clinical scenario
   - History
     - Useful to determine etiology of lesion
     - Increased risk of melanoma or non-melanoma skin cancer
       - Age >60
       - Fair skin
       - Chronic repeated sun exposure
       - History of radiation
     - Length of time lesion has been present
       - Chronic lesion- likely malignant in adults
     - History of previous skin cancer
     - Family history of malignancy
       - Melanoma
     - Trauma
     - Prior surgeries
   - Physical Exam
     - Examine parts involved
       - Partial or full-thickness
       - Skin mobility of tumor

- External ear breakdown into 3 areas
  - Superior 3rd
  - Middle 3rd
  - Lower 3rd
- Anatomy of the ear
  - 1st branchial arch
    - Superior helix
    - Tragus
    - Root of the helix
  - 2nd branchial arch
    - Antihelix
    - Antitragus
    - Lobule
- Check for old scars
- Evaluate
  - Lymphadenopathy of neck
  - Parotid gland
- Look for concomitant lesions
- You should be capable of drawing an ear template with all the critical parts
- Work-up
  - Same as tumor work-up in lip, nose, eyelid reconstruction
    - Tumor cases
      - Biopsy to determine etiology
      - Consider if imaging needed to determine extent of disease
    - Staging of malignant lesions
    - Consider need for:
      - Chest x-ray
      - CT scan head and neck/abd/pelvis r/o visceral metastasis
      - MRI
      - PET scan
- Trauma
  - ATLS protocol
  - R/O concomitant injuries
- Congenital
  - R/O other medical problems
    - Especially renal: Kidneys develop at the same time as the ear in utero

- Cardiac
- Consultants
  - Radiation Oncology
- Resection margins
  - Moh's reliable
  - Permanent sections are the gold standard
- Must know etiology of lesion/defect prior to reconstruction
  - Benign lesions can be less aggressive with margins, better prognosis
- Types of skin cancer review sections in eyelid chapters

2. Consider reasonable goals in diagnosis and management *(Management and treatment, surgical indications, operative procedures and anesthesia)*

- Tumor management/Resection margins
  - Basal cell carcinoma (BCC)
    - 2mm acceptable
    - 3-5mm better if possible without major aesthetic deformity
  - Aggressive BCC
    - 7mm margin + radiation or
    - Moh's resection
  - Squamous cell carcinoma (SCC)
    - Minimum of 1cm margin
    - Radiation ineffective as only modality for squamous cell
    - Use as only modality if patient is high risk for surgery
  - Melanoma management
    - >1mm Sentinel node biopsy
    - 1-4mm elective lymph node dissection vs. sentinel node biopsy
    - >4mm no benefit to lymphadenectomy
    - All patients treated with chemotherapy and surgery
  - Only proceed with reconstruction after confirmed negative margin by Moh's or permanent section.
  - Acceptable to do single stage excision and closure after Moh's resection
- Reconstruction based on:
  - Tumor location

- Site of the wound
- Thickness of defect partial vs. full thickness
- Segmental vs. complete defect
- Topographical regions
  - Antihelix/Antitragus
  - Helical rim (upper 1/3)
  - Conchal bowl (middle 1/3)
  - Lobule (lower 1/3)
- Reconstructive ladder
  - Healing by secondary intention
  - Primary closure
  - Skin grafting
  - Most commonly used reconstructive options
    - Wedge resection and closure
    - Direct advancement and closure
    - Reconstruction with chondrocutaneous flaps
  - Central defect with intact cartilage
    - Healing by secondary intention or
    - Skin graft split or full thickness
  - Helical rim defects <2.5cm
    - Advancement flap of helical rim- Antia-Buch flap
  - Upper 1/3 (Helical rim)
    - Direct closure <2cm
      - Undermine after wedge resection, decreased vertical height
    - Rotation flap
    - Antia-Buch flap
      - In defects not amenable to primary closure
    - Cartilage graft
      - With peri-auricular flap coverage if extensive
  - Larger defect <25% of total ear
    - Star-shaped excision or
    - Anterior composite Burrow's triangle excision
      - Redistribute tension to avoid cupping with primary closure
  - Partial thickness defects
    - Full thickness skin graft
      - Periauricular

- Neck
- Supraclavicular areas
    - Can skin graft on perichondrium of freshly created surgical excisions
  - Helical defect 25-50%
    - Antia-Buch
      - Free helix from scapha incision is carried through cartilage
      - Skin undermined above perichondrium
      - Close without tension
      - Excision of Scapho-fossa may ease closure
  - Lesion >50% Framework
    - Requires rib cartilage graft
    - Coverage with
      - Postauricular skin followed by elevation and skin graft or
      - Temporo-Parietal Fascia (TPF) flap with STSG
    - Old school option
      - Tube flap for significant middle helical defects
      - Inadequate if not used with rib graft for support
- **Defects with more than two dimensions involved requires rib graft for adequate reconstruction as per Firmin.**
  - Large full thickness defects of helix and antihelix
    - Composite free graft of up to 1.5cm wide from contralateral ear
    - Full thickness wedge 1/2 size of defect
    - Returns symmetry to both ears
  - Middle and lower 1/3 defects
    - Direct closure
    - Composite grafts
    - Local flap reconstruction
  - Composite defect of conchal bowl
    - Often amenable to direct closure with or without helical advancement
    - Secondary healing
    - Full thickness skin graft coverage
    - Retroauricular subcutaneous island flap

- Choice depends on soft tissue structures involved
  - Exposed cartilage will desiccate
    - Management:
      - Local flap closure
      - Cartilage excision and skin graft
  - Large composite defects
    - More extensive reconstruction needed
    - Structural support rib framework and vascularized skin cover
    - TPF flap and skin graft if local skin not available
- Other flap options
  - Preauricular flap for small antehelical defect coverage
    - Can be done as a 2-stage procedure
    - Design flap at junction of ear and face
    - Blood supply based on either superior or inferior pedicle
  - Postauricular flap
    - Versatile flaps
  - Larger lateral ear defect
    - Pedicled postauricular flap
      - Can be done as 2-stage procedure
      - Flap designed and placed over defect
      - Flap division and closure done with donor site coverage

3. Select appropriate options in diagnosis and management

- Decide on reconstructive plan based on diagnosis and presented defect
- Be familiar with the steps and anatomy of commonly used flaps for ear reconstruction
- Be prepared to discuss steps of total ear reconstruction
- Have follow-up plan for skin cancer patients
  - Close f/u of skin in all patients
    - >50% new cancer within 5 years
  - Sun avoidance - sunscreen

4. Understand risks and benefits of various approaches

- Be prepared to discuss the advantages and disadvantages of different approaches; defend your choice
- Any preventative measures to avoid complications?

5. Address complications and unexpected problems adequately

- Hematoma
- Skin necrosis with cartilage exposure
    - Exposure
        - <1cm may heal with local care- risk of resorption
        - >1cm local skin flap for coverage
        - TPF flap with skin graft in large defect
- Infection
    - How do you manage chondritis?
        - Admit
        - IV Antibiotics
        - Debridement
        - Sometimes radical debridement
        - Reconstruct after wound stablized
- Irregularities in ear shape
- Recurrent tumor
- Graft loss
- Pneumothorax if lung injured during harvest
- Thoracic deformity in total ear reconstruction
- How do you manage abnormal scarring, post-op deformities or bulky flap?

6. Demonstrate ability to structure alternative plan

- Backup plan for failed flap
- Patient refuses treatment for melanoma
- Positive margin on final pathology after your reconstruction

Chapter Twenty-Four

Upper Lip Reconstruction

24
Upper Lip Reconstruction

1. Identify General Problem/Diagnosis/Planning
   (Describe photo, working diagnosis, key problems, evaluates patient)

   - Describe photo
     - Detail location of lesion
     - Size of defect
     - Note in detail what is missing
       - Skin
       - Muscle
       - Mucosa
     - Specific anatomic structures involved
       - Philtrum
       - Nasolabial fold
       - Tubercle
       - Vermilion
       - Comminures
       - White roll
       - Wet-dry border
       - Other
   - Give your working diagnosis
     - Etiology of lesion based on presentation
       - Tumor
       - Trauma
       - Burn injury
       - Congenital
       - Other
   - Discuss key problems of reconstruction
     - Aesthetic and reconstructive concerns

   - History
     - Non-healing lesion
       - Age of patient
       - How long has lesion been present?
       - Chronic sun exposure?
     - Concern for cancer
       - Past history of cancer

- Immunocompromised (transplant recipient vs. other)
- Crusting or bleeding
- Recent change in lesion
- Prior radiation
        - Medical history
            - HTN
            - DM
            - Anticoagulation
            - Cardiovascular disease/CHF
            - Immunosuppressant's
            - Steroid use
            - Other
    - Physical Exam
        - Look for separate metachronous lesions, common finding
        - Examine
            - Lips
            - Oral cavity
                - Teeth
                - Tongue
                - Alveolus/Gums
                - Mandible
                - Maxilla
            - Mobile vs. Fixed lesion
            - Lymphatics
                - Neck
                - Submental- central lesions
                - Submandibular- ipsilateral lesions
                - Parotid
            - Local scars?
                - May affect reconstructive options
            - Note location of lesion
                - Mobile or fixed
                - Involves mandible?
                - Direct extension
                - Perineural invasion
                - Lymphatic spread
        - Anatomy of the lip
            - Consider subunits involved
            - Lateral and medial elements

- Central portion philtral dimple
- Bound by two curvilinear philtral columns
- Commissure
- Parts
  - Skin
  - Wet/dry vermilion
  - Muscle
  - Mucosa
        - Size of defect breakdown
          - 1/3 of the lip
          - 1/3-2/3 of the lip
          - Subtotal or total lip
          - Size of defect dictates ideal reconstructive management
    - Establish diagnosis
      - Is the lesion benign vs. malignant?
        - Affects margins and post-op treatment plan
      - Biopsy
        - Incisional or excisional depending on size of the lesion
    - Skin cancer risk factors
      - Fitzpatrick I and II
      - Males
      - Age >50
      - Chronic sun exposure (farmer classic)
        - Most important risk factor
    - Key problems
      - What is missing?
      - Staging
        - Is there lymphatic involvement?
        - Is there Mandibular/Maxillary involvement?
          - < 4cm segment
            - Bone graft acceptable
          - > 4cm segment
            - Vascularized flap
        - Consider vascularized flap if post-op radiation is anticipated
    - Work-up
      - Biopsy to determine pathology
      - Determine extent of disease
        - PE findings
        - +/- imaging as indicated (eg. fixed lesion)

- CT scan or MRI
- Determines extent of disease
- If bony involvement (mandible/maxilla suspected) imaging is needed
  - CT scan or panorex (for mandibular involvement)
  - <2% of cases will have distant metastasis
- Consultants
  - Oncology
  - ENT or Oral surgery for primary resection
- Staging Skin Cancers
  - Non-Melanocytic
    - Stage 0- In-situ
    - Stage I- <2cm
    - Stage II- >2cm
    - Stage III- Below skin to lymph node/cartilage/muscle/bone
    - Stage IV- Metastasis
  - Melanocytic
    - Based on Breslow Classification- Thickness of lesion
      - Stage 0- In-situ 5mm or less
      - Stage I- Up to 1.5mm, no lymphadenopathy
      - Stage II- >1.5mm, no lymphadenopathy
      - Stage III- (+) lymphadenopathy
      - Stage IV- Metastasis
  - About the lip
    - Prone to cancer because vermillion lacks pigmentation layer which protects from UV rays
    - Lip comprises 25% of all oral cavity tumors

2. Consider reasonable goals in diagnosis and management *(Management and treatment, surgical indications, operative procedures and anesthesia)*

- Tumor type dictates necessary margins and post-op care plan
  - Basal cell carcinoma
    - 2mm margin for resection
  - Recurrent basal cell

- Moh's resection best choice
- Squamous cell carcinoma
  - 1-2cm margin
- Melanoma
  - In situ: 5mm margin
  - 1mm thickness: 1cm margin
  - 1-2mm thickness: 1-2cm margin
  - >2mm thickness: 2cm margin
- Operative procedures
  - Local with sedation an option in most adults for most reconstructions
    - Infraorbital nerve block
    - Blocks upper lip
    - Infraorbital foramen 5mm from infraorbital rim generally along medial limbus
  - Can use general anesthesia for more extensive procedures or if that is surgeon's preference
  - If white roll is involved in excision always mark prior to injection with local.
- Treatment
  - Based on:
    - Histologic diagnosis
    - Resection with tissue specific margins
  - Reconstruction goals
    - Sensate lip
    - Functional sphincter
      - Watertight seal
    - Adequate opening for food and dental care
    - Aesthetic appearance
    - Good apposition of lower and upper vermilion
  - In sub-total and total reconstruction all goals cannot be satisfied.
  - Prior to reconstruction
    - Resection with appropriate margins and tissue diagnosis
    - If necessary delay closure until definitive margins known by:
      - Permanent section OR
      - Moh's
- Management of Vermilion Lesions
  - May require excision of white roll

- Mark prior to infiltration with local
  - Make all incisions perpendicular to vermilion
  - Small lesions
    - V-Y advancement may be effective
  - Large lesions
    - Vermilion advancement flaps
    - Mucosal V-Y advancement
    - FAMM flaps for large vermilion defects
      - Subtotal or total lip loss cases
- Management Options
- Up to 25% defect
  - Excise and close primarily
  - Older patients defects up to 1/3 may be excised and closed, more laxity in the elderly
  - Philtral distortion may occur in central wedge
- Lesions across mucocutaneous border
  - Partial or full-thickness wedge excision
  - Excellent outcomes
- Be sure to align:
  - Vermilion
  - White roll
  - Orbicularis muscle
- Defects that ablate philtrum, consider:
  - Abbe flap
  - Full thickness skin graft
  - Composite graft
  - Cross Lip Flaps
    - Criteria
    - Lower lip must have adequate volume
    - 14-21 days before division
      - Can be as short as 7-10 days
  - Division time dependent on:
    - Flap size
    - Size of mucosal attachment
    - Maintenance of axial vessel
    - Longer delay better blood supply
- Defects 1/3-2/3 of lip
  - Primary closure results in tight oral stoma
    - Uses local tissue from cheeks
    - Tissue is advanced with or without compensatory excisions of healthy skin and subcutaneous tissue

- Revision often necessary
- Flap closure is best choice in 1/3-2/3 defects
  - Generally local tissue is available for flap closure
  - Abbe flap
    - Based on labial artery
    - Primarily for central upper lip defects
  - Reverse Estlander Flap
    - Based on lateral elements of lower lip which are rotated into upper lip
    - Downside: commissure distortion
    - Can be full thickness or cutaneous flap only
      - Flap used depends on defect
        - Full thickness vs. partial thickness
  - Webster flap
    - Vermilion advancement to reconstruct mucosa
    - Flap of lower lip skin and muscle rotated to reconstruct the remaining defect
  - Bilateral nasolabial flaps
    - Superiorly based
    - Borrow tissue from behind nasal sill if available OR…
    - Cheek can be advanced into upper lip with donor site in lateral cheek and closed with skin graft in large defects
  - Bilateral lower cheek flaps
    - Inferiorly based counterparts of nasolabial flap
    - Kazanjian/Converse
  - Reverse Gilles Fan Flap
    - Rotates lateral tissue into defect
    - Compensates donor site by placing z-plasty at base of rotation
    - Random blood supply, rarely used
  - Reverse Karapandzic flap

- Circumoral incision of remaining upper and lower lip
- Divides skin, muscle and mucosa while preserving facial nerve branches and axial to preserve function vessels
- Risk of microstomia due to extensive incisions
    - McGregor Flap
        - Full thickness lateral cheek tissue
        - Rotated around fixed commissure
    - Nakajima Flap
        - Same as McGregor flap but preserves vessels and nerves
- Defects > 2/3's
    - May require microvascular free-tissue transfer especially if upper and lower lip is involved in defect
    - Generally though even subtotal defects can be reconstructed with local tissue.
        - Bernard-Weber flaps
    - Options in free tissue transfer
        - Radial forearm + palmaris longus tendon
            - Sensate but static
        - Gracilis + STSG
            - Potential for motor function
            - Beneficial in younger patients <50
            - Will need PT/OT to learn to use muscle
    - Mucosal reconstruction
        - Healing by secondary intention ("small" defects)
        - Primary closure
        - Mucosal advancement flaps
        - FAMM flaps for large defects
        - STSG

3. Select appropriate options in diagnosis and management

- You must be thoroughly comfortable with the execution of these flaps:
    - Local anatomy

- How to draw them, practice drawing
- Nuances
  - What size to make flap based on defect
  - Blood supply
  - How to optimize outcome
- Know 2 or 3 flap options for each type of lip defect based on size and location (central, lateral, commissure, extensive)
    - Must choose best option based on clinical presentation
      - Primary factor size of defect and what is missing
    - In isolated vermilion and mucosal defects local recon is best
    - Don't underestimate need for mucosal lining- significant contracture may ensue if inadequate!
    - Have a long-term post-op plan based on etiology of defect, most especially for tumor cases.

4. Understand risks and benefits of various approaches

   - Primary risks- microstomia, insensate flaps
   - Think about the reconstructive ladder
   - What is the anticipated aesthetic outcome?
   - Best way to optimize function?
   - Why choose one option over another?
   - What do you anticipate as the outcome?
     - Level of difficulty getting there

5. Address complications and unexpected problems adequately

   - Post-op Management
     - Microstomia regimen
       - Lip stretching by appliances and dentures
       - To collapse during insertion and removal
   - Decreased sensation- drooling, injury from hot foods
   - Decreased elasticity
   - Full thickness nasolabial tissue may denervate upper lip muscle
   - Problems with anesthetic lip or poor sulcus depth
     - Drooling tendency
     - More often problem in lower lip reconstruction
     - Tx:
       - Deepen vestibular trough
       - Reposition frenulum

- Broaden zone of attached gingival tissue
- Infection- Rare
- Wound dehiscence
- Flap loss- uncommon, secondary to inadequate blood supply
    - Avoid by:
        - Avoiding scar tissue at base of flap
        - Minimize tension
        - Gentle handling of tissue

6. Demonstrate ability to structure alternative plan

- Backup plan for flap failure or preferred donor tissue not available
- Plan for management of flap complications
    - Abnormal aesthetics
    - Pin cushioning
    - Hypertrophic scarring
    - Severe microstomia
- Management protocol for failing free flap
- Elderly patient who refuses cancer treatment
- Patient who is belligerent with office staff

Chapter Twenty-Five

Lower Lip Reconstruction

25
Lower Lip Reconstruction

1. Identify General Problem/Diagnosis/Planning
   (Describe photo, working diagnosis, key problems, evaluates patient)

   - Describe photo
     - Detail location of lesion
     - Size of defect
       - Note in detail: What is missing and specific anatomy involved
   - Discuss key problems of reconstruction
     - Aesthetic and reconstructive concerns
   - Differences from upper lip:
     - Lower lip can sustain greater tissue loss without distortion
     - Can donate larger amounts of tissue for upper lip recon
   - History
     - Age of patient
     - Non-healing lesion?
     - How long has lesion been present?
     - Chronic sun exposure?
     - Concern for cancer
       - Past history of cancer
       - Immunocompromised
         - (transplant recipient vs. other)
       - Crusting or bleeding
       - Recent change in lesion
       - Prior radiation
     - Medical history
       - HTN
       - DM
       - Anticoagulation
       - Cardiovascular disease/CHF
       - Immunosuppressant's
       - Steroid use
   - Physical Exam

- Look for separate metachronous lesions, common finding
- Examine
  - Lips
  - Oral cavity
  - Lymphatics
    - Neck
    - Submental- central lesions
    - Submandibular- ipsilateral lesions
    - Parotid
  - Local scars?
    - May affect reconstructive options
- Note location of lesion
- Mobile or fixed
  - Involves mandible?
    - Direct extension
    - Perineural invasion
    - Lymphatic spread
- Anatomy of the lip
  - Consider subunits involved
  - Lateral and medial elements
  - Commissure
  - Parts
    - Skin
    - Wet/dry vermilion
    - Muscle
    - Mucosa
  - Size of defect breakdown
    - 1/3, 1/3-2/3, Subtotal, total
    - Size dictates management

- Establish diagnosis
  - Is the lesion benign vs. malignant?
    - Affects margins and post-op treatment plan
    - Biopsy: Incisional/excisional depends on size
  - Skin cancer more common in the following:
    - Fitzpatrick I and II
    - Males
    - Age >50
    - Chronic sun exposure (farmer classic)
      - Most important risk factor

- Key problems
  - What is missing?
  - Staging- lymphatic involvement
  - Mandibular/Maxillary involvement
    - < 4cm segment- bone graft acceptable
    - > 4cm segmental vascularized flap
    - Consider vascularized flap if post-op radiation is anticipated
- Work-up
  - Determine extent of disease
    - PE findings
    - +/- imaging as indicated (eg. fixed lesion)
      - CT scan or MRI
  - If bony involvement (mandible/maxilla suspected) imaging is needed
    - CT scan or panorex (for mandibular involvement)
    - <2% of cases will have distant metastasis
  - Consultants
    - Oncology
    - ENT or Oral surgery for primary resection
- Staging Skin Cancers
  - Non-Melanocytic
    - Stage 0- In-situ
    - Stage I- <2cm
    - Stage II- >2cm
    - Stage III-Below skin to lymph node/cartilage/muscle/bone
    - Stage IV-Metastasis
  - Melanocytic
    - Based on Breslow Classification - thickness of lesion
      - Stage 0-In-situ 5mm or less
      - Stage I-Up to 1.5mm, no lymphadenopathy
      - Stage II- >1.5mm, no lymphadenopathy
      - Stage III-(+) lymphadenopathy
      - Stage IV-Metastasis
- About the lip
  - Prone to cancer because vermillion lacks pigmentation layer which protects from UV rays

- o 25% of all oral cavity tumors

2. Consider reasonable goals in diagnosis and management *(Management and treatment, surgical indications, operative procedures and anesthesia)*

    - Treatment: Resection, spare uninvolved structures
    - Primary treatment modalities
        - o Radiation
            - Only used for patients that are poor risk for surgery, rarely needed
        - o Surgery
            - Surgery can often be done under local with some sedation avoiding general anesthesia
        - o Radiation and surgery are equivalent in early lesions (<3 cm)
            - 90-95% cure @ 5 years
    - Determine type of tumor: dictates margins and post-op care plan
        - o Basal cell carcinoma
            - 2mm margin for resection
        - o Recurrent basal cell
            - Moh's resection
        - o Squamous cell carcinoma
            - 1-2cm margin
            - Lower lip squamous cell carcinoma
            - 1-1.5cm lesions- margin 7-10mm
        - o Melanoma
            - In situ: 5mm margin
            - 1mm thickness: 1cm margin
            - 1-2mm thickness: 1-2cm margin
            - >2mm: 2cm margin
    - Operative procedures
        - o Local with sedation an option in most adults for most reconstructions
        - o Upper lip can be blocked by bilateral mental nerve block
            - 2nd Bicuspid- approximately 1cm lateral to canine in lower buccal sulcus
        - o If white roll is involved in excision always mark prior to injection with local
    - Treatment

- Based on:
  - Histologic diagnosis
  - Resection with tissue specific margins
- Reconstruction goals
  - Sensate lip
  - Functional sphincter
    - Watertight seal
  - Adequate opening for food and dental care
  - Aesthetic appearance
  - Good apposition of lower and upper vermilion
- In sub-total and total reconstruction all goals cannot be satisfied.
- Prior to reconstruction
  - Resection with appropriate margins and tissue diagnosis
    - If necessary delay closure until definitive margins known by permanent section or Moh's

- Management of Vermilion Lesions
  - May require excision of white roll
  - Mark prior to infiltration with local
  - Make all incisions perpendicular to vermilion
  - Small Lesions
  - Small V-Y advancement may be effective
  - Large Lesions
  - Vermilion advancement flaps
  - Mucosal V-Y advancement
  - FAMM flap
    - In subtotal or total lip loss cases
- Management Options
- Defect <30%
  - Shield shaped excision extending to not crossing labio- mental fold
  - Use z-plasty if incision crosses labio-mental fold
- Defect 30-65%
  - Borrow upper lip tissue:
    - Lip switch flap
    - Cheek advancement flap
    - Oral circumference advancement (Karapanzic flap)
    - Innervated composite flaps

- Step reconstruction appropriate for central defects
- Abbe flap
  - Based on labial artery
  - Flap from medial or lateral upper lip, avoid central upper lip
  - 2-stage procedure
  - Initially denervated sphincter function returns later
  - 3rd stage can do vermilion reconstruction if needed
- Bernard procedure
  - En bloc tumor excision
  - Incisions extend from commissure
- Estlander flap good for defects involving commissure although commissure will still be distorted
- Gilles Fan Flap
  - Extended Estlander flap
  - Carries commissure and lower lateral lip inward
  - Results in distortion of commissure

- Defect >65%
  - Bilateral cheek advancement
  - Bilateral oral circumferential advancement
  - Bilateral innervated composite flaps
  - If adequate tissue not available locally
    - Radial forearm free flap +/- palmaris longus tendon
    - Gracilis free flap + skin graft
  - In local flaps exceeding 2:1 ratio in random skin flaps may increase risk for distal necrosis (rare)
  - Mucosal reconstruction
    - Healing by secondary intention ("small" defects)
    - Primary closure
    - Mucosal advancement flaps
    - FAMM flaps for large defects
    - STSG

3. Select appropriate options in diagnosis and management

    - You must be thoroughly comfortable with the execution of these flaps:
        - Local anatomy
        - How to draw them, practice drawing
        - Nuances
            - What size to make flap based on defect
            - Blood supply
            - How to optimize outcome
        - Know 2 or 3 flap options for each type of lip defect based on size and location (central, lateral, commissure, extensive)
    - Must choose best option based on clinical presentation
        - Primary factor defect and what is missing
    - In isolated vermilion and mucosal defects, local recon is best
    - Don't underestimate need for mucosal lining- significant contracture may ensue if inadequate!
    - Have a long-term post-op plan based on etiology of defect, most especially for tumor cases

4. Understand risks and benefits of various approaches

    - Consider risks benefits of different approaches in different clinical scenarios.
    - What are the upsides and downsides of different procedures?
    - What is your anticipated outcome?
    - Any preventative measures for microtomia, poor sensation, drooling, other?

5. Address complications and unexpected problems adequately

    - Tight inverted upper lip
    - Postop microstomia
        - Tx:
            - Lip stretching exercises
            - Appliances, Dentures
    - Decreased sensation
    - Decreased elasticity
    - Drooling
        - Tx:
            - Deepen trough

- - Reposition frenulum
    - Broaden zone of attached gingival
- Infection- infrequent
- Wound dehiscence
- Flap necrosis
- Recurrent tumor

6. Demonstrate ability to structure alternative plan

    - Cancer patient refuses treatment
    - Residual tumor in resection margin
    - Failed flap back-up plan
    - Alternative donor sites
    - Alternative treatment based on type of cancer

Chapter Twenty-Six

Cheek Reconstruction

26
Cheek Reconstruction

1. Identify General Problem/Diagnosis/Planning
   (Describe photo, working diagnosis, key problems, evaluate patient)

   - Describe photo
     - Detail and classify
       - Defect, Anatomy, Structures involved
   - Working diagnosis
     - Key problems present
   - Anatomy of the cheek
     - Boundaries
       - Medial- Buccal mucosa
       - Anterior- lips
       - Posterior- Pterygomandibular raphe
       - Superior- upper alveolar ridge
       - Inferior- lower alveolar ridge
   - Cheek functions
     - Mastication
     - Deglutition
     - Communication
   - Hx
     - Age of patient
     - Non-healing lesion
     - How long has lesion been present?
     - Chronic sun exposure?
     - Concern for cancer
       - Past history of cancer
     - Immunocompromised (transplant recipient vs. other)
     - Crusting or bleeding
     - Recent change in lesion
     - Prior radiation
     - Medical history
       - HTN
       - DM
       - Anticoagulation
       - Cardiovascular disease/CHF
       - Immunosuppressants

- Steroid use
- Physical Exam
    o Comprehensive head and neck exam
    o 3 distinct zones or aesthetic units of the cheek
        - Suborbital
            - Anterior to sideburn to nasolabial line
            - Lower eyelid to gingival sulcus
        - Preauricular
            - Supero-lateral junction of helix and cheek to mandible
        - Buccomandibular
            - Remaining area of the cheek
    o Note the status of the facial nerve
        - Facial palsy suggests malignancy
    o Facial nerve exam
        - Raise brows
        - Close eyes
        - Symmetrical smile
        - Show teeth
        - Tense neck muscles
        - Check for lymphadenopathy
- Work-up
    o As in other skin lesions, most defects are secondary to tumors
    o Establish diagnosis
        - Biopsy
            - Resection with clear margin by Moh's or permanent section
            - Follow with reconstruction
        - Estimate and determine extent of disease
        - Metastatic work-up if warranted
    o Consultants
        - Oncology, oral surgery, ENT surg onc
    o Medical optimization prior to surgery
        - Controlled HTN
        - DM
        - CAD
        - Anticoagulants
    o Additional work-up to consider when malignancy is present:
        - Basal Cell Carcinoma (BCC)

- CXR
  - Generally not needed
  - Low incidence of metastasis
- LFT's
  - If metastasis suspected
  - Rare in BCC
- Squamous Cell Carcinoma (SCC)
  - CXR- indicated in large tumors
  - LFT's- indicated in large tumors
  - CT scan to confirm if bony involvement present only if suspected
  - MRI- evaluates perineural invasion
- Melanoma
  - CXR
  - LFT's
  - CT scan for stage III and IV disease
    - Brain
    - Lung
    - Abdomen/Pelvis

2. Consider reasonable goals in diagnosis and management *(Management and treatment, surgical indications, operative procedures and anesthesia)*

- Treatment options
  - Basal cell carcinoma:
    - Radiation- if poor candidate for surgery
    - Surgery
      - Topical antineoplastic agents in diffuse cases: 5-FU
  - Squamous cell carcinoma
    - Radiation
    - Surgery
    - Chemotherapy in metastatic cases
  - Melanoma
    - Surgery +/- sentinel node +/- lymphadenectomy
    - Stage III- interferon alpha-2B
    - Role for radiation not well defined
    - Clinical trials important
- Reconstruction

- o Options based on:
  - Location
  - Extent of tissue loss
  - Functional loss
  - Comorbidity
- o Considerations
  - Skin coverage (external requirement)
  - Lining
  - Involvement of parotid gland
    - Stenson's duct
- o Goals of reconstruction
  - Aesthetic reconstruction
  - Resumption of oral diet
  - Normal speech
  - Re-establish:
    - Oral sphincter
    - Vermilion for sensory function
    - Prevent drooling
  - In cases of the loss of motor function
    - Use fascial sling to decrease drooling and re-establish commissure
  - Adequate surgical margin in the case of malignancy
  - May require excision of underlying structures:
    - Cartilage
    - Bone
    - Parotid superficial and/or deep
    - Lymph nodes
  - If facial nerve sacrificed
    - Sural and other nerve grafts
- Reconstructive Options
  - o Primary closure
    - Small superficial defects
  - o Defect > 3cm
    - Random local tissue transfer or mucosal flap
    - Skin graft or pedicled musculocutaneous flap
  - o Goal: minimize contracture leading to trismus
  - o Defect of entire buccal mucosa
    - If reconstructed with insensate grafts:

- Xerostomia
- Numbness
  - Rehabilitation for speech and swallow may be needed
- Large defect may need transfer of sensate lubricating free grafts to improve function
- Free flaps
  - Potential for sensation or lubrication
  - Flaps with nerve for sensation are ideal
- Common local flap options
  - Rhomboid flaps
  - Rotation advancement flaps
  - Transposition flaps
- Pedicle flap muscle skin
  - Pectoralis major
  - Latissimus dorsi
  - Upper Trapezius
  - Temporalis
- Free flaps - ideal for large defects
  - Choice based on "what's missing"
  - Superior aesthetic and functional outcomes
    - Radial forearm
      - Pliable, thin sensate
      - Coapt to lingual nerve or inferior alveolar nerve
    - Transverse colon
      - Can be used as mucosal free-flap
      - Adequate pedicle, durable
    - Anterior lateral thigh flap
    - Rectus abdominis flap
      - Versatile standby flap
      - Skin and muscle
      - Muscle will mucosalize
    - Latissimus dorsi
      - Skin and muscle
    - Fibula free flap +/- second flap for skin coverage
      - If mandibular reconstruction required
- Lining Management/Buccal defects
  - Small mucosal resection

- Primary closure only
  - Larger resection
    - Mucosal flap or skin graft
  - Defect of entire buccal mucosa may need skin and/or muscle to decrease trismus or xerostomia
  - Cervical pedicle myocutaneous flap
    - Good option for small to larger defects
    - Platysma myocutaneous flap
      - Wide arc of rotation
      - Thin pliable
      - Buccal mucosal defects up to 5-7cm
    - Sternocleidomastoid myocutaneous flap
- Full thickness defect considerations
  - Decreased sensation
  - Lubrication
  - Facial motor function
  - Mandibular continuity
- Guides for surgical margins
  - Basal cell carcinoma: 2mm
  - Squamous cell carcinoma: 1cm minimum
  - Melanoma- Breslow classification
    - In situ 0.5mm or less- 1cm margin
    - 0.5 to 1 mm thickness- 1cm margin
    - 1mm-2mm- 1-2cm margin
    - 2mm-4mm- 2cm margin
    - >4mm- 2-3cm margin
- Melanoma management
  - >1mm thickness- sentinel node biopsy
    - Performed 2-4 hours after radionucleotide injection
  - 1-4mm thickness lesions
    - Elective lymph node dissection
    - 20% risk of spread to nodes
  - >4mm
    - No benefit to lymph node dissection

3. Select appropriate options in diagnosis and management

- Make your reconstruction plan based on:
  - Etiology of defect
  - Size of defect
  - What is missing

- - o Available donor sites
  - Take into consideration primary goals of reconstruction and what can be achieved.

4. Understand risks and benefits of various approaches

   - Surgical considerations
     - o Local tissue gives good color match
     - o Design of local flaps should be slightly smaller than defect allows incorporation of surrounding tissue
     - o Management of redundant tissue
       - Excise
       - Remove dog-ears
   - Disadvantages of pedicled muscle flaps
     - o Contracture of base of flap
     - o Excessive bulk
     - o Not ideal for functional purpose
   - Be able to discuss the risks and benefits of various approaches
     - o Eg: Skin Graft vs. Local Flap vs. Pedicled Flap vs. Free Flap
   - Preventative measures to avoid possible complications?

5. Address complications and unexpected problems adequately

   - Trismus
   - Xerostomia
   - Drooling
   - Bleeding
   - Infection- uncommon
   - Ectropion
     - o Management:
       - Scar massage 6-9 months
       - If persistent- flap revision
         - Scar release and reconstruction
   - Facial nerve injury
   - Parotid gland/Stenson's duct management
   - Flap necrosis
   - Incomplete tumor resection and recurrence
   - Recurrent tumor
   - Microsurgical complications
   - Have a management plan for various potential complications

6. Demonstrate ability to structure alternative plan

    - Cancer patient refuses treatment
    - Residual tumor in resection margin
    - Failed flap back-up plan
    - Timing of redo surgery
    - Alternative donor sites
    - Alternative treatment based on type of cancer

Section Five
Facial Fractures

Chapter Twenty-Seven

Facial Fracture Overview

27
Facial Fracture Overview

1. Identify General Problem

    - Describe photo
    - Give working diagnosis
    - Key problems
    - Evaluate patient
    - Diagnosis/Planning
    - Go through ABC's of trauma management
    - Brief relevant medical and surgical history
    - Control airway, bleeding, resuscitation
    - GCS assessment of neurosurgical prognosis
    - How do you manage uncontrolled facial bleeding?
        - Scalp
        - Nasal
        - From soft tissue
        - From facial fractures
    - Give accurate evaluation of fractures and anticipated clinical problems. Be prepared to read CT scans. Make plans and assessment based on what is shown. DO NOT ASK FOR MORE VIEWS, YOU WON'T GET ANY.
    - Classify specific fracture type(s)
        - Frontal sinus (anterior, posterior)
        - NOE
        - Orbit
        - Maxilla
        - Mandibular (condyle, coronoid, ramus, body, symphysis)
    - Detail your systematic craniomaxillofacial exam
    - Need for additional work-up or consultants?
    - Ophthalmology for all orbital fractures: Dilated Eye Exam
    - Neurosurgery
    - CT scan (Thin cut axial/coronal/sagittal view) +/- 3D Recon
    - Panorex
    - Angio for uncontrolled bleeding

2. Consider reasonable goals in diagnosis and management

    - Management and treatment
    - Surgical indications
    - Operative procedures and anesthesia
    - Surgical goals of ORIF
        o Restoration of occlusion and aesthetic appearance
        o Maintain height and width of face
    - Management of significant bone loss
        o Indications for bone grafting
    - Timing of your surgery
    - Prevent complications
        o Mucocele
        o Tear duct obstruction
        o Enophthalmos
        o Ectropion
        o Malocclusion
    - Discuss standard treatment based on fracture type
    - Points of fixation
    - Plate type and size
    - Incisions and approach
    - Orbital floor reconstruction techniques
    - What kind of exposure is needed and why?
    - Soft tissue defects?
    - 3-4 point fixation in all ZMC fractures

3. Select appropriate options in diagnosis and management

    - Give your choice of surgical approach and why?
    - Sequence of reconstruction
    - Post-op management
    - Closure technique
    - Preventative measures- Frost suture
    - How is procedure performed?
    - Key steps of surgery
    - Markings and relevant anatomy

4. Understand risks and benefits of various approaches

    - Discuss risks, benefits of various approaches
        o Subciliary vs. Transconj vs. Orbital rim incision

- o Reconstruction bar vs. miniplates
- o Risdon incision vs. intraoral percutaneous techniques
- o Titanium vs. resorbable plates
    - Indications for external fixation of mandible
    - Indications for splinting of mandible

5. Address complications and unexpected problems adequately

    - Be prepared to manage and know the causes of:
        - o Enophthalmos
        - o Ectropion
        - o Malocclusion
        - o Mucocele
        - o Tear duct obstruction
        - o Loose hardware
        - o Malunion
        - o Nonunion
        - o Inadequate reduction
    - What if multiple concurrent injuries?
    - GCS of 3 and guarded prognosis?

6. Demonstrate ability to structure alternative plan

    - Does approach change based on medical status, age of patient, time since injury 1week vs. 10 weeks?
    - Why did complications occur?
    - Timing of revision or re-operation (osteotomies needed)

Chapter Twenty-Eight

Facial Fractures

———

28
Facial Fractures

1. Identify General Problem/Diagnosis/Planning
   (Describe photo, give working diagnosis, key problems, evaluates patient)

   - Describe photo, note and classify all fractures seen in radiologic studies
   - Note key plastic surgery related problems
   - Before initiating plastic surgery related procedures:
     o Evaluate patient by standard ATLS Protocol
     o Primary survey:
       - Airway
         - Stridor
         - Presence of blood
         - Air hunger
       - Breathing
         - Adequate ventilation
         - End tidal CO2
       - Circulation
         - Control any active bleeding
         - Check pulses, BP, HR
         - IV access
     o Secondary survey:
       - Intracranial and/or C-spine injury
       - Thoracic trauma
         - Pneumothorax
         - Hemothorax
         - Aortic dissection
       - Spinal cord injury
       - Intraabdominal trauma
       - Pelvic fractures
       - Long bone fractures
       - Maxillofacial trauma
     o Look for sources of significant blood loss (scalp laceration, etc.)
     o Note if facial fracture is impacting the airway or ventilation secondary to:
       - Displacement of fractures

- Indirectly from hemorrhage
- History
    - Ample history
    - Cause of trauma
    - Pre-existing medical conditions
    - Medications and allergies
    - Loss of consciousness at the scene
        - May indicate brain injury
        - Obligates head CT
    - MVA?
        - Where was patient sitting?
        - Restrained or ejected?
        - Steering wheel or dashboard deformed
        - Windshield cracked
    - Immunized for tetanus
    - Past eye or nasal surgeries
    - Previous surgical procedures
    - Smoker?
    - Drug abuse
- Physical Exam
    - Glascow Coma Scale
    - C-spine injury exam
    - Ocular trauma
    - Occlusion
    - Sensibility
    - Focus on systematic maxillofacial exam:
    - Memorize the same systematic examination (scalp to chin or chin to scalp your preference):
        - Craniomaxillofacial exam
            - Scalp to chin:
            - Point tenderness or crepitus at fracture sites
            - Palpate bony prominences
            - Palpable step-offs?
                - Cranial vault
                - Forehead
                - Orbits
                - Midface
                - Mandible
            - Bimanual palpation for facial mobility

- Assessment for Lefort I, II or III fractures
  - Anterior maxilla and nasion
- Check sensibility
  - Forehead
  - Cheek
  - Chin
  - Supra- and infraorbital nerve distribution inferior alveolar nerve
  - Mental nerve
- Note facial edema
- Intraoral exam
  - Lacerations
  - Dental injury
    - Fractured, missing or loose teeth in fracture line (mandibular or maxillary fractures)
  - Occlusion
  - Wear facets
- Intranasal exam
  - Septal hematoma
  - Lacerations
  - CSF
- Ocular exam
  - Gross vision
  - Marcus-Gunn pupil
  - Absence of pupillary constriction of unilateral pupil afferent visual pathway
- Is trachea midline?
- Enophthalmos
  - Not always immediate
  - Frequent follow-up post-op to check
- Facial nerve function
- Mandible specific

- Clinical diagnosis followed by Panorex
- PE findings- intraoral and extraoral examination
- Malocclusion (primary finding)
    - Any change in occlusion is clinically significant
    - Edema
    - Crepitation
    - Trismus
    - Neurosensoral changes
    - Check the quality of and status of dentition
  - DOCUMENT- sensory exam (infraorbital nerve and inferior alveolar nerve, facial nerve function) especially in Casebooks!
- Work-up
  - Trauma Labs
    - CBC
    - Chem 7 + LFT's
    - PT, PTT
    - Type and cross
  - X-Rays
    - C-spine
    - T & L-spine
    - CXR
    - Pelvis
  - Maxillofacial CT scan
    - 2-D axial and coronal and sagittal
    - 1.0mm to 2.0mm cuts
    - 3-D Reconstruction for fracture pattern optional
  - PANOREX
    - Mandatory for all mandible fractures
    - In isolated mandible fracture- Panorex and plain films adequate for work-up
    - In complex mandible fractures- CT scan occasional adjunct to Panorex
- Basic Trauma Management:
  - 2 large bore IV's 16 gauge
  - IV fluids Lactated Ringers (LR) for resuscitation
  - Oxygen

- o Foley for extensive injury
- o Orogastric tube avoid intracranial placement of NGT in extensive facial fracture
- o Analgesics and sedatives if airway stable
- o Keep patient warm to avoid hypothermia
- Management of uncontrolled bleeding from facial fractures:
  - o Nasal packing
  - o Foley catheter inflate balloons
  - o Emergent angiogram for embolization
- Consultations:
  - o Trauma surgery
  - o Neurosurgery
  - o Ophthalmology
    - Posterior chamber exam pre-op in all orbital fractures
- Most Common Etiologies of Facial Fractures
  - o MVA
  - o Gunshot/Altercations
  - o Sports
  - o Other
- Components of Craniofacial Region
  - o Break up into thirds:
    - Superior 1/3:
      - Frontal Region
      - Orbits
      - NOE- superior portion
    - Middle 1/3:
      - NOE- inferior portion
      - Nose
      - Zygomatico-maxillary
    - Inferior 1/3:
      - Mandible

- Note frontal sinus fractures: higher incidence of CNS injury

2. Consider reasonable goals in diagnosis and management *(Management and treatment, surgical indications, operative procedures and anesthesia)*

- Operative Management and Goals Based on Fracture Site
- Frontal Bone and Sinus Fracture
- Goals:

- o Aesthetics recontour forehead
- o Repair dura and obliterate frontal sinus if indicated to prevent mucocele
- Consider status of:
  - o Anterior table
  - o Posterior table
- Early CT scan
  - o R/O associated head injury (high incidence)
  - o Check for pneumocephalus
- Non-displaced anterior table or posterior table w/o CSF leak
  - o OBSERVATION only
- Displaced anterior table only
  - o Reduce and fixate
- Displaced anterior and posterior table + CSF leak
  - o Repair dura- neurosurgery consultation
  - o Cranialization
  - o Obliterate mucosa by technique of choice:
    - Burring
    - Strip and cauterization
    - Fat grafting
    - Pericranial flap
    - Other
- If nasofrontal duct fractured: Work-up
  - o Fluorescein dye
  - o Methylene blue
  - o Check for dye in nasal airway
- If fractured:
  - o Obliterate
  - o Remove sinus mucosa
    - Dye with methylene blue
    - Burr
    - Fill with:
      - Morcelized bone
      - Fat
      - Muscle
      - Galea
      - Artificial material
  - o Cranialization- prevents mucocele
- Frontal sinus fracture management
  - o Gold standard:
    - Coronal approach
    - Exception

- Substantial open laceration that will give adequate exposure
  - Reconstruction Options
    - Plating system 1.5 or 1.6mm plates
    - Wires 25 gauge or smaller
    - Resorbable plates
- Orbital floor fracture
  - Anatomy
  - 7 bones
    - Maxilla, Zygoma, Frontal, Palatine, Lacrimal, Ethmoid, Sphenoid
  - Roof:
    - Frontal, Sphenoid (Lesser wing)
  - Medial wall:
    - Ethmoid, Lacrimal, Maxilla (frontal process), Sphenoid (body)
  - Floor:
    - Maxilla, Zygoma, Palatine
  - Lateral wall:
    - Zygoma, Sphenoid (greater wing)
  - Inferior orbital margin
    - Maxilla, Zygoma
  - Orbital floor fracture
    - Osseous defect with fat herniation and potential ocular muscle entrapment
- Pathophysiology of Orbital fractures Controversial (2 theories):
  - Transmission of mechanical energy
    - Absorbed by globe and loss of resistance through dynamic compression of osseous walls
  - Direct impact
    - Explosion of osseous walls frequently medial wall and floor
    - This protects the globe
  - Either way enophthalmos may result
  - Blow out fracture
    - Pure
    - Isolated fracture of floor or medial wall in absence of a fracture of the orbital margin
    - Etiology
    - Medium or low impact

- Altercations or sports related
      - Blow in fracture
          - Floor fracture with proptosis
- Work-up
  - Requires CT scan with coronal views
  - Coronal view evaluates the floor
- Indications for surgery
  - Moderate displacement
  - Risk of enophthalmos
  - Acute enophthalmos (sunken eye)
  - Defect >1cm on coronal CT
  - Mechanical muscle entrapment
- Surgical goals
  - Adequate fracture exposure
  - Adequate reduction and fixation
  - Discreet incisions
- Approaches
  - Transconjunctival
    - Lowest risk for post-op ectropion
    - May encounter inferior rectus during exposure
  - Transcaruncle
    - Adjunct to transconjunctival in medial wall fractures
    - Avoid medial canthus, lacrimal sac
  - Subciliary
    - Highest risk for post-op ectropion
  - Orbital rim
- Approach based on fracture location
  - Orbital roof
    - Coronal approach
    - Eyebrow
    - Risk of supraorbital n./supratrochlear n. injury
    - More difficult exposure
  - Medial wall
    - Transcaruncle
    - Upper eyelid
  - Lateral wall
    - Lateral brow
  - Floor
    - Transconjunctival +/- lateral canthotomy

- - - Subciliary
    - Infrapalpebral (Orbital rim)
  - Options for orbital floor reconstruction
    - Autologous
      - Fracture fragments if not comminuted
      - Cranial bone graft (outer table calvarium)
        - Harvest in-situ or via craniotomy (neurosurgeon)
      - Rib, Iliac crest
    - Alloplastic
      - Resorbable plate
      - Titanium mesh
      - Porous polyethylene (Medora Plates)
      - Silicone rubber
      - Gel film (may augment repair if small residual defects present)
    - Fixation
      - Rigid or semi-rigid
      - Wire or microplates (1.5mm, 1.6mm or smaller)
  - Procedure
    - Expose orbital floor in subperiosteal plane
    - Reduce herniated contents
    - Define margins of defect
    - Optic nerve 47mm from edge of inferior orbital rim
    - Bridge defect with autologous bone or alloplastic material
    - If simple reduction guarantees stability no need to do more
    - Forced duction test before you leave the room
  - Naso-orbital-ethmoid (NOE) fracture
    - History
      - High-energy mechanism
      - Horse kick to face
      - Face against steering wheel in MVA
    - Physical Exam
      - Traumatic telecanthus
      - May ask review old photographs of patient
      - Depression of nasal dorsum with elevation of nasal tip and shortening of columella
      - Epiphora
      - Enophthalmos

- NOE Classification
    - 3 types- graded by comminution and relation of fragments to medial canthal tendon
    - Grade I: Large fragment, medial canthus attached
    - Grade II: Small fragment, medial canthus attached
    - Grade III: Highly comminuted nasal bones, medial canthus completely detached
- Approach
    - Gold standard: Coronal incision
    - Exception: wide-open laceration with excellent exposure
    - +/- transconjunctival incision for further exposure
- Areas to expose
    - Medial orbit
    - Medial canthus
- Goals
    - Correct telecanthus
    - Correct enophthalmos
    - Restore nasal projection (immediate cantilever bone graft may be needed)
- Reduction dependent on amount of available bone
    - If medial canthus is attached to a large fragment
        - Reduce and plate
        - >75% of cases can be reduced and plated
    - If medial canthus is detached
        - Transnasal wiring
        - Awl and drill to contralateral side
    - In severe fractures dorsal nasal support may be needed
        - Cantilever bone graft
        - Prefer:
            - Rib with cartilage in tip
            - Fix bone to frontal sinus via burr hole or miniplates
            - Cranial bone graft or iliac crest can be used

- Nasolacrimal duct injury

- o Initial management
  - Probe or cannulate if possible
  - If lacerated suture over Crawford tube and leave tube minimum 4-6 months
  - If unsafe to probe or uncertain, observe
  - If no resolution of epiphora in 3-6 months
    - Explore
    - May have to manage with dacryocystorhinostomy (DCR)
  - Do not perform DCR in setting of acute trauma
- Nasal Fracture
  - o Clinical diagnosis in isolated nasal fracture
  - o PE
    - R/O septal hematoma
    - Drain septal hematoma early to prevent septal necrosis, which may result in a secondary saddle nose deformity
  - o Timing of intervention
    - Immediate reduction within first 24 hours
    - Allow edema to resolve minimum 2-3 days
    - In early fractures
      - May attempt closed reduction within first 1-2 weeks
      - Re-create injury pattern
      - Splint
    - If closed reduction fails
      - Osteotomy after healing
    - Delayed repair
      - Use standard rhinoplasty techniques including osteotomy
    - Immediate osteotomy is acceptable, delayed repair is the more conservative option
- Zygomaticomaxillary Complex (ZMC) Fracture
  - o Management
    - Requires minimum of:
    - 3 points of fixation for adequate stabilization in quadripod fx
    - 2 of 3 points in tripod fx
    - Use lateral orbital wall as a guide to alignment

- 4 Points of Fragility In ZMC fractures (Quadripod fx)
  - Zygomatic arch
  - Frontozygomatic suture
  - Orbital floor
  - Lateral buttress of maxilla
  - When zygomatic arch is preserved- considered tripod fracture
- Points of Fixation
  - Orbital rim
  - Zygomaxillary suture
  - Zygofrontal suture
  - Nasomaxillary suture
- The zygomatic arch
  - Relates the temporal bone to the body of the zygoma
  - Lateral-inferior wall of the orbit joins to zygomatic process of maxilla
- Approach
  - Exposure usually requires a combination of incisions
    - Gingivobuccal sulcus
    - Upper Lid
    - Lower Lid
      - Orbital Rim
      - Subciliary
      - Transconjunctival
    - Brow
    - Gillies
      - Approach for isolated zygomatic arch fractures
      - Especially greenstick fractures can reduce without fixation
    - Coronal
      - Reserved for generally severe cases
      - When wide exposure of lateral wall and arch needed
- ORIF is the preferred method of treatment
  - Miniplate (2.0mm or microplates 1.6mm)
- Indications for intervention

- Visible deformity
- +/- trismus
- Functional occlusion problems
- Maxillary Fracture
    - Middle 1/3 of the face
    - Classify by Lefort fracture system
        - Lefort I: Fracture through base of piriform aperture, pterygoid plates
        - Lefort II: Fracture through junction of the nasofrontal junction
        - Lefort III: Craniofacial dysjunction, fracture through nasofrontal junction and zygomatic-frontal suture
    - Goal
        - Restore proper vertical sagittal dimensions
    - Approach
        - Place first in MMF for occlusion
        - Use vertical buttresses for support
            - Nasomaxillary
            - Zygomaxillary
        - Bone gap of buttress >1.5cm requires bone grafting
            - Cranial bone
            - Iliac crest
            - Rib
        - High Comminution Injuries
            - Use maxillary suspension with wires to cranially stable region
            - Zygomatic arch or lateral orbital wall OR
            - Can use autogenous bone grafts
        - Ultimate intervention depends on the stability of the fracture
            - Unstable fracture
            - Loss of vertical height
        - ORIF is appropriate in all patients including pediatric population
            - Pediatric avoid tooth buds when placing plates
    - Access Incision
        - Gingivolabial sulcus (Caldwell-Luc)
        - Miniplates 2.0mm or microplates 1.6mm

- Plates placed on vertical buttress
  - Zygomaticomaxillary
  - Nasomaxillary
- Mandible fracture
  - Clinical Indication
    - Malocclusion
  - Panorex is the critical work-up study in mandible fractures
    - Evaluates entire mandible including condyles
  - Goal
    - Accurate dental occlusion
    - Establish pre-injury occlusion
      - Wear facets useful guide
      - Not infrequently patient is not Angle Class I pre-injury
  - Classify Fracture Based On
    - Anatomic location
      - Symphyseal- between canines
      - Body- between canine and 2nd molar
      - Angle- 2nd molar and ascending mandible
      - Ramus- between angle and sigmoid notch
      - Coronoid
      - Condylar
    - Direction of fracture and muscular function
      - Favorable
      - Unfavorable
    - Dental elements
    - Severity of damage
      - Displaced
      - Non-displaced
      - Comminuted
      - Non-comminuted
    - Relation between fracture site and external environment
      - Open
      - Closed
  - Management
    - Non-displaced fracture

- Maxillo-mandibular fixation (MMF) 4-6 weeks or…
- ORIF to allow early function
  - ORIF may be better in unreliable patients
- Favorable fractures
  - Non-comminuted and closed
  - MMF for 4-8 weeks
- Unfavorable fractures
  - Complex
  - Comminuted
    - Exposed bone: E.g. Gunshot
  - Treatment
  - ORIF with rigid or semi-rigid fixation
  - Compression zone at base of mandible
  - Tension zone at level of alveolus
  - High comminution- "bag of bones"
    - External fixation recommended
- Approach, Operative
  - Place in arch bars, i.e. MMF
  - Align fracture
  - Reduce and plate
  - Standard 2.0 mm mandibular plate with bicortical screws on compression zone or
  - Reconstruction plate 2.4mm bicortical screws on compression zone
  - PLUS
  - Tension band- arch bar or monocortical plate in tension zone, level of alveolus
  - Then compression, lower border plate
  - In comminuted fractures mandibular reconstruction plate useful
  - ALTERNATIVE
    - Lag screws
    - After fixation
    - MMF removed and alignment checked

- If occlusion is okay elastics may be used 2-4 wks postop
  - The Teeth
    - If teeth interfere with alignment
      - Have periodontal involvement
      - Then extract: Prefer to preserve the teeth if possible
      - Teeth help to stabilize fragments
  - Exposure/Incisions
    - Open wound?
      - Can be used if adequate exposure
    - Risdon
      - Extraoral
      - Safe conservative approach to any mandibular fracture
      - Acceptable post-op scar
      - Submental placement for parasymphyseal fracture
      - Submandibular for body, angle or ramus fractures
    - Preauricular/Temporal
      - Condylar fractures
    - Intraoral- Gingivolabial
      - Symphyseal/Body fractures
    - Percutaneous with trocars
- Condylar fractures
  - Head
  - Subcondylar: High, Low, Basal
  - Management controversial
  - Conservative therapy preferred if possible
    - WHY?
    - Manipulation of condyle may cause Temporomandibular joint ankylosis
  - Absolute Indications for ORIF
    - Dislocation into middle cranial fossa
    - Inability to attain premorbid occlusion via closed reduction
    - Lateral extracapsular dislocation of condyle
    - Bilateral condylar fracture
    - Foreign body in TMJ joint
  - Relative Indications

- Bilateral edentulous patient
- Patients with relative contraindication to MMF
  - Seizure Disorder
  - Psychiatric patients
  - Bilateral condylar fracture with other fractures
    - Approach
- Extraoral- preauricular incision
  - Beware facial nerve
- Endoscopic
  - In experienced hands, reduction and plating are possible

3. Select appropriate options in diagnosis and management

- Detail your operative plan based on fractures present
  - Your operative approach
  - Your sequence of repairs
- Timing of intervention based on clinical status
  - Repair can be early within 24 hours
  - Delayed 5-7 days to allow for decreased edema
- Intervention and timing in critically ill/head injured patients controversial
  - If medically stable and can tolerate general anesthesia:
  - Probably better to proceed with repair
  - If waiting longer than 3 weeks osteotomies will be needed
  - Minimal initial intervention
    - Repair lacerations
    - Put patient in maxillomandibular fixation
- Be familiar with size of plates in plating systems
  - Which size plate to use in different types of fractures
  - Indications for reconstruction plate in mandible fractures
- Resorbable vs. Titanium plates vs. Wires
- Post-op management plan
  - Especially in mandibular fractures

4. Understand risks and benefits of various approaches

- Why would you choose various incisions for exposure?
  - Based on precise diagnosis of fracture pattern
  - Fracture type and pattern should dictate surgical approach
  - What are the benefits and downsides of different approaches?
- Treatment plan based on:
  - Location of fracture
  - Direction of fracture line
  - Dislocation of fragments
  - Comminution
  - Bone gaps
  - Dental elements
- ORIF is considered the standard of care for all facial fractures
  - Miniplates- titanium
- Pre-op ophthalmology exam
- Choice of plating systems
  - Adults- generally titanium
  - Peds- resorbable plates and screws okay
- Complication rate
  - Generally related to complexity of fracture pattern
  - Difficulty of reduction
- Fracture specific complication patterns

5. Address complications and unexpected problems adequately

- Frontal sinus fractures
  - Meningitis
  - Osteomyelitis
  - Mucopyocele
- NOE fractures
  - Telecanthus
    - In treated or missed fractures
- Wound infection
- Hardware exposure
- Visual disturbances
  - Diplopia
  - Ocular injury
- Ectropion - lid retraction
  - Less common in transconjunctival approach

- Enophthalmos- frequent checks post-op to check for potential evolving enophthalmos
- Malocclusion
- Malunion or nonunion
  - More common in mandibular fractures
  - Accurate reduction and rigid fixation decreases the risk

6. Demonstrate ability to structure alternative plan

- Back-up plan if initial reconstruction fails
- Alternative methods of fracture fixation (e.g. indications for lag screws, Champy plate)
- How do you manage non-compliant patients?
- What will you do in severely head injured patients?
- What if fractures heal prior to early fracture management?
- ADDITIONAL THINGS TO THINK ABOUT IN FACIAL FRACTURES
-
- MANDIBLE
  - Muscle Function
  - Anterior Mandible
    - Floor of mouth
    - Base of tongue
    - Inserts on chin
  - Fixation points of the muscles of mastication
    - Mandibular Angle: Masseter
    - Coronoid process: Medial pterygoid
    - Condyle: Lateral pterygoid, Temporalis
  - Direction of function and muscle function
    - Is the fracture site under compression? i.e. favorable
    - Is the fracture displaced by the muscles? i.e. unfavorable
    - This predicts success of treatment by MMF only
    - Favorable fractures may be successfully treated with MMF
    - All unfavorable fractures require rigid fixation
- PEDIATRIC CONSIDERATIONS
  - Increased incidence of associated fractures

- Avoid metal fixation if possible
- WHY?
  - Transcranial migration
  - Infrequent clinical consequences
  - Growth disturbances, growth restriction
- Mandible fractures
  - Goal: Restore pre-injury occlusion with minimal growth disturbance
  - Treatment
  - MMF
    - Via creative means
    - Minimal space between teeth, small teeth hard to seat wires for arch bars makes MMF difficult
    - Splinting may be needed
  - Piriform suspension wires
  - Circumandibular wires
  - MMF prior to ORIF to avoid injury to tooth buds
  - Effect on facial growth uncertain
  - Potential for restricted or inhibited facial growth
  - Minor malocclusion well tolerated
    - Definitive treatment can be done later
    - Orthodontics vs. orthognathics surgery in teen years
  - Favorable, non-displaced mandible fracture in pediatric patient
    - Treatment: Soft diet, good oral hygiene
- Condylar head fracture
  - Treatment: Therapeutic PT
- Orbital Fractures
  - If no enophthalmos or entrapment
  - Treat vertical orbital dystopia
  - Treat persistent diplopia
  - Can consider non-operative management
- Maxillary and midface fractures
  - Rare
  - Conservative treatment if minimally displaced

- - Correct occlusion later
- Nasal fractures
  - No clear guidelines
  - Conservative approach
  - Reduce and stabilize if necessary
- ZMC
  - Conservative treatment
- Many texts recommend conservative treatment for pediatric fractures, they can be treated by ORIF if significant displacement present. Craniofacial trained surgeons tend to be more aggressive. Surgery seems to be tolerated well despite classic teachings of conservative management.

Section Six
Facial Paralysis

Chapter Twenty-Nine

Facial Paralysis Overview

29
Facial Paralysis Overview

1. Identify General Problem

   - Describe photo
   - Give working diagnosis
   - Key problems
   - Evaluate patient
   - Diagnosis/Planning
   - Classify and specify deficits
     - Forehead/Brow, Eyelids, Nose, Mouth/Smile
   - Which nerves are involved?
   - Age of patient important
   - Time of injury or period of time with loss of function
   - Etiology of paralysis
     - Idiopathic, Tumor, Trauma, Infection, Congenital
   - Previous surgery
   - Bell's reflex intact?
   - Detail your exam and what your are looking for
   - Medical status
     - HTN, DM, CAD, Anticoagulants
   - Pertinent positives and negatives in H&P
     - Drooling, Eye irritation, Poor smile, Breathing problems
   - What bothers the patient?
   - Need for additional work-up or consultants?
     - Imaging studies, Nerve studies, Ophthalmology, Neurology

2. Consider reasonable goals in diagnosis and management

   - Management, Surgical indications
   - Operative procedures and anesthesia
   - Specify clinical concerns based on area of paralysis
     - Brow ptosis, Eyelid closure
     - Lower lid ptosis- obstruction, irritation, corneal abrasion
     - Nasal obstruction, Breathing issues
     - Mouth- drooling, smile

- Consider surgical options, timing, staging, priorities
- Planning and intervention based on:
    - Etiology of paralysis
    - Length of time paralysis present (motor end plates)
    - Age of patient
    - Functional deficit

3. Select appropriate options in diagnosis and management

    - Give your surgical plan and why?
    - Timing and goals of surgery
    - Steps of operation
    - Details of graft, flap harvest, gold weight selection, etc.
    - Anatomic factors of surgery
    - Post-op management (biofeedback)
    - How is procedure performed?
    - Key steps of surgery
    - Markings and relevant anatomy

4. Understand risks and benefits of various approaches

    - Discuss risks, benefits of various static and dynamic procedures
    - How you determine which intervention?
        - Etiology of paralysis
        - Time of injury
        - Patient age
        - Patient preferences

5. Address complications and unexpected problems adequately

    - Be prepared to manage complications and explain causes
        - Gold weight erosion
        - Inadequate excursion
        - Failing free flap

6. Demonstrate ability to structure alternative plan

    - Lifeboat or back-up plan if initial therapy fails
    - Patient compliance

Chapter Thirty

Facial Paralysis

30
Facial Paralysis

1. Identify General Problem/Diagnosis/Planning
   (Describe photo, working diagnosis, key problems, evaluate patient)

    - Give detailed description of findings in photo
    - Give your working diagnosis
        o Most likely etiology of facial paralysis
        o Your best guess based on presented clinical scenario
    - Note key problems:
        o Dry eye, risk of corneal keratopathy
        o Nasal breathing
        o Drooling, ability to eat, smile
        o Aesthetic problems
        o Synkinesis
        o Detail affected structures and facial appearance
    - History
    - Note length of time of paralysis
    - Determine etiology
        o Idiopathic (Bell's Palsy)
        o Congenital causes
            - Moebius
            - Hemifacial microsomia
            - Goldenhar syndrome
            - Birth injury
        o Traumatic injury
        o Iatrogenic
        o Neoplastic
        o Horner's syndrome
        o Primary or secondary acoustic neuroma
        o Parotid tumor
        o Infections
        o Metabolic
        o Hyperthyroidism
    Note, it is important to know:
        o How and when paralysis occurred
        o Presentation pattern
            - Considered chronic if onset or time of paralysis > 1 year

- Treatment of chronic facial nerve paralysis is surgical
  - Age of patient
    - Influences surgical options if surgery is indicated
    - Age <40 better response to nerve repairs and facial reanimation by free flap
  - Duration of deficit
    - Impacts surgical options
  - History of previous surgery?
    - May impact surgical options
    - Iatrogenic etiology of paralysis?
  - Ocular symptoms
    - Dry eyes
  - Oral compensation
    - Difficulty eating
    - Drooling present
  - Facial distortion with smile
    - Significant concern
  - Breathing difficulty
- PE
- Check for intact Bell's phenomenon, why?
  - Protective for eye during sleep
  - If positive, need for intervention less urgent
- Focus on major branches of facial nerve:
  - Raise brow- temporal branch
  - Close eyes tightly- zygomatic branches to orbicularis
  - Smile symmetry- zygomatic and buccal branches to zygomaticus major muscle, buccal branches to buccinator contributes to smile
  - Tooth show with smile- marginal mandibular branch
    - Depressor angularis muscle
  - Tense neck muscles- cervical branches
  - Check tongue movement
    - Hypoglossal nerve XII may be needed for reanimation surgery
- Check sites of preexisting scars
- Are donor sites available if needed?
  - Primary source for nerve grafts: Sural nerve
- Look for synkinesis
- ***Review House-Brackmann Classification of facial function**

- Work-up
  - Level of motivation of the patient
    - Intense rehab needed postop (eg. Biofeedback training)
    - Rehabilitation after reanimation requires motivated patient
  - Electromyogram (EMG)
    - Polyphasic motor unit potentials (MUP)- expression of regeneration
    - Fibrillations- sign of poor regenertion
      - Intervention based on timing of injury
      - May benefit from neurorrhaphy
    - Silence- sign of long term denervation
      - Requires reconstruction
  - Minimal and maximal stimulation tests (MST)
  - Electroneuronography (ENog)
  - Nerve conduction velocity (NCV)
    - Determine extent of paralysis
    - Prospect for recovery
    - Assists in surgical planning prior to muscle atrophy
  - If history of malignancy
    - Use preop imaging studies to rule out residual or recurrent tumor prior to proceeding with surgery
  - Preop Consultation
    - PT/OT for biofeedback to retrain nerves
    - ENT to help determine timing of tx
  - Ophthalmology
    - Globe exam and treat corneal exposure
- Additional facts
  - Spontaneous release of acetylcholine gives resting tone to muscle after denervation of muscle after 2-3 weeks
  - Extrajunctional sensitivity to acetylcholine develops fibrillations on EMG
  - Fibrillations are pathognomonic for denervation
  - Absence of fibrillations does not rule out viability
  - Facial muscles are capable of renervation several months after injury, unlike other skeletal muscle

2. Consider reasonable goals in diagnosis and management *(Management and treatment, surgical indications, operative procedures and anesthesia)*

- Dry eyes: Initial treatment:
    o Liberal lubrication with saline drops
    o Eye taping during sleep
    o In severe cases tarsorrhaphy may be needed to avoid corneal or scleral injury or assist in healing
- Timing of intervention
    o May intervene when it is determined that there is no potential for improvement in function
    o Timing >9-12 months all comers even idiopathic cases (Bell's palsy) surgical intervention warranted
    o Must be free of malignancy
- Goals of treatment
    o #1 protect cornea from exposure
    o #2 restore oral competence
    o #3 normal resting balance; create dynamic symmetrical smile (challenging)
- Surgical options
    o Immediate nerve repair +/- nerve graft
        - Direct repair if no tension
        - Grouped fascicular technique first choice
        - Tension increases scar formation which hinders axonal regeneration
    o Delayed repair
        - Use interpositional nerve grafts to avoid tension
    o Graft donors
        - Sural nerve
        - Great auricular nerve
        - Medial cutaneous antebrachial nerve
        - Ansa hypoglossi (available during exposure for parotidectomy)
    o Regrowth of nerve 1mm/day
        - Track with Tinel sign
    o Gold weight (small 1-1.2gm)
        - Assists in closure of affected upper lid
        - Place pretarsal via lid crease under local with sedation
        - Choose weight pre-op

- Weighs lid down by gravity, does not affect eye opening
  - Oculomotor n. (CNIII) innervates levator muscle
- Does not protect cornea when patient is supine (sleeping)
  - Eye must be taped during sleep
- Cross-face nerve grafting
  - Donor facial nerve on unparalyzed side
  - Cannot do if contralateral facial nerve abnormal
  - Identify usable branches by intra-op electrical stimulation
  - Expose via rhytidectomy incision
  - Duplicate branches supplying zygomaticus major are used
  - 1st stage
    - Usable branch transected and repaired to proximal end on normal side
    - Graft tunneled to paralyzed side
  - 2nd stage
    - Distal end repaired to stumps of paralyzed muscle in 6-9 months
      - Up to 3 grafts can be used
    - Muscles to reinnervate
      - Zygomaticus major
      - Orbicularis oculi
      - Depressor labii muscle
- Hypoglossal-Facial nerve transfer
  - After surgery improvement in tone over 4-6 months
  - Technique: partial transfer end to side coaptation
  - Decreases tongue morbidity
  - Can combine with cross-face nerve graft as a babysitter procedure
    - Babysitter procedure prevents atrophy of muscle while awaiting innervation of cross facial nerve graft

- - - Dr. Zucker no longer uses this babysitter procedure
  - Static Procedures
    - Brow Lift
      - Endoscopic
      - Coronal
      - Open
    - Eyelid Surgery
      - Upper lid blepharoplasty
      - Lower lid surgery
        - Wedge resection of lid
        - Tarsal Strip to tighten lid
        - Lateral canthopexy to tighten lid
    - Facial slings
      - Support and reposition midface and lower lip
      - Does not provide smile but controls drooping, improves symmetry
      - Options
        - Fascia lata
        - Temporalis fascia
        - Gortex
    - Partial cervicofacial rhytidectomy
      - Can improve facial symmetry
  - Lower Lip Reconstruction
    - Wedge resection
    - Digastric transposition
  - Dynamic Muscle Transfer
    - Temporalis muscle
    - Masseter muscle
    - Digastric muscle can reproduce action of the depressor anguli muscle
    - Indicated for reanimation smile primarily
      - Improve symmetry
      - Provide some function
  - Temporalis
    - Central 1/3 reflected inferiorly
    - With or without fascial graft or periosteal strip to provide length
    - Inset at modiolus (i.e. corners of upper and lower lips)
    - Overcorrect at time of surgery

- Masseter muscle transfer
  - Pulls in a more lateral vector
- Botox of opposite depressor anguli muscle can be done if only symmetry is needed
- Free Muscle Transfer
  - Indicated in cases of long periods of denervation of mimetic muscle
  - Congenital cases (Moebius, severe hemifacial microsomia)
  - Generally if muscle not innervated for greater than 18 months clear indication. Can be done if muscles are out for 9 months or more
  - Single stage or two-stage procedure
  - Frequently done as cross-face nerve graft
- Neurotization Options
  - Proximal stump of facial nerve if available
  - Combine with 1st stage cross-face nerve graft when proximal stump not available
  - Hypoglossal or masseteric nerve as babysitter
  - Masseter motor nerve (Moebius or other case when bilateral facial nerve not available)
- Muscle choices
  - Gracilis most popular choice
    - Obturator nerve, medial circumflex vessels
    - Less bulky than other muscle options
    - Can be split for multiple sites of insertion
  - Serratus anterior- has 2-3 slips with long thoracic nerve
    - Can be place in multiple vectors
  - Latissimus dorsi- thoracodorsal nerve and vessels
    - Bulky muscle
  - Pectoralis minor
    - Difficult to harvest
- Single stage

- - - Simultaneous cross-face nerve graft and free muscle transfer
    - Two stages
      - Cross-face nerve graft followed by free muscle transfer
  - Be familiar with a technique of your choice to correct various problems presented by facial paralysis.
  - Include static and dynamic techniques
  - Know relevant anatomy

3. Select appropriate options in diagnosis and management

   - Many options, tailor to treat patient
     - Based on:
       - Age
       - Medical condition
       - Etiology of paralysis
       - Treatment objectives
       - Experience and technical expertise of operating surgeon
   - Deficit > 1year
     - Cannot reanimate with nerve graft or primary repair
       - Why? End plates deactivated by the time nerve regeneration will occur
     - Renervation not reliable if nerve regeneration will be >18 months
     - Will need free muscle transfer or static procedures
   - Immediate nerve repair +/- nerve graft
     - If injury discovered at the time of injury, iatrogenic cases
     - Immediate reconstruction at time of tumor resection
   - Nerve graft indicated for proximal facial nerve transection
     - 2 cable grafts for upper and lower axonal groups
   - Cross-face nerve grafting
     - Indicated when ipsilateral facial nerve stump is not available
     - Eg. Post acoustic neuroma resection
     - Distal stumps must be available and can be renervated
   - Hypoglossal-facial nerve transfer
     - Indicated if proximal central stump is unavailable for transfer

- No proximal stump available but extracranial facial nerve is intact and facial muscle still available for renervation
- Contraindicated in contralateral hypoglossal nerve or vagus deficit
- Weaker muscle function but potentially functional
- Static Procedures
    - Generally indicated for older patients age >50
    - Frequently require bilateral correction
    - Can be used as adjunctive or touch-up procedure after dynamic reconstruction
- Static slings
    - Always overcorrect
    - Some relapse will occur
- Dynamic muscle transfer
    - Improves symmetry and function of smile
- Free muscle transfer
    - Primary indication young patients
    - Denervated facial muscles > 9-12 months
    - Improvement common, improved symmetry with animation and at rest
    - Spontaneous smile unlikely
    - Improvement in 94% of patients
    - Failure rare
- Postop management in nerve repair and facial reanimation
    - PT/OT and biofeedback in optimizing reanimation
    - Significant training in biofeedback needed to train patient to use transferred muscle
    - PT/OT teaches:
        - How to innervate and use the muscle
        - How to increase muscle strength

4. Understand risks and benefits of various approaches

- General considerations that dictate risks and benefits:
    - Age of patient
    - Etiology of paralysis
    - Timing of paralysis
    - Medical status of patient (can tolerate multiple procedures)
    - Patient goals

- Relevant issues reviewed in sections 2 and 3.
- Why would you do one intervention plan over another?
- Downsides and upsides of any intervention?

5. Address complications and unexpected problems adequately

- Most frequent complications of nerve rehabilitation:
    - Synkinesis
    - Facial Spasm
    - Mass Movement
- Hypoglossal nerve post-op complications
    - Synkinesis- involving grinning with tongue movement
    - Articulation errors of speech
    - Ophthalmologic problems (dryness, irritation)
    - Absence of spontaneous facial movement
- Temporalis muscle transfer
    - Post-op problems
        - Hollowing in temporal region- can correct with implant
        - Abnormal bulk over zygomatic arch
        - Dyskinesia- activated while eating
- Free muscle transfer
    - Post-op problems
        - Weak smile
        - Poor symmetry
        - Hematoma
        - Seroma
        - Failed free flap
- Most frequent complications
    - Inadequate axonal regeneration and distal muscle atrophy
    - Result: inadequate muscle pull, weak smile
    - Poor axonal regeneration
- Failure of renervation
    - Secondary to poor repair or tension across nerve repair
    - Synkinesis- mass movement of muscle
        - Occurs frequently
        - Secondary to cross innervations
        - More proximal injuries greater synkinesis
    - Overly active pull of transferred muscle can occur

- Secondary to fibrosis and contracture
- Options for management:
  - Synkinesis/Hyperkinesis
    - Botulinum toxin therapy
      - Repeat every 3 months
      - 5-10 Units for eyebrow spasm
      - 10-20 Units for injections in area of zygomaticus major muscle
      - Adjust dose according to response
    - Static procedure if dynamic ones fail
    - Revision of nerve repairs, evaluate for neuroma formation
    - PT/OT
- What will you do for complications including common surgical complications such as hematoma, infection, wound dehiscence, donor site problems?

6. Demonstrate ability to structure alternative plan

- Must be able to manage patients by facial paralysis algorithm taking into account age, etiology of facial paralysis and length of time of paralysis.
- Have back up options for failures
- Management of free flap postop
- Examiners may change the scenario: age of patient, timing of paralysis, etiology and what nerves are available for management in order to test your complete understanding of facial paralysis management. Have a set algorithm.

Section Seven
Cosmetic Face

Chapter Thirty-One

Cosmetic Face Overview

———

31
Cosmetic Face Overview

1. Identify General Problem

   - Describe photo
   - Give working diagnosis
   - Key problems
   - Evaluate patient
   - Note pertinent positives and negatives in history
   - Previous surgery
   - Note pre-op visual problems
     - Dry eye
   - Check for ptosis
   - Note hairline
   - Classify areas to be addressed
   - Reiterate healthy patient, non-smoker, no DM, CAD or HTN
   - Relevant medications especially anticoagulants
   - Have an algorithm for facial analysis
   - Need for additional work-up for operative planning?
   - Be sure patient has "pure" motives for surgery
   - What are the patient's expectations?

2. Consider reasonable goals in diagnosis and management

   - Management and treatment
   - Surgical indications
   - Operative procedures and anesthesia
   - Surgical plan
   - All options to address areas for rejuvenation including non-surgical
   - Note potential problems, risks
   - Anticipated outcome and patient satisfaction
   - Note what does the patient want
   - Hypertension control pre and postop
   - Periop pain control and nausea management?
   - Preventative measures and preparation for laser resurfacing?
     - Acyclovir
     - Topical skin therapy

3. Select appropriate options in diagnosis and management

    - What option would you choose and why?
    - What will you do to prevent complications especially in lower lid bleph?
    - How do you do cervicoplasty, blephs, rhytidectomy, brow lifts etc.?
    - Key steps of surgery
    - Markings and relevant anatomy
    - Your post-op management

4. Understand risks and benefits of various approaches

    - Note benefits and risks of various approaches
    - Manage patient desires and expectations
    - Anticipate your expected outcome.

5. Address complications and unexpected problems adequately

    - Be prepared to manage all potential complications
        o Note your timing for any intervention
        o Will you bill the patient?
        o Your billing policy for complications or dissatisfaction with outcomes?
    - How do you manage?
        o Hematoma
        o Skin slough
        o Facial nerve injury
        o Ectropion
        o Extra-ocular muscle injury
        o Inadequate correction
        o Great auricular nerve injury
        o A-frame deformity- excess fat removal from upper lid
        o Retrobulbar hematoma
        o Other

6. Demonstrate ability to structure alternative plan

    - What if patient doesn't agree with your proposal?
    - Patient unsatisfied requests money back
    - Do you bill for early revisions?

Chapter Thirty-Two

Non-operative Facial Rejuvenation

32
Non-operative Facial Rejuvenation

1. What if the patient requests non-surgical rejuvenation?

   - You must have an understanding of the role of:
     - Chemical peels
     - Injectables
     - Fillers
     - Lasers

   - Chemical peel
     - A form of skin care
     - Controlled removal of:
       - Stratum corneum
       - Epidermis
       - Superficial dermis
     - Improves skin texture and pigmentation
     - Superficial peels
       - Mild exfoliation of stratum corneum
     - Medium depth
       - Affects stratum corneum, epidermis, superficial dermis
       - Trichloroacetic acid
       - Improves facial dyspigmentation
     - Deep peel
       - Affects skin to level of deep dermis
       - Phenol improves superficial facial rhytids, but, produces skin lightening
     - Contraindicated in systemic tretinoin treatment in previous 6 months or as a treatment for keloids
     - Estrogen replacement predisposes to hyperpigmentation
       - Discontinue 3-6 months prior to procedure
     - Indications fair complexion patients
       - Dyspigmentation- best indication
       - Poor skin texture
     - Relative contraindications

- Dark skin (Fitzpatrick type IV and higher)
  - Risk of hypopigmentation
- Retinoids within past year
  - Reduces activity of sebaceous glands
  - Increases susceptibility to hypertrophic scarring
- Radiated skin
  - Contraindications
    - Hypersensitivity to skin peels
    - Keloid formation within 6 months after cessation of oral retinoids
    - Evidence of poor healing

- Fillers
  - Primary indication
    - Nasolabial folds
    - Marionette lines
    - Glabellar folds
  - Indications
    - Nasolabial fold prominence (Lemperle Scale)
    - Marionette lines and secondary smile lines
    - Perioral lines
    - Paramental soft tissue atrophy
    - Tear trough atrophy
    - Temporal and buccal fat loss
    - Generalized cheek atrophy
    - Crow's feet
    - Glabellar lines
    - Combination therapy with laser, chemical peel or facelift
  - Contraindications
    - Positive skin allergy test
    - Known sensitivity to planned injectable
    - Severe skin disease
    - Active acne
    - History of connective tissue disease
    - Recent use of NSAID's or anticoagulants
    - Previous lumps/nodules in area of injection
    - Dense scar tissue
  - Hyaluronic acid- glycosaminoglycan

- Restylane, Perlane, Juvederm, Captique, Hyalform
  - History of cold sores in lips
    - Use herpes prophylaxis; day of injection
    - Injection can reactivate latent infection
  - Injection technique
    - Threading
    - Fanning
    - Serial droplet
    - Crosshatch
  - Complications
    - Pain
    - Erythema
    - Swelling
    - Bruising
    - Inflammation
    - Asymmetry
    - Hematoma
    - Allergy
    - Early resorption
    - Nodularity and purulence
  - Post op care
    - Monitor in office 15 min post injection
      - Observe for hematoma
      - Cold compress
    - Check for nodularity, palpability
    - No dressing required
    - Make-up may be applied
    - Refrain from vigorous activity 7 days (No scientific basis for this)
    - Re-eval in 2 weeks
    - Pre- and post-op photos
    - Long-term care minimal

- Botulinum Toxin A
  - Brow elevation
    - Depends on relative weakness of:
      - brow elevators vs. brow depressors
    - Lower frontalis greatest effect on brow rise
  - Dose based on muscle mass, not rhytid depth
  - Avoid antiplatelet meds, NSAID's prior to injection

- Threading technique more effective than common point technique
- Cooling skin prior to injection minimizes discomfort
- Over injection of mentalis- witch's chin deformity
- Most frequently performed cosmetic procedure
- Type A- causes presynaptic nerve blockade (acetylcholine receptors)
- Initial use blepharospasm and strabismus 1977
- First publication Alan Scott 1980
- Duration of Action
    - Response excellent first 3.5-4 months
    - 6-7 months for clinical effect to fade
    - Longer duration of action with repeated injection
- Reconstitution package 2.5ml non-preserved saline, can use 4ml
- FDA approval
    - Glabellar rhytids in patients under 65
    - All other use is off-label
- Indications
    - Glabellar rhytids
    - Complications from aesthetic procedures
        - Can treat incomplete corrugator or procerus resection post browlift
        - If excessive pull early postop early, treat by maintaining brow elevation
        - Disinsertion of mentalis after chin aug and skin dimpling
        - Overly elevated brows post browlift, can be dropped with aggressive frontalis injection
        - Prolonged spasm post breast aug, inject lower pec
        - Facial nerve injury after surgery or trauma- weaken unaffected side for symmetry
            - Especially marginal mandibular nerve injury post facelift inject contralateral depressor anguli oris
    - Hyperhydrosis

- Contraindications
  - Disorders of neuromuscular transmission
  - Aminoglycoside antibiotics (potentiates effects)
  - Pre-pregnancy, pregnancy, breast feeding (No evidence to suggest potential harm)
- Effect is not all or none, fine control is possible
- Dosing
  - Men require higher doses
  - Optimum dose varies patient-to-patient, muscle-to-muscle
  - No true standard doses
- Understanding functional anatomy of face is the key to good results
- Must analyze each face, discern which portions of which muscles dominate
- Anatomic Regions
- Glabella
  - Median dose 17.5 units women/20 units men
  - Use minimal volume and dose avoids eyelid ptosis
- Forehead
  - Median range 3.75-30 units
  - Most injections 5-7.5 units
  - Muscle targeted not the rhytids
  - Complications
    - Smooth artificial appearance
    - Brow, Lid ptosis
  - Observe normal animation
- Crow's Feet and Lower Eyelid
  - Weaken lateral and inferior orbicularis oculi m. to diminish crow's feet and lower lid rhytids
  - There are different patterns of crow's feet
  - Dose 3.75 to 5 units per side
  - Inject the most dynamic area
  - Upper lateral orbicularis oculi- brow depressor, lower lateral portion important cheek elevator.
  - Complications
    - Deer in the headlights look
    - Cheek ptosis

- Frank ectropion or lower lid retraction
- Exaggerate and hasten fat 'bags"
- Lymphedema
  - Brow Elevation
    - Botox can easily and reliably elevate brows 6mm
    - By concentrating on areas that depress the brow allows brow to rise
    - Weakening the muscle that lifts it, muscle reacts to weakened muscle by increasing its pull
    - Individualize injection pattern
  - Neck
    - Improves horizontal 'necklace' rhytids
    - 15-30 units avg. 20 units
  - Nasolabial fold
    - Can affect medial nasolabial fold
    - Changes smile pattern
    - Levator labii superioris alaeque nasi muscle
  - Perioral rhytids, dimpled chin, downturned oral commissures

- Laser Facial Resurfacing and Dermabrasion
  - Fitzpatrick type IV and higher risk of hyperpigmentation, pre-treat with hydroquinone or other bleaching agent
  - Peri-orbital area corneal shield
  - Protect airway, avoid O2 (fire hazard)
  - No more than three passes
    - Deep damage at third pass
  - A few Fitzpatrick I or II may have delayed hypopigmentation resistant to treatment
  - ACCUTANE
    - Avoid laser resurfacing or dermabrasion within 6 months of use, preferably a year
  - Ideal areas for laser resurfacing
    - Periorbital
    - Perioral
    - Not improved by facelift procedures
  - Can repeat treatment after 3-6 months, result additive

- Pretreat with tretinoin (speeds re-epithelialization) and skin bleaching Fitzpatrick IV or higher
- Prophylactic antibiotics and antivirals
- Complications
    - Hyperpigmentation: Treat with tretinoin, bleaching agents
    - Delayed hypopigmentation
    - Inclusion cysts or milia
    - Infection
- Other applications
    - Laser blepharoplasty
- Options
    - CO2 laser
        - Prolonged healing time
    - Erbium
    - Intense pulsed light
    - Fractionated lasers

Chapter Thirty-Three

Facial Rejuvenation
(Facelift/Necklift/Brow Lift/Blepharoplasty/Nonsurgical)

33
Facial Rejuvenation
Facelift, Necklift, Brow Lift, Blepharoplasty, Nonsurgical

1. Identify General Problem Diagnosis/Planning
   (Describe photo, give working diagnosis, key problems, evaluates patient)

   - Describe photo in detail
   - Break up face into thirds or fifths with attention to:
     - Forehead
     - Eyebrows, eyelids, ptosis (brow and upper lids)
     - Periorbital skin and soft tissue
     - Nasolabial creases
     - Jowls
     - Neck
   - History
   - Determine motivation for surgery
     - Avoid patients with:
       - Spur of the moment decisions
       - Recent displeasing life event
       - Ask for:
         - Patient specific complaints
         - Perception of existing problems
     - (Will likely be clinical findings that you see on photo)
   - Assess emotional stability
   - Medical suitability (ASA II or less)
     - DM
     - Steroids
     - HTN
     - CAD
     - Smoking
       - Increased risk of skin slough
       - Avoid nicotine patch
     - Anticoagulant's including NSAID use
     - Easy bleeding or bruising
     - History of keloids, avoid surgery

- o   Herbal meds: some are anticoagulants
- Special medical conditions
    - o   Cutis laxa- rhytidectomy beneficial
    - o   Ehlers Danlos- rhytidectomy contraindicated
- Previous surgery
    - o   Cosmetic procedures
    - o   Existing facial scars
- Physical Exam
- Note skin quality
    - o   If preexisting sun damage
        - Consider preop skin regimen
            - Laser, Chemical Peel
    - o   Periorbital rhytids
        - Consider simultaneous skin resurfacing
    - o   Condition of pretragal skin
        - Decide pretragal vs. post tragal incision
- Skin Type Fitzpatrick Classification
    - o   Important in use of skin peels or laser
    - o   Fitzpatrick I or II good response, V or VI poor candidates
- Associated skin lesions/skin cancer address prior to elective cosmetic procedures
    - o   Biopsy any suspicious lesions
- Preexisting scars
- Consider hairline and sideburns
    - o   Avoid abnormal elevation of these
- Earlobe position (attached or hanging)
    - o   Must recreate at closure
- Facial shape
    - o   Round vs. angled
    - o   Poorer results in round faces, note pre-op
- Upper face (hairline to glabella)
    - o   Address position of brow
    - o   Position of hairline (forehead and temples)
    - o   Need for eyelid procedures?
        - Resurfacing only vs. bleph with skin +/- fat excision
    - o   Ptosis correction?
    - o   Glabellar region rhytids
        - Neuromuscular blockade (botulinum tox. A)
        - Deep furrows: Fillers (fat vs. other)

- o Relax forehead with deep wrinkles prior to choosing procedure
  - Smile
  - Close eyes and slowly open
- o Forehead profile contour
  - Note bossing or other irregularities
- Midface (Glabella to subnasal)
  - o Brow position
  - o Eyelids
  - o Eyebrows
    - Upper border of eyebrows should be at least 2.5cm above mid pupil on straight gaze
    - Medial end caudal to lateral extreme
    - Highest portion of arch at junction of the lateral 1/3 with medial 2/3
      - Lateral limit of limbus in straight gaze
  - o Eyebrow ptosis causes crowding in orbital region
  - o Normal intercanthal distance (medial canthi) 31-33mm
  - o Check for eyelid ptosis
    - Normal upper lid position 1mm below limbus
  - o Supratarsal fold
    - Normally 3-4 mm above lid margin
    - May be absent in Asian eyelids
    - Levator dehiscence
      - Tarsal show is increased with a more cephalad supratarsal crease
      - Check levator function to determine procedure
  - o Presence of Bell's Phenomenon
    - Ask pt hold eyes shut tight, attempt to open, does globe
    - Roll cephalad?
      - Yes-Positive Bell's
        - o Protection post op if complication occurs
      - No-Negative Bell's
        - o Increased risk of dry eye complication from corneal exposure

- Pleasing lower lid
  - Located at caudal limit of limbus or slightly overlaps
  - Excess scleral show
    - Sign of lower lid laxity
  - If scleral show or negative vector is present
    - Conservative bleph surgery
    - Use adjunctive canthoplasty or canthopexy
    - Give extra lid support
- Lid snap
- Ideal mobility of lateral canthus less than 7-8 mm
- Eyelid edema
  - Maybe a symptom of thyroid dysfunction
- Cheek descent?
  - Descent of malar cheek pad requires midface lift
- Nasolabial folds
  - Rhytidectomy may worsen fold
  - Address with fillers or direct excision
- Depression in nasojugal area or cephalad to infraorbital rim may necessitate soft tissue repositioning or fat grafting
- Nasal skin
  - Thick or very thin poor rhinoplasty candidate
- Nasal show
  - On frontal view should have some nostril show
    - Inadequate show
      - Long nose, or caudally positioned ala
    - Excess show
      - Short nose or retracted alar rims
  - Exaggerated with smile
- Alar base distance
  - Should be slightly wider than intercanthal distance
- Lower face (Subnasal to chin)
  - Hypoplastic chin
    - Chin augmentation vs. Sliding genioplasty

- Can be combined with rhytidectomy to improve facial balance
  - Lip incompetence
    - Contraindication to chin augmentation
  - Consider tooth alignment and need for orthodontic procedures
  - Excess submental fat
    - Direct excision and/or liposuction
    - Goal improve obtuse mandibular-cervical angle
  - Consider subplatysmal fat
  - Jowls
  - Platysmal bands
    - Prominent, divergent bands may need direct reapproximation
    - Via submental incision (actual incision, distal to crease to prevent witch's chin deformity)
  - Prominent submental salivary glands
    - Point out preop may be prominent postop
  - Pleasing neck 100-degree angle between chin/neck
  - Beware obtuse neck angle
    - Excess skin
    - Excess supra-platysma fat
    - Excess sub-platysma fat
    - Prominent neckbands
- Hypertrophic anterior belly digastric muscles or submandibular gland
    - Ptotic submandibular gland
- Overhead view
- Internal nasal exam
- Preop Work-up
  - Minimal in healthy patients
  - Labs based on medical history
  - CXR/EKG may need for pts >50 in some facilities
  - Review current standards
  - Age over 50
  - Full medical checkup especially exercise tolerance
  - Ophthalmologic exam within one year if eyelid surgery contemplated
- Photos: AP, Lateral, Oblique
- Lateral cephalogram if chin augmentation is planned

- Consults
    - Cardiology clearance may be needed
    - Primary medical physician should review med hx, current meds and exercise tolerance
- Be sure surgeon and patient expectations are the same!
- Comprehensive Health form
- Informed Consent
    - Risks of complications
    - Surgical and non-surgical options
    - Preferred technique vs. patient preference
    - More than one meeting prior to surgery
- R/O Body Dysmorphic Disorder-
    - Sees deformity that does not exist or sees a great deal more than is present
    - Preoccupation with perceived defects
    - Complaints may be specific or vague
- Risk factors for DRY EYES:
    - Pre-existing lower lid laxity
    - Loss of lower lid tone
    - Negative vector (malar soft tissue prominence behind cornea)
    - Borderline tear production
    - Symptoms of dry eyes
    - Conservative surgery: canthopexy or canthoplasty

2. Consider reasonable goals in diagnosis and management *(Management and treatment, surgical indications, operative procedures and anesthesia)*

- Preop skin regimen
    - Retinoids, Bleaching creams (hydroquinone)
- Improved skin appearance adds to overall result of surgery
- Isolated wrinkling around eyes not addressed by rhytidectomy
- Periop
    - Meds to alleviate anxiety or minimize postop complications
    - Sedatives night before and morning of surgery
    - Antiemetic (Zofran 4mg IV)
- Give patient's own antihypertensives
- Consider periop clonidine (0.1 to 0.3mg 1 hour preop) to decrease risk of hematoma

- Consider periop steroids decrease swelling, augments the effects of other meds
- Modern rhytidectomy
- Primary goal
    - Facial shape modification via repositioning facial fat key to excellent result. Not a simple stretching and pulling of the skin.
- Youthful face
    - Round, full with soft curves and full midface and malar region.
- Options
- Facelifts
    - Skin only: Oldest and simplest
    - Address descent of deeper structures by redraping skin and repositioning composite flap of cheek fat and SMAS layer
        - SMAS plication
            - Sutures placed anterior to retaining ligaments of cheek and malar complex
        - SMAS elevation
            - Develop SMAS and platysma to reshape
            - Extended SMAS, high SMAS, auto cheek augmentation
        - SMASectomy
            - Excision of a strip of SMAS
    - Deep plane facelift
        - Elevates forehead, eyelids and SMAS in continuity
    - Subperiosteal facelift
- Consider Adjuvant procedures
    - Browlift, Blepharoplasty, Rhinoplasty, Chin augmentation
- Other
    - Laser resurfacing
    - Chemical Peel
    - Fat Injections
    - Botox injection
- Can be body procedures as well:
    - Mastopexy
    - Abdominoplasty

- Single stage vs. multiple stages

3. Select appropriate options in diagnosis and management

    - See options under each procedure/facial region above.
    - Select from the available options and create your own operative plan based on the presented clinical photo.
    - Main considerations
    - Candidate for surgery based on medical history and other factors?
    - Preoperative or nonoperative options to optimize surgical outcome
    - Safety measures
    - Postoperative concerns
    - Anticipated potential complications
    - What is your operative approach and technique?
        - Your cervicoplasty, rhytidectomy
    - What are the anatomic considerations?

4. Understand risks and benefits of various approaches

    - See types of procedures in 2.
    - Note advantages, disadvantages of different types of facelifts
    - What are the general complications of cosmetic face surgery?
    - How long do you anticipate results will be maintained?

5. Address complications and unexpected problems adequately

    - Discuss all possible common complications preop.
    - Hematoma
        - Primarily related to HTN post and periop
        - Pain sign of hematoma, generally pain is minimal
        - Early recognition and drainage key to prevent skin necrosis
        - Drains do NOT prevent hematoma
        - Small (2-20ml) not apparent until edema subsides
            - Occurs in 10-15%
            - Liquefies at 7-10 days can aspirate or drain manually

- Can result in skin firmness, irregularity, discoloration that persists several weeks to months
- Discoloration- from hemosiderin deposits
                - Expanding hematoma
                    - Occurs in 1-8%
                    - Twice as common in males
                    - Most frequently in first 6-8 hours postop
                    - Surgical emergency
                    - Causes
                        - Inadequate preop eval
                        - Inadequate hemostasis/management of BP, nausea, pain
                    - Preop Clonidine (0.1 to 0.3mg) lasts 10 hours
                    - Intra op labetalol or vasotec
                    - Treatment (Tx):
                        - Remove dressings and evaluate for bluish discoloration and hardness
                        - Bedside removal of sutures prior to return to OR
                        - In OR remove all clots, cauterize for hemostasis
        - Postop Edema
            - Elevate head of bed
            - Postop steroids
        - Ecchymosis
        - Nerve Injury- most dreaded complication
            - Great auricular nerve
                - Most frequently injured
                - Sensory nerve loss, avoidable
                    - Sensation to lower 2/3 of ear, preauricular area, cheeks
                - Anatomy
                    - With head turned 45 degrees to opposite direction
                    - The nerve crosses the superficial surface of the sternocleidomastoid muscle; below its fascia 6.5cm below the caudal edge of the bony external auditory canal

- Just posterior to external jugular vein
- Deep to SMAS/Platysma level
  - Typically, some numbness first 2-6 weeks post op
  - Repair if injury recognized during surgery
        - Facial nerve Injury (Incidence 0.9% or higher)
          - Frontal branches
            - Anatomy
            - Emerges from beneath parotid on a line extending from 0.5cm below the tragus to 1.5cm above the lateral brow.
            - Passes deep to SMAS over zygomatic arch
            - Long lasting weakness >4 months
          - Buccal branch- most commonly injured
            - Expected return of function 3-4 months
          - Permanent injury rare
          - If transection detected during surgery immediate repair
          - If not wait for recovery, camouflaging procedures if full recovery does not occur
    - Hypertrophic scar- rare but does occur
        - Most frequently at preauricular incision
        - Cause
          - Flap compromise
          - Excess skin tension
        - Tx:
          - Small volume kenalog
          - Scar massage
          - Silicone sheets
          - Pressure garment therapy
    - Superficial Slough
        - Usually heals uneventfully
    - Full thickness slough
        - Some residual permanent scarring will be present
        - Most frequently postauricular and mastoid areas
          - Thinnest skin
          - Most distant circulation
        - Incidence of skin slough 1-3%

- Causes
  - Undiagnosed hematoma
  - Thin skin flaps
  - Excess tension at closure
  - Smoking (12X's risk)
- Tx:
  - Careful observation NOT surgery!
  - Will contract dramatically
  - Resulting scar usually much better than would be anticipated
  - Scar revision if necessary after complete healing
- Seroma
  - Aspirate
- Contour irregularities
  - Cause
    - Improper defatting of platysma
    - Must leave 5-7mm of fat on skin flaps
- Wound infection- Rare <1%
  - S. aureus most common organism
- Hyperpigmentation from hemosiderin deposits
- Apposition of ear/hairline issues
- Patient dissatisfaction
  - How do you manage a dissatisfied patient?

6. Demonstrate ability to structure alternative plan

- What if the patient requests non-surgical rejuvenation?
- You must have an understanding of the role of injectables, fillers, lasers and chemical peels.

Neck Rejuvenation

1. Identify General Problem, Diagnosis/Planning
   (Describe photo, give working diagnosis, key problems, evaluates patient)

   - PE
   - Candidates
   - Moderate to severe laxity of submental region
     - Not likely to improve after submental lipectomy
   - Key features
     - Platysmal banding
     - Pre and subplatysmal fat deposits
     - Skin laxity
     - Protruding anterior belly of digastric
     - Submandibular gland ptosis
   - Note loss of neck contour in initial exam
   - Evaluate cervicomandibular angle
   - Exam
   - Front view, Profile view
   - Chin and face held in repose and tilting down
   - Palpate the neck assess submandibular glands
   - Assess platysma
   - Ask patient to tighten neck
     - If tightens:
       - Dynamic bands respond to surgery or botox
     - If no tightening:
       - Skin folds will need skin tightening
   - Assess submandibular gland and anterior belly of digastric for hypertrophy/ptosis

2. Consider reasonable goals in diagnosis and management
   (Management and treatment, surgical indications, operative procedures and anesthesia)

   - Goals
   - Even, smooth platysmal layer
   - Interventions frequently adjuncts to rhytidectomy
   - Correct obtuse cervicomental angle
   - INDICATIONS
     - Young patient with obtuse cervicomental angle

- Neck as prominent part of facial aging
- Patients undergoing other aesthetic facial procedures which accentuate neck laxity
- Submandibular gland suspension
  - Glandular ptosis
- Submandibular gland resection
  - Glandular hyperplasia
- CONTRAINDICATIONS
  - Cardiopulmonary dysfunction
  - Bleeding disorders
  - Connective tissue disease
  - Wound healing problems
- SURGERY
  - IV sedation of general
  - Neck exposure 3.5cm submental incision posterior to submental crease
  - Lateral neck via traditional rhytidectomy post auricular exposure see Facelift section
- OPTIONS
- SMAS suspension and platysmal plication
  - In combo with rhytidectomy
    - Transpose vertical strip of SMAS to tighten platysma
    - Free anterior platysma through submental incision
    - Separated platysma brought together in midline
    - Subplatysma fat may be resected if necessary
    - Frequently combined with other procedures
  - SUBMANDIBULAR GLAND SUSPENSION AND RESECTION
    - Performed through submental incision
    - Dissection subplatysmal
    - Submandibular gland is marked preop
    - Suspension can be performed transorally
    - Formal excision can be performed

3. Select appropriate options in diagnosis and management

- Make decision on your surgical intervention based on presented scenario.

4. Understand risks and benefits of various approaches

    - Be aware of risks and benefits of various approaches. What is your anticipated outcome?

5. Address complications and unexpected problems adequately

    - Submandibular gland resection risks marginal mandibular branch injury, but, can be done safely indicated in some patients
    - Hematoma
    - Infection
    - Seromas
    - Irregularities
    - Salivary fistulas
    - Dryness of mouth if preexisting xerostomia or borderline dryness

6. Demonstrate ability to structure alternative plan

    - Other options if patient doesn't agree with your proposed plan
    - Interventions for inadequate correction

Chapter Thirty-Four

Forehead Rejuvenation

34
Forehead Rejuvenation

1. Identify General Problem Diagnosis/Planning
   (Describe photo, give working diagnosis, key problems, evaluates patient)

   - Addresses ptotic brow assess for eyelid ptosis as well
   - May be subconscious compensatory elevation of eyebrows
   - Smiling reduces compensation
   - Anatomy
     o Supraorbital nerve exits supraorbital foramen 2.7cm from midline
     o Supratrochlear nerve 1.7cm from midline, 0.8cm anterior to supraorbital n.
   - Botox can treat frontal migraine headaches
   - Senescent changes
     o Glabellar lines
     o Eyebrow ptosis
     o Deep frown lines
     o Elongation of forehead
     o Deep horizontal lines
   - Preop assessment
     o Forehead length
     o Eyebrow position
     o Male pattern baldness
     o Frown lines- tired, angry appearance
   - Differentiate eyebrow vs. eyelid ptosis
   - Check for frontalis compensation
     o Smiling eliminates frontalis compensation
     o Tightly close eyes then gradually open till patient can see examiner
   - Discuss all finding with patient preop
     o Length disharmony or receding hairline
     o Frontal bossing
     o Glabellar flattening
     o All wrinkles
     o Eyebrow ptosis
     o Misshapen eyebrow arch
   - Hx: Headaches?- may be secondary to frontalis migraine

- **MANTRA FOR COSMETIC PATIENTS**
  - Discuss options for treatment
  - Let patient choose procedure
  - If potentially suboptimal adequately discuss
- **ANATOMY**
  - Frontalis
    - Arises from skin and subcutaneous tissue inserts into galea
    - Expresses attention
    - Elevates eyebrows
    - Causes transverse wrinkles
  - Orbicularis oculi
    - Orbital portion- depresses eyebrow
    - Palpebral portion- contains preseptal and pretarsal portions
  - Corrugator supercilii muscle
    - Small pyramidal muscle located at medial end of eyebrow, deep to frontalis and orbicularis
    - Originates from supraciliary arch inserts into skin of forehead deep surface, creates vertical lines

2. Consider reasonable goals in diagnosis and management *(Management and treatment, surgical indications, operative procedures and anesthesia)*

- Emphasis minimize incisions and long-term side effects
- **INDICATIONS**
  - Forehead wrinkles but does not want surgery
    - BOTOX A
    - Fat injection- longer lasting than BOTOX
    - May augment invasive techniques
  - Transpalpebral corrugator resection
    - Significant glabellar frown lines and corrugator hyperactivity
    - Minimal or no eyebrow ptosis
    - Proptosis and deep frown lines
    - For those who do not want full forehead rejuvenation
  - Endoscopic forehead rejuvenation

- Procedure of choice:
- Patients with optimal or borderline forehead length
- Eyebrow ptosis
- Hyperactive forehead muscles without deep horizontal forehead lines
  - Subcutaneous forehead rhytidectomy
    - Better choice:
    - Borderline to mild forehead elongation
    - Receding hairline
    - Extensive deep wrinkles
    - Deep lines in forehead that cannot be eliminated by endoscopic alone or endoscopic with laser resurfacing
  - Scalp advancement with or without forehead lift
    - Superior choice for patient with significant forehead elongation

3. Select appropriate options in diagnosis and management.

   Treatment options
   - Fat injection
     - Can eliminate facial lines
     - Forehead dynamic zone, activity of frontalis causes wrinkles
       - Frontalis- horizontal lines
       - Corrugator- vertical lines
       - Depressor supercilii- oblique lines in medial eyebrow area
       - Procerus- creases at root of nose
     - Technique
       - Lido/epi
       - Hyaluronidase 3units
       - Lower abd or gluteal region
         - Localize
         - Aspirate 14 gauge cannula/1ml syringe
         - Centrifuge
       - Inject with 18 gauge needle on Coleman cannula

- - - Release fibrous bands to get 4-5mm area under deep portion of frown line
      - Inject fat with multiple passes
    - Minimal postop care
  - Fat Graft
    - Large grafts volume loss 50%
    - Graft thinner than 1cm better graft take
    - Works well for glabellar frown lines- high success rate
    - Adjuvant in forehead rejuvenation
    - Fat alone or with dermis (risk of cyst formation)
    - Technique
      - Lido/epi
      - Hyaluronidase 3units
      - Stab incision
      - Develop pocket for insertion (needle or scissors)
      - Do not overcorrect
      - Close pocket with 6-0 plain, fast
  - Transpalpebral corrugator excision
    - Results in disappearance of frown lines
    - Adjunct to endoscopic or blepharoplasty
    - Predictable and reliable
    - Technique

    In bleph
      - After skin resection
      - Retract orbital septum caudal, muscle cephalad
      - Expose depressor and corrugator
      - Protect supratrochlear nerve and supraorbital nerves
      - Excise muscle with coagulation: Aggressive excision to avoid irregularities
      - Avoid excess excision of procerus: Excess elevation of medial brow can occur
      - Fat graft to fill depression
        - Does not affect brow ptosis, may elevate medial brow
  - Endoscopic forehead lift
    - Advantage:
      - Avoids large incisional scars

- Reduced chance of forehead elongation
- Reduced surgery related alopecia
- Technique
  - IV with sedation or general anesthetic
  - Braid hair
  - Localize forehead and hair bearing scalp
  - Midline radial incision 0.5cm behind hairline at widow's peak
  - Two incisions in temple area
    - 7cm and 10 cm from midline
    - 1.5-2cm behind the hairline
    - 1.2-1.5cm in length
  - Most lateral incision to deep temporal fascia, expose deep temporal fascia
  - Make space above deep and superficial temporal fascia for endoscopic assist device at each incision site
  - Subperiosteal dissection in central forehead/superficial to deep temporal fascia in temporal region
  - At supraorbital rim arcus marginalis and periorbita are released until orbital septum visible
  - Complete release of periorbita essential to procedure
  - Excise corrugator as radically as possible
  - Preserve supratrochlear and supraorbital nerves
  - Glabellar area periosteum not transected unless significant medial eyebrow ptosis
  - Meticulous hemostasis throughout
  - Fat graft corrugator site-from deep temporal fascia above zygomatic arch if no other procedure performed
  - Fascia suspension sutures placed minimum of one on each side (3-0 PDS) through superficial temporal fascia
  - Scalp retracted as far posteriorly as possible
  - Two burr holes for suture fixation
  - Screws (require later removal) or absorbable devices can be used

- Drain (remove at 2 days) and skin closure (absorbable sutures)
  - Disadvantages
    - Deep horizontal lines not as effectively addressed as with open technique
      - Can combine with laser resurfacing
    - Not optimal for elongated forehead
    - Inadequate or excessive eyebrow elevation
    - Under- or overcorrection
    - Persistent anesthesia
    - Temporal branch facial nerve injury- usually transient
    - Persistent itching
- Open forehead lift with/or without forehead shortening
  - Quicker operation
  - Bloodless plane of dissection
  - Good technique to begin learning forehead facial rejuvenation
  - Technique
    - Braid hair
    - Localize
    - Coronal incision curvilinear (Stealth)
      - 5cm behind hairline, temple to temple directly above the ear
    - Lateral dissection
      - Superficial to deep temporal fascia
    - Medial dissection
      - Supraperiosteal to orbital rim
    - Arcus marginalis and fibrous bands along lateral orbital wall released
    - Expose corrugator and depressor supercilii, radical excision
    - Fat graft
    - Hemostasis
    - Central conservative skin excision, no tension
    - Drains
    - Two layer closure PDS and chromic
  - Disadvantages
    - Most common mistake, aggressive elevation of the eyebrows, esp. medially
    - Long incisions

- Elongates forehead
- Most serious complication hair loss
- Under- or overcorrection
- Parasthesia or permanent anesthesia in forehead area
- Infection and hematoma rare
- Temporal branch injury
- Scarring
- Intense itching of scalp 3-6 months
- Forehead tightness 12-18 months
  - Postop
    - Antibiotic ointment 5-7 days
    - Drain removal at 2 days
    - Shampoo third postop day
    - Avoid hair dryers/curling irons 2 weeks due to hypoesthetic scalp
    - No hair coloring for 2-3 weeks
- Forehead Rhytidectomy with pretrichial incision
  - Eliminates crow's feet and forehead wrinkles
  - Avoids post op hair loss
  - Scalp sensation well preserved
  - Long forehead shortened (mild or mod elongation)
  - Can expose depressor supercilii and corrugator
  - Technique
    - IV sedation or general
    - Incision design critical to visibility
    - Curvilinear, 1cm behind exaggerated widow's peak
    - Localize
    - Dissection between subq and frontalis or submuscular or subperiosteal
    - Excise corrugators
    - Fat graft
    - Excise redundant skin
    - No tension on closure
- Shortening Elongated Forehead
  - If elongated >1.5-2cm aesthetically pleasing scalp advancement can be performed
  - Can be combined with forehead lift
  - Technique
    - Posterior supraperiosteal dissection is performed to occipital notch

- One to three relaxing incisions made in galea 4cm apart
  - Each incision 1-1.5cm advancement
- Bone tunnels made for scalp fixation, safety guard 5mm
  - Two holes 3-4mm apart, 3-0 PDS
  o Complications: patchy alopecia

4. Understand risks and benefits of various approaches

   - Leave periosteum of glabellar area intact prevents excess medial elevation of eyebrow
   - Lateral brow and periosteal release critical in fixation
   - If proptosis present conservative eyebrow lift
   - Smokers submuscular dissection is safer

5. Address complications and unexpected problems adequately

   - Fat injection complications
     o Unpredictability
     o Does not eliminate muscle function
   - i.e. area of volume loss will recur over time
     o Over- or under-injection
     o Blindness-Rare- via emboliztion to retinal artery
   - Tx: Ophthalmology consultation
   - Fat graft complications
     o Irregularities
     o Infection
     o Hematoma
     o Generally good outcomes
   - Transpalpebral corrugator excision
     o Induration
     o Asymmetric corrugator function
     o Permanent numbness
     o Scar hypertrophy
   - Wound complications
   - Inadequate correction

6. Demonstrate ability to structure alternative plan

   - Consider other options based on clinical presentation

Chapter Thirty-Five

Eyelids/Blepharoplasty

35
Eyelids/Blepharoplasty

1. Identify General Problem/Diagnosis/Planning
   (Describe photo, give working diagnosis, key problems, evaluates patient)

   - Determine exact patient desires and expectation
   - Ophthalmology exam within 1 year of surgery
     - Assess for:
       - Dry eye
       - Unrecognized corneal disorders
       - Visual defects
       - Glaucoma
   - Strict control: HTN, DM
   - Avoid anticoagulant meds, NSAIDS, herbal supplements that affect coagulation
   - History:
     - Graves, bleeding disorders
     - CV
     - Renal disease
     - Other
     - Previous eyelid surgery
     - Trauma
     - Inflammation
     - Allergies
     - Ptosis
   - Physical Exam
     - Evaluate frontalis contribution
       - May mask eyelid ptosis!
       - May cause asymmetric eyebrow position
     - Margin reflex distance (MRD) ideally 4-5mm
     - Lower lid laxity
       - Consider need for canthopexy or –plasty
     - Check for negative vector
       - Most prominent area of globe anterior to orbital rim, increased risk of dry-eye syndrome
     - Lacrimal gland prolapse
     - Redundancy of skin

- o Reduction of visual field
- o Eyelashes in visual axis
- o Normal upper lid overlaps limbus 1-2mm
- o Assess levator function
  - Ruler next to eyes
  - Head immobilized
  - Look down
    - Level of eyelid noted on ruler
  - Look upward
    - Gain noted on ruler
  - Repeat to get reliable number
  - Difference is levator excursion
    - Normal - 15mm or more
    - Excellent - 10-15 mm
    - Good - 8-10 mm
    - Fair - 5-7 mm
    - Poor - 4mm or <
  - Aponeurotic ptosis usually excellent levator function, congenital ptosis usually poor
- o Aponeurotic ptosis
  - Higher supratarsal crease may be noted
- o Lacrimal gland ptosis
  - May be evident as fullness in lateral portion of upper lid
- o Lateral upper lid fullness may be from ROOF (retroorbicularis oculi fat)
- o Lower lid
  - Usually touches lowest portion of limbus
  - Scleral show undesirable
    - May indicate lower lid laxity
- o Evaluate infraobital rim (malar groove) or nasojugal area
- o Check for hyperpigmentation
- o Check Bell phenomenon
  - If negative increased risk for exposure keratitis postop
  - Close eyes forcefully, examiner tries to open eyes
  - Globe normally rotates cephalad
- o Check snap back and pinch test
  - Snap back

- Good tone if resumes position in a fraction of a second
    - Pinch test
        - Lower lid should not move more than 6mm from globe
  - Negative vector
  - Gross visual exam with vision chart
  - Consider- Schrimer's test- <10mm abnormal
    - Tear break time
- Anatomy
  - Lower lid, three fat pads
    - Medial
    - Central
    - Lateral
  - Upper lid, two fat pads
    - Medial
    - Central
    - Lacrimal gland
  - Supratarsal crease 8-10mm above upper lid margin
    - Absent in Asians
  - Orbicularis m. two portions
    - Orbital- overlies orbital rims
    - Palbebral- preseptal and pretarsal
  - Retroorbicularis oculi fat pad
    - Between orbicularis and septum upper lid
  - Suborbicularis oculi fat pad
    - Same structure in lower lid
  - Preaponeurotic fat pad
    - Between levator m. and orbital septum
  - Blood supply
    - Ophthalmic branch of internal carotid
    - Supplemented by abundant collaterals from external carotid
  - Sensation
    - Trigeminal nerve VI- ophthalmic branch
    - Lower lid primarily infraorbital nerve V2
  - Main lacrimal gland
    - Lateral horn of levator transects it
    - Dividing into orbital lobe and palpebral lobe
  - Asian eyelid may have caudal attachment of levator aponeurosis with prolapse of fat between levator and orbital septum

- Senescent changes periorbital region
  - Brow ptosis
  - Excess skin of upper lid
  - Protrusion orbital fat upper and lower lids- weakening of septum
  - Involutional eyelid ptosis (aponeurotic ptosis)
- Blepharochalasia- idiopathic recurrent swelling
- Dermatochalasis- excess eyelid skin

2. Consider reasonable goals in diagnosis and management *(Management and treatment, surgical indications, operative procedures and anesthesia)*

- Full informed consent discuss all risks and potential complications
  - High rate of complication with lower lid bleph upwards of 20%
- Conservative fat excision
- Consider repositioning fat especially in lower lid
- Conservative skin excision in lower lid
- Indications
  - Excess skin upper or lower
  - Steatoblepharon- fat protrusion upper or lower lids
  - Ptosis or drooping of upper lids
  - Eyelid hyperpigmentation
- Contraindications
  - Severe dry eyes
  - Facial palsy- avoid eyelid excision
  - Lagophthalmos- exception removal or repositioning of fat at time of correction of lagophthalmos
  - Corneal disease- bleph may exacerbate this
  - Will not completely treat dynamic rhytids
  - Will not treat static rhytids- laser or chemical resurfacing
- CAUTION
  - Tendency tower lower lid ectropion
  - Eyelid retraction
  - Lagophthalmos preop
  - Keratitis sicca
  - Recurrent erosion
  - Keloid formation

- - - Graves
  - - Note: Preexisting asymmetry

3. Select appropriate options in diagnosis and management

   - Upper Lid Blepharoplasty
     - Local with sedation
     - Inject after marking
     - Caudal portion of incision at or slightly below (older pts) eyelid crease
     - Cephalic portion marked and skin preserved to allow lid closure via pinching
       - Best to pinch in supine position/avoid excess excision
     - Mark fat compartments
     - With traction incision is made caudal first through skin and subq, then cephalic incision
     - Skin excision/may include orbicularis
       - AVOID orbicularis excision to avoid injury to levator aponeurosis
       - Fine tip cautery
     - Fat excision
       - Medial fat pad/preaponeurotic temporal fat pad
       - Via incision in septum
       - Conservative fat excision to avoid hollowing
     - Meticulous hemostasis- cauterize vessels in fat
     - Skin closure 6-0 fast-gut
     - Consider lacrimal gland suspension if it protrudes beyond orbital rim
       - Via 6-0 nonabsorbable suture to periobita
     - Rarely, ROOF excess laterally, consider excision
     - Perform canthoplasty prior to lateral skin closure if planned as part of upper lid bleph
   - Lower Lid Blepharoplasty
     - Jelks NO TOUCH LOWER LID BLEPH
     - Avoid violating:
       - Pretarsal orbicularis
       - Midlamellar region centrally
     - Prevents:
       - Orbicularis oculi paresis

- Midlamellar scar which is common- prevent with frost suture
- Lower lid malposition
  - Use lateral upper lid incision for access
    - Get in submuscular plane/preseptal
    - Incise periosteum
    - Excise lateral fat pad as indicated
  - Then lateral canthoplasty can be performed
    - Use inferior retinacular component of lateral canthus
    - Suture to interior lateral orbital rim
    - Closes distance of soft tissue to orbital rim
    - OVERCORRECT
  - Use transconjunctival approach to access medial fat pads
  - Incision made 8mm below tarsus
  - Use traction sutures
  - Vertically incise capsulopalpebral fascia (retains function)
    - Give access to arcus marginalis, inferior orbital rim
  - Excess fat can then be removed, leave thin edge of fat
  - Complete release of arcus marginalis/place fat in this space, no sutures needed
    - This improves tear trough deformity
  - Tie down canthoplasty
  - Last step skin pinch
    - Conservative skin excision
    - Incision placed 1-2mm caudal to eyelashes
  - Inferior retinacular canthoplasty
  - Decide preop if canthoplasty needed
  - Traditional Bleph
    - Incise 1-2mm below lower lid margin (subciliary incision)
    - Incise skin and muscle flap
    - Incise septum and excise medial, lateral, central fat compartments as indicated
    - Release arcus marginalis and position SOOF (suborbicularis oculi fat)
    - Perform canthoplasty/pexy
    - Drape skin and conservative excision

- Close
- Meticulous hemostasis
            - Transconjunctival Bleph
                - Can be done if no skin excision needed
                - Augment with laser resurfacing
            - Address ptosis if present brow or eyelid
        - POST OP CONSIDERATIONS
            - Control BP
            - Monitor in RR 2 hours prior to discharge
            - Treat nausea/vomiting aggressively Zofran
            - Cold pack 24-48 hours
            - Ophthalmic abx ointment to incisions
            - Frost suture 24 hours
            - No strenuous exercise 2-3 weeks

4. Understand risks and benefits of various approaches

    - Review above
    - AVOID
        - Upper lid bleph/ptosis correction in patient with dry eyes
    - Options to address lower lid laxity:
        - Canthopexy or –plasty
        - Minor wedge excision of lateral tarsus
    - If orbicularis skin flap performed, resuspend to canthopexy/canthoplasty
    - Measures to prevent ectropion

5. Address complications and unexpected problems adequately

    - Minor temporary post-bleph lagophthalmos common, even more so after levator approach to ptosis surgery
    - Postop frequent lubrication and ophthalmic ointment, lid exercises
    - Risks
        - Blindness 1:2K-5K
        - Retrobulbar hemorrhage
        - Clinical signs: proptosis, pain, mydriasis (pupil dilation)
            - Tx:
                - Open incision, drain hematoma
                - Lateral canthotomy and cantholysis

- High dose steroids (Dexamethasone 10mg)
- Emergent ophthalmology eval
- Surgical exploration and decompression
- Mannitol
- Common complications
    - Slight dryness of eyes
    - Conjunctivitis
    - Chemosis
    - Excessive ecchymosis
    - Conjunctival ecchymosis 2-3 weeks to resolve
- Less common
    - Infection
    - Hematoma
    - Wound dehiscence
    - Exacerbation of dry eye syndrome
    - Lagophthalmos
    - Hypertrophic scars and keloids
    - Epiphora
    - Protracted hyperpigmentation
    - Residual bags
    - Asymmetry
    - Hollow lower eyelids
    - Lid retraction
    - Eyelid ptosis
- Rare complications
    - Ectropion
    - Loss of vision- exceedingly rare
- Intraop excessive bleeding
    - Check coags
    - If persistent give DDAVP
    - Check BP and control HTN (systolic BP >130mmHg treat)
        - Clonidine hydrochloride 0.1 or 0.2mg
- Diplopia- may be from injury to inferior oblique, inferior rectus or superior oblique
    - Tx:
        - Observe, muscle dysfunction usually transient
        - If persistent refer to ophthalmology for strabismus surgery eval- poor outcomes

- Lid retraction/Ectropion
  - Tx:
    - Eyelid massage
    - Severe cases surgical correction
    - See Ectropion (Chapter 21)
- Dry eye
  - Tx:
    - Lubrication
    - Ophthalmology consultation
- Chemosis
  - Tx:
    - Lubrication
    - Ophthalmic steroid
    - Severe cases temporary tarsorrhaphy
    - May be prevented by temporary tarrsorhaphy

6. Demonstrate ability to structure alternative plan

- Consider management of complications
- Inadequate correction
- Over resection of fat pads
- Plan for simultaneous bleph and ptosis surgery
- Adjunctive measures for skin
- Unsatisfied patient

Chapter Thirty-Six

Rhytidectomy and Cervicoplasty

36
Rhytidectomy and Cervicoplasty

1. Identify General Problem Diagnosis/Planning
   (Describe photo, give working diagnosis, key problems, evaluates patient)

   - Describe photo in detail
   - Break up face into thirds or fifths with attention to:
     o Forehead
     o Eyebrows, eyelids, ptosis (brow and upper lids)
     o Periorbital skin and soft tissue
     o Nasolabial creases
     o Jowls
     o Neck
   - History
   - Determine motivation for surgery
     o Avoid patients with:
       - Spur of the moment decisions
       - Recent displeasing life event
       - Ask for:
         • Patient's specific complaints
         • Perception of existing problems
     (Will likely be clinical findings that you see on photo)
   - Assess emotional stability
   - Medical suitability (ASA II or less)
     o DM
     o Steroids
     o HTN
     o CAD
     o Smoking
       - Increased risk of skin slough
       - Avoid nicotine patch
     o Anticoagulant's including NSAID use
     o Easy bleeding or bruising
     o History of keloids: avoid surgery
     o Herbal meds: Some are anticoagulants
     o Special medical conditions

- Cutis laxa- rhytidectomy beneficial
- Ehlers Danlos- rhytidectomy contraindicated
  - Previous surgery
    - Cosmetic procedures
    - Existing facial scars
- Physical Exam
  - Note skin quality
  - If preexisting sun damage
    - Consider preop skin regimen
      - Laser
      - Chemical Peel
  - Periorbital rhytids
    - Consider simultaneous skin resurfacing
  - Condition of pretragal skin
    - Decide pretragal vs. post tragal incision
  - Skin Type Fitzpatrick Classification
    - Important in use of skin peels or laser
    - Fitzpatrick I or II good response, V or VI poor candidates
  - Associated skin lesions/skin cancer address prior to elective cosmetic procedures
  - Biopsy any suspicious lesions
  - Preexisting scars
  - Consider hairline and sideburns
    - Avoid abnormal elevation of these
  - Earlobe position (attached or hanging)
    - Must recreate at closure
  - Facial shape
    - Round vs. angled
    - (poorer results in round faces note pre-op)
  - Upper face (hairline to glabella)
    - Address position of brow
    - Position of hairline (forehead and temples)
    - Need for eyelid procedures?
    - Resurfacing only vs. bleph with skin +/- fat excision
    - Ptosis correction?
    - Glabellar region rhytids
      - Neuromuscular blockade (botulinum toxin A)
      - Deep furrows
      - Fillers (fat vs. other)

- Relax forehead with deep wrinkles prior to choosing procedure
  - Smile
  - Close eyes and slowly open
- Forehead profile contour
  - Note bossing or other irregularities
- Midface (Glabella to subnasal)
  - Brow position, Eyelids, Eyebrows
    - Upper border of eyebrows should be at least 2.5cm above mid pupil on straight gaze
    - Medial end caudal to lateral extreme
    - Highest portion of arch at junction of the lateral 1/3 with medial 2/3
    - Lateral limit of limbus in straight gaze
    - Eyebrow ptosis causes crowding in orbital region
    - Normal intercantal distance (medial canthi) 31-33mm
  - Check for eyelid ptosis
    - Normal upper lid position 1mm below limbus
  - Supratarsal fold, normally 3-4 mm above lid margin
  - Levator dehiscence- tarsal show is increased with a more cephalad supratarsal crease
  - Check levator function to determine procedure
  - Presence of Bell's Phenomenon
    - Ask pt hold eyes shut tight, attempt to open, does globe roll cephalad?
    - Yes-Positive Bell's, protection postop if complication occurs
    - No-Negative Bell's, increased risk of dry eye complication from corneal exposure
  - Pleasing lower lid- located at caudal limit of limbus or slightly overlaps
  - Excess scleral show
    - Sign of lower lid laxity

- If scleral show or negative vector is present
- Conservative bleph surgery
- Use adjunctive canthoplasty or canthopexy
- Give extra lid support
  - Lid snap
  - Ideal mobility of lateral canthus less than 7-8 mm
  - Eyelid edema: Maybe a symptom of thyroid dysfunction
  - Cheek descent?
    - Descent of malar cheek pad requires midface lift
    - Nasolabial folds
    - Rhytidectomy may worsen fold
    - Address with fillers or direct excision
    - Depression in nasojugal area or cephalad to infraorbital rim may necessitate soft tissue repositioning or fat grafting
  - Nasal skin
    - Thick or very thin poor rhinoplasty candidate
  - Nasal show
    - On frontal view should have some nostril show
    - Inadequate show
    - Long nose, or caudally positioned ala
    - Excess show
    - Short nose or retracted alar rims
    - Exaggerated with smile
    - Alar base distance
    - Should be slightly wider than intercanthal distance
- Lower face (Subnasal to chin)
  - Hypoplastic chin
  - Chin augmentation vs. Sliding genioplasty

- Can be combined with rhytidectomy to improve facial balance
- Lip incompetence
- Contraindication to chin augmentation
- Consider tooth alignment and need for orthodontic procedures
- Excess submental fat
  - Direct excision and/or liposuction
- Goal improve obtuse mandibular-cervical angle
- Consider subplatysmal fat
- Jowls
- Platysmal bands
  - Prominent, divergent bands may need direct reapproximation
  - Via submental incision (actual incision, distal to crease to prevent witch's chin deformity)
- Prominent submental salivary glands
  - Point out preop may be more prominent post op
- Pleasing neck 100-degree angle between chin and neck
- Beware obtuse neck angle
  - Excess skin
  - Excess supra-platysma fat
  - Excess sub-platysma fat
  - Prominent neckbands
- Hypertrophic anterior belly digastric muscles or submandibular gland
- Ptotic submandibular gland
- Overhead view
- Internal nasal exam
- Preop Work-up
    - Minimal in healthy patients
    - Labs based on medical history
    - CXR and EKG may require in pts over 50 in some facilities
    - Review current standards
    - Age over 50
        - Full medical checkup especially exercise tolerance

- Ophthalmologic exam within one year if eyelid surgery contemplated
  - Photos: AP, Lateral, Oblique
  - Lateral cephalogram if chin augmentation is planned
  - Consults
    - Cardiology clearance may be needed
    - Primary medical physician should review: med hx, current meds, exercise tolerance
  - Be sure surgeon and patient expectations are the same!
  - Comprehensive health form
  - Informed Consent
    - Risks of complications
    - Surgical and non-surgical options
    - Preferred technique vs. patient preference
    - More than one meeting prior to surgery R/O Body Dysmorphic Disorder: Patient sees a deformity that does not exist or sees a great deal more than is present, preoccupation with perceived defects, complaints may be specific or vague
  - Risk factors for DRY EYES:
    - Pre-existing lower lid laxity
    - Loss of lower lid tone
    - Negative vector (malar soft tissue prominence behind cornea)
    - Borderline tear production
    - Symptoms of dry eyes
  - Conservative surgery: canthopexy or canthoplasty only

2. Consider reasonable goals in diagnosis and management *(Management and treatment, surgical indications, operative procedures and anesthesia)*

   - Preop skin regimen
     - Retinoids
     - Bleaching creams (hydroquinone)
     - Improved skin appearance adds to overall result of surgery
     - Isolated wrinkling around eyes not addressed by rhytidectomy

- Periop
  - Meds to alleviate anxiety or minimize postop complications
  - Sedatives night before and morning of surgery
  - Antiemetic (Zofran 4mg IV)
  - Give patient's own antihypertensives
  - Consider periop clonidine (0.1 to 0.3mg 1 hour preop) Decreases risk of hematoma
  - Consider periop steroids
    - Decreases postop edema
    - Augments the effects of other meds

- Modern rhytidectomy
  - Primary goal
    - Facial shape modification via repositioning facial fat- key to excellent result
    - Not a simple stretching and pulling of the ski.
  - Youthful face
    - Round, full with soft curves
    - Full midface and malar region

Facelifts
  - Skin only: Oldest and simplest
    - Address descent of deeper structures by redraping skin and repositioning composite flap of cheek fat and SMAS layer
  - SMAS plication
    - Sutures placed anterior to retaining ligaments of cheek and malar complex
  - SMAS elevation
    - Develop SMAS and platysma to reshape
    - Extended SMAS, high SMAS, auto cheek augmentation
  - SMASectomy
    - Excision of a strip of SMAS
  - Deep plane facelift
    - Elevates forehead, eyelids and SMAS in continuity
  - Subperiosteal facelift
  - Consider Adjuvant procedures
    - Browlift
    - Blepharoplasty

Chapter Thirty-Seven

Facelift Principles and Surgery

37
Facelift Principles and Surgery

1. No universal technique

2. PRINCIPLES

    - Surgery should divert tension away from skin to superficial musculoaponeurotic system (SMAS) and platysma. Unless other deeper structures are addressed.
    - Skin has a covering function not supporting function. When used as support abnormal tension leads to:
        o Poor scars
        o Tragal retraction
        o Ear lobe malposition
        o Tight and unnatural appearance
    - SMAS should be used to lift sagging facial tissues, can give support
    - Midface lifts may fail to address other areas of atrophy
        o Views anterior upper cheek as sole area of sagging
        o Frequent disappointing outcomes
    - Most patients who need midface lift also need a facelift:
        o Must address sagging in cheek and jowl
    - Midface lift may be best as an adjunct to other procedures than as stand alone procedures.

3. INDICATIONS

    - Aging and breakdown of skin surface
    - Facial sagging
    - Skin redundancy
    - Loss of youthful facial contour
    - Facial wasting
    - Atrophy and age-related lipodystrophy
    - Assess patient priorities, time, trouble and expense willing to endure to obtain desired result.
    - Surface aging concerns?
    - Address with surface treatments:
        o Peels
        o Laser resurfacing

- - Chemodenervation
    - Fillers and fat grafts
  - Concerned with facial sagging and excess skin, loss of facial contour?
    - Not fully addressed by surface treatments
    - Require formal surgical lifts
      - Reposition tissue
      - Excise redundant tissue
    - Facial atrophy and age-related facial wasting
      - Need volume replacement in addition to the above
  - Pan-facial rejuvenation
    - Stress to patient facelift does not address all areas
    - Especially upper face
    - Caution in patients requesting surgery in only one area

4. TECHNIQUES

  - Conventional low cheek SMAS elevated below zygomatic arch
    - Drawback:
    - Does not affect midface and infraorbital tissue planes not opened
    - Higher flap along superior border of zygomatic arch overcomes this problem and improves the result.
  - High SMAS
    - Readily combined with midface fat injections
    - Midface and infraorbital plans are not opened
    - Averts the need to perform complex and potentially problematic procedures in which orbital fat is transposed, orbital septum 'reset' or free grafts placed
  - Lamellar dissection
    - Skin and SMAS two separate layers
    - Allows advancement in separate vectors
    - Suspension under differential tension
  - Plan incisions to avoid
    - Disruption of hairline
    - Tragal distortion
    - Abnormal earlobe placement
    - Sideburn elevation

- o Occipital hairline notching
- ▪ SMAS elevation
    - o Gives more natural appearance
    - o Improves scars
    - o Improves longevity of the procedure

6. Numerous techniques

- ▪ Skin only
    - o Skin tension
    - o Simple procedure
    - o Flattens contour
- ▪ SMAS Plication
    - o No midface affect
- ▪ SMASectomy
- ▪ Strip of SMAS excised obliquely over anterior parotid
- ▪ Cut edges reapproximated to support jawline and lateral perioral region
    - o No subSMAS dissection needed
    - o Skin and SMAS can be placed in different vectors
    - o Wide undermining
    - o Some risk to facial nerves
    - o Minimal midface effect
- ▪ Deep Plane
    - ▪ High risk to facial nerves
    - ▪ Dissection deep to SMAS
    - ▪ Skin and SMAS elevated as one layer
    - ▪ Less time, good blood supply
    - ▪ Increased risk to facial nerves
    - ▪ Abandoned by Hamra for composite
- ▪ Composite
    - ▪ Deep plane that includes orbicularis oculi- raises lid-cheek junction
    - ▪ Midface can be elevated by medially vectored flap of orbicularis
    - ▪ Skin and SMAS unidirectional
    - ▪ Prolonged periorbital edema
- ▪ Lamellar SMAS dissection and bidirectional
    - o Skin and SMAS elevated as different layers
    - o Advanced along different vectors
    - o Can place in different vectors

- Minimizes skin only problems of skin tension, hairline displacement, objectionable wrinkle shifts
- More time consuming
- Risk of facial nerve injury due to subSMAS dissection
- Extended SMAS
    - Improves midface, infraorbital region, increased support of lower eyelid- Stuzin, Baker, Gordon
    - Separate skin and SMAS flaps
    - SubSMAS dissection in area of upper cheek and midface to release retaining ligaments and free up malar fat pad
    - Improved midface and infraorbital region effect
- High SMAS
    - Restores youthful upper cheek contour
    - Increased lower lid support
    - Improved nasolabial fold correction
- Modified low cheek SMAS
    - Flap planned along superior border of zygomatic arch
    - Extended dissection medially mobilizes midface tissues
    - Exerts effect on midface and infraorbital region
    - Performed as two layer lamellar technique or as one
    - Can combine with midface fat injection because midface and infra-orbital tissue planes are not opened
    - Generally averts need for midface procedure
    - Theoretical increased risk to frontal branch
- Subperiosteal
    - Theoretical advantage for repositioning sagging tissue
    - But periosteum is densely adherent to bone unlikely to sag with aging
    - Hard to improve jaw line
    - Requires concomitant use of suspension sutures
- Endoscopic
    - Does not allow for skin excision
    - No technique as of this time
    - May be applicable to midface elevation

7. Midface Lifts

- Fraught with complications
    - Lid retraction
    - Ectropion

- o Canthal displacement
- o Dry eye
- o Disappointing results
- Inverted triangular area over anterior upper cheek
- Borders
  - o Zygomaticus major m. laterally
  - o Nasolabial fold medially
  - o Infraorbital rim superiorly
- Midface ptosis occurs with aging
  - o Isolated midface lifts not perfected
  - o Steep learning curve
  - o Procedure elevates lid-cheek junction only
  - o No correction of nasolabial fold
  - o May not address whole face, many patients would benefit from facelifting
- Complications
  - o Lid retraction
  - o Ectropion
  - o Canthal displacement
  - o Dry eye problems
- To prevent problems combine with:
  - o Canthoplasties
  - o Canthotomies
  - o Orbicularis oculi m. suspension
- Suspension suture
  - o No predictable support
  - o Infections
  - o Extrusion
  - o Traction dimples
  - o Visible bowstrings
  - o Nerve injuries
  - o Palpable suture knots
  - o Choking sensation
- MACS (Minimal Access Cranial Suspension)- Tonnard
  - o Combines short scar with suture suspension of deep tissue
  - o Diverts tension from skin to deeper layers- improved scar quality
  - o Suspension by gathering and microplication of SMAS
  - o Targets midface, cheek, jowl, lateral neck
  - o Incision is on temporal hairline

- - - o Does not require SMAS dissection
  - Short scar
    - o Skin redundancy is a problem, compromises improvement
    - o Limited access to deep structures
    - o Gathered skin along incision
    - o Postauricular scar is shortened
    - o Questionable value, requires sideburn scar
  - Mini-lift
    - o Simple skin excision
    - o No SMAS modification

8. THE FACELIFT- SURGICAL CONSIDERATIONS

  - PLAN TEMPORAL INCISION
    - o Place in temporal scalp if cheek skin redundancy is small and there is ample temple and sideburn hair.
      - Causes minimal sideburn elevation and temporal hairline retrodisplacement
      - Best choice in young and/or mild cheek laxity only
  - Incision along hairline
    - o If larger skin shift planned
    - o If patient has sparse temple hair
    - o Otherwise significant displacement of hairline may occur
  - Factors for incision placement
    - o Patient preference after informed consent
    - o Distance between lateral orbit and anterior aspect of temporal hairline
      - Increases with age
      - Shorter distance more temporal hair available and temporal incision okay
    - o Distance
      - Young patients 4-5cm
      - Shorter in older patients
    - o Estimate of skin redundancy
      - Upper cheek
      - Measure by pinching
      - Estimates best site for temporal incision
    - o Use temporal incision if:

- - - Temporal hairline will stay within 5cm of lateral orbit
    - Incision placed within 4-5cm of lateral orbit
  - Use hairline incision
    - If predicted hairline will be more than 5cm from lateral orbit
    - Or if sideburn hair will be shifted above ear scalp junction
- PLAN PREAURICULAR INCISION
  - Traditional vs. retrotragal incision
  - Traditional preauricular well anterior to border of helix and tragus
    - Works well only if cheek tragus is good skin color match unusual
    - Later obvious mismatch
  - Retrotragal incision
    - Probably best used in most cases
    - Incision goes along posterior margin of tragus rather than pretragal sulcus
    - Properly executed
      - Tragal retraction or other anatomic irregularity will not occur
      - In male patients intraop destroy beard follicles
      - Do not place truly retrotragal but along posterior margin of tragus
    - Incision stays in creases of ear especially at junction of anterior lobule and cheek
  - PERILOBULAR INCISION
    - Preserve natural sulcus between earlobe and cheek
    - Incision 1-2 mm below this junction not directly in sulcus
- POSTAURICULAR INCISION
  - Traditionally goes over posterior surface of concha
  - Should be marked in auriculomastoid groove
  - And turned posteriorly at the level of the anterior crus of antihelix
  - Ear must be in natural resting position
- OCCIPITAL INCISION

- Plan as in temporal incision consider final placement of hairline and scar visibility
- Traditionally arbitrarily placed transversely
- 2cm or less skin excess
- Traditional incision over mastoid extending into scalp at mid-ear
- Postauricular flap should not be advanced and returned to original position
- \>2cm skin excess
  - Place along occipital hairline, turn incision inferiorly at junction of thick and thin hair at nape of neck
- **SUBMENTAL INCISION**
  - Place posterior to submental crease
    - Avoids double chin or witch's chin deformity
    - Parallel 3.5-4.5cm in length
- **THE TECHNIQUE**
  - Skin flap elevation sharp under direct vision
  - Preserve anterior platysma-cutaneous ligaments
  - Anterior dissection ends posterior to perioral region, malar area
  - Bevel to preserve hair follicles
  - SMAS traced high over midpoint of zygomatic arch
    - Outer malar area to superior portion of tragus
    - Turned inferiorly and carried over preauricular portion of parotid
- **SMAS flap**
  - Incise over zygomatic arch first
  - Frontal branch should be deep to fibrous fat which should be preserved
  - Preauricular incision made
    - Dissection ends at anterior border of sternocleidomastoid muscle
  - Scissors dissection for SMAS elevation
    - Limited in pre-parotid cheek
    - More extensive over zygoma and upper mid-face
- **SMAS Suspension**
  - Posterosuperior vector parallel to long axis of zygomaticus major m.

- o Superior margin can be trimmed or used for volume augmentation of cheek
- o Suture 3-0 suture over zygomatic arch directly to deep temporal fascia
- o No suturing at level of zygomatic arch
- o Some trimming of posterior margin of SMAS flap then approximated to preauricular remnant

Drains used routinely
- o 10 French placed in cervical skin
- Skin flap positioning
    - o Excise redundancy, do not tighten
    - o More posterior less superior direction than SMAS flap
    - o Cheek skin vector roughly parallel to nasolabial fold
    - o Postauricular skin parallel to mandibular border
- Two key points of suspension
    - o Supra-auricular area where ear joins scalp, cheek skin as above
    - o Postauricular crease- anterosuperior aspect of occipitomastoid incision as above
- Incision for exteriorization of lobule
    - o Incrementally performed with care
    - o Apex of incision should sit snugly against inferormost portion of conchal cartilage beneath lobule
- Skin flaps trimmed and closed
    - o Postauricular area first
    - o Occipital incision
    - o Preauricular area
- Inset lobule last step
- Temporal incision closure
- Submental incision closure

9. POSTOP

- Iced compresses 3 days
- No dressing
- Oral analgesics
- Antiemetics
- Ophthalmic ointments
- Sleep flat without pillow 2 weeks, neck roll okay
    - o To avoid neck flexion

- Shower and wash incisions
- Drains for 4-5 days
- Suture removal at 1 week
- 2-3 weeks to recover from surgery

10. COMPLICATIONS

- Objectionable temple, sideburn
- Occipital hairline displacement
- Scarring related to inappropriate skin tension
- Poor planning of incisions or performance of surgery itself
- Alopecia
- Skin flap necrosis
- Hematoma/infection/nerve damage

Section Eight
Rhinoplasty

Chapter Thirty-Eight

Rhinoplasty Overview

38
Rhinoplasty Overview

1. Identify General Problem

    - Describe photo
    - Give working diagnosis
    - Key problems
    - Evaluate patient
    - Give specific diagnosis regarding what needs to be addressed
    - Note pertinent positives and negatives in history
        - Previous surgery, any airway issues?
    - Specify anatomic areas to be addressed
    - Briefly reiterate healthy patient, non-smoker, no DM, CAD, HTN
    - Relevant medications especially anticoagulants
    - Have an algorithm for facial analysis
    - Detail specifics of your nasal physical exam
        - External exam
        - Internal exam
        - Note skin type
        - Specifics related to male vs. female patient
    - Be prepared for any nasal deformity
        - Bulbous tip
        - Boxy tip
        - Dorsal hump
        - Poor projection
        - Nasal show
        - Other
    - Your airway assessment and evaluation
    - Assess chin
        - Will orthognatic intervention add to facial balance?
    - Need for additional work-up for operative planning?
        - Cottle test
        - Vasoconstriction
        - Speculum exam in office
    - Assess the motivation of the patient
    - SIMON vs. SYLVIA

2. Consider reasonable goals in diagnosis and management

    - Management and treatment plans
    - Surgical indications
    - Operative procedures and anesthesia
    - Surgical plan
    - Options to address areas for improvement
    - Note potential problems, risks, anticipated outcome and patient satisfaction
    - Note what does the patient want

3. Select appropriate options in diagnosis and management

    - What option would you choose and why?
    - What will you do to prevent complications especially post-op airway obstruction?
    - How do you do your rhinoplasty?
        - Specify steps of procedure
        - Sequence
        - Grafts you would use and suturing techniques
    - Post-op management
        - Splinting
        - Packing?
        - Timing of suture and packing removal
        - Return to activity
    - Follow-up (short-term and long-term)
    - Focus strongly on:
        - How is procedure performed?
        - Key steps of surgery
        - Markings and relevant anatomy

4. Understand risks and benefits of various approaches

    - Note benefits and risks of various approaches.
    - Manage patient desires and expectations
    - What is your anticipated outcome?

5. Address complications and unexpected problems adequately

    - Be prepared to manage all potential complications
        - Note your timing for any intervention
        - Will you bill the patient?

- Management of:
  - Hematoma
  - Persistent bleeding
  - Inadequate correction
  - Polybeak deformity
  - Airway obstruction
  - Under or over resection of dorsum
  - Visible grafts
  - Persistent crooked nose
  - Saddle nose
  - Inverted V
  - Other

6. Demonstrate ability to structure alternative plan

   - What if patient doesn't agree with your proposal?
   - Patient unsatisfied requests money back
   - Do you bill for early revision?
   - Secondary revision plan
   - Septum not available for cartilage harvest?

Chapter Thirty-Nine

Rhinoplasty

39
Rhinoplasty

1. Identify General Problem/Diagnosis/Planning
   (Describe photo, working diagnosis, key problems, evaluates patient)

   - Describe photo in detail
     - Break up face in thirds or fifths
     - Note your findings
     - Note facial balance
     - Detail any and all nasal deformities
   - Identify patient motivation
   - Specific complaints about appearance
     - Aesthetic (precise specific regarding size, shape, contour)
     - Functional
   - Hx (thorough, unrushed history):
     - Previous nasal surgery
     - History of nasal trauma?
     - Symptoms of airway obstruction
       - Exam: Determine Structural vs. Medical Causes
       - Allergic and reactive airway symptoms may be worsened by surgery
     - Allergies
     - Sinus problems
     - Medical history regarding airway
     - Past interventions
     - Decongestants- helpful in allergic symptoms
     - Septal deviation, may have improvement on affected side with breath-right strips
       - Improvement may signify middle vault collapse
     - Smoker
     - Illicit drug use (cocaine)
     - Medications
     - Cyclical pattern to breathing
   - Delineate patient aesthetic goals
     - Allows patient to communicate desired result

- - Evaluates appropriateness of patient for surgery
  - PATIENT SCREENING DANGER SIGNS
    (Applicable to all cosmetic patients)
    - Minimal disfigurement
    - Delusional distortion of body image
    - Identity problem; sexual ambivalence
    - Confused or vague motives for rhino
    - Unrealistic expectation of change in life situation as result of surgery
    - Hx of poorly established social; emotional relationships
    - Unresolved grief or currently in crisis situation
    - Present misfortunes blamed on appearance
    - Older neurotic man overly concerned about aging
    - Sudden dislike for one's anatomy, esp. older man
    - Hostile blaming attitude toward authority figures
    - Hx of seeing physicians and being dissatisfied with them
    - Paranoid thoughts
    - SIMON (single immature males overly expectant narcissistic)
    - Men have poorer understanding of deformity than women
  - PE

    - Focus on any deviation from "normal" aesthetics
    - Include evaluation of whole face:
    - Especially:
      - Chin
      - Facial skeleton
      - Break into thirds:
        - Hairline to Brow/nasal base/menton
        - Upper third least important
  - INTRANASAL EXAM
    - Examine inside of nose with and without nasal decongestant
    - Key to exam
    - Strong light source
    - Nasal speculum
    - Vasoconstriction
    - Evaluate:
    - Nasal mucosa

- Size and position of turbinates
  - Hypertrophy (congenital vs. acquired)
- Position of septum
- In secondary cases check for residual septal cartilage
- Internal nasal valve for collapse or scarring
- Examine nose with breathing
  - Middle vault and alar rims for collapse
  - Get feedback from patient
  - Cottle maneuver in all patients
    - Asymptomatic patients will get some improvement
    - Symptomatic patients get dramatic improvement
- Examine Dorsum and upper 2/3 of nose
  - Dorsal height (often too low or too high)
  - Specific attention to location of radix
  - Deviation of nasal dorsum
  - Follow dorsal aesthetic lines
  - Width of dorsum
    - If too narrow may indicate internal nasal valve collapse
- Examine tip and lower 1/3 of nose
  - Check projection
    - Distance of nasal tip from face on lateral view
    - Overprojected tip appears large
    - Underprojected appears small
  - Check rotation
    - Position of tip to lip and face
    - Over-rotated
    - More obtuse columellar-labial angle
    - Increased nasal show from anterior view
    - Under-rotated
      - More acute columellar-labial angle
      - Droopy with undesirable amount of nostril show
  - Check tip support- difficult to quantify
    - Strength of medial crura and connection to septum
    - Evaluate by palpating tip for ease of displacement
- One or more tip defining points

- - -
    - ○ Symmetry comes from the paired lower lateral cartilages
    - ○ Boxy tip if superior asymmetry with poor tip definition
    - ○ Pinched tip if narrow angle at the domes
    - ○ Wide alar base may cause flaring
  - Examine the skin
    - ○ Thick vs. thin skin
    - ○ Thin skin postop irregularities may be more obvious
    - ○ Very thick skin
      - Rhinophyma may be better treated with skin treatments
    - ○ Fitzpatrick Classification
  - Anatomic features
    - ○ Nasal length (radix to tip) equal to stomion to menton distance
    - ○ Lip-chin relationship
      - Vertical line dropped from half nasal length tangential to vermillion of upper lip
      - Lower lip no more than 2mm behind this line
      - Discrepancies
        - Consider genioplasty vs. orthognathic surgery
  - Nasal features
    - ○ Frontal view
      - Nasal deviation address septum
      - Dorsum check aesthetic lines
      - Relationship bony base 80% normal alar base
      - Alar base 2mm wider than intercanthal distance (width of one eye)
        - Wide?
        - Increased interalar width- nostril sill resection
        - Alar flaring- alar base resection
      - Osteotomies narrow dorsum
      - Tip
        - Supratip break
        - Tip defining points
        - Columellar-lobular angle

- - Outline of alar rims and columella (resembles seagull)
  - Basal view
    - Teardrop-like geometry
    - Lobule to nostril ratio 1:2
  - Lateral view
    - Radix- position and depth of nasal root at nasofrontal angle
      - Apex between upper lid eyelashes and supratarsal fold
      - Ideal angle
        - 134 degrees female
        - 130 degrees male
  - Perceived nasal length and tip projection altered by position of nasofrontal angle
    - If anterior:
      - Nose appears elongated
      - Nasofacial angle decreased
      - Tip projection diminished
    - If posterior:
      - Nose shorter appearing
      - Tip more projecting
  - Tip projection
    - Draw line form alar-cheek junction to tip of nose
      - If 50-60% of line if anterior to a vertical line adjacent to most projecting part of lip then NORMAL projection
      - OVERPROJECTION- >60% of line anterior to reference line
      - UNDERPROJECTION- <50% of line anterior to reference line- augmentation needed
    - OR
    - Compare line drawn from alar base to alar base width
      - Should be equal
    - Compare ratio of nasal length (RT) to tip projection (alar base-to-tip)
      - Ideal tip projection 0.67 x RT

- Dorsum
  - Ideal nasal dorsum
    - 2mm behind and parallel to line from radix to tip-defining points in women
    - Slightly higher in men
- Supratip break
  - Check when nasal tip projection and dorsum evaluated
  - Slight tip break preferred in women not in men
  - Gives more definition, distinguishes dorsum from tip
- Tip rotation
  - Naso labial angle determines degree of tip rotation
  - Angle between line coursing through most anterior and posterior edges of nostril and plumb line dropped perpendicular to natural horizontal plane
    - 103-105 degrees in women
    - 95-100 degrees in men
- Alar-columellar relationship (lateral and frontal views)
  - Line drawn through long axis of nostril and a perpendicular line alar rim to columellar rim that bisects this axis
  - Assess columellar show
    - Increased
    - Decreased
- Features of Male Nose
  - More square
  - Less rounded appearance
  - Stronger more pronounced features
  - Dorsum straighter, wider
  - Decreased concavity at superciliary ridges
  - Nasal dorsal profile 1mm or less
  - No supratip break
  - Tip rotation slightly less (95-100 vs 103-105)
  - Less nostril show
  - Stronger chin abutting plumb line

- Broader, more bulbous, nasal tip
- Thicker skin

- Standard photos with eight views
    - Frontal
    - Lateral
    - Oblique
    - Lateral smiling
    - Worm's eye
- Document surgical plan, specific maneuvers that will address problems, used as guidelines.
- Rhinoplasty can be exploratory, modification to surgical plan may be needed.
- Plan on second consultation visit prior to surgery
- Consultations
    - No specific consultations needed
    - Consider ENT in severe medical airway patients.
- Consider computer imaging, no guarantee
- PRE-OP INSTRUCTIONS
    - No NSAID'S two week prior to surgery
    - No smoking 4 weeks before surgery
    - Notify surgeon if active cold sores before surgery

2. Consider reasonable goals in diagnosis and management *(Management and treatment, surgical indications, operative procedures and anesthesia)*

    - Know your personal limitations
    - Formulate specific plan before OR
        - Modify based on intraop findings
    - Review plan with patient before OR
    - Goals
        - Balanced harmonious nose in relation to the rest of the face
        - Functional nose (preserve function or improve with surgery)
    - Causes of poor results:
        - Poor evaluation of original problem
        - Poor execution of surgical plan
        - Misguided surgical planning
        - Patient misconception of the goal of rhinoplasty
    - INDICATIONS

- - Functional
    - Nasal airway obstruction (congenital, traumatic)
  - Reconstructive
    - Posttraumatic
    - Congenital
  - Cosmetic
    - Desire to change shape of nose
      - To change self-image
      - To create more nasal harmony
- ANATOMIC CONSIDERATIONS IN RHINOPLASTY
  - External skin and soft tissue
  - Underlying framework (bony and cartilaginous)
  - Ligamentous support
  - Relevant muscles
    - Levator labii alaeque nasi
      - Maintains patency of external nasal valve
    - Depressor septi nasi
      - Can alter upper lip length and tip projection
      - May require dissection and transposition
  - Enhances tip-lip relationship
  - Relative upper lip lengthening
  - Relative fullness to upper lip
  - Maintenance of tip rotation/projection on animation
  - Blood Supply
    - Branches of ophthalmic and facial arteries
    - In open approach columellar vessels are transected
      - Lateral nasal and dorsal arteries, remaining blood supply
    - AVOID extended alar resections which can injure the lateral nasal vessels
  - Caution with debulking nasal tip
  - Preserve musculoaponeurotic layer by supraperichondrial dissection
  - Nasal Vaults
    - Three:
      - Bony
      - Upper cartilaginous

- Lower cartilaginous
  - Keystone area:
    - Nasal bone overlap of upper lateral cartilages 4-6mm
  - Over-resection dorsal hump in upper cartilaginous vault
  - Result:
    - Inverted-V deformity OR
    - Disruption of dorsal aesthetic lines
    - Component dorsal septal reduction avoids this
- Septum
  - AVOID iatrogenic injury to cribriform plate during rhino can cause CSF leak
- Turbinates
  - Inferior turbinate greatest effect on nasal airflow
  - 2/3 total airway resistance
  - Over-resection:
    - Crust formation
    - Bleeding
    - Nasal cilia dysfunction
- Internal nasal valve
  - Can contribute up 50% of total airway resistance
  - Narrowest segment of nasal airway
  - Angle formed by:
    - Intersection of nasal septum
    - Caudal margin of upper lateral cartilage 10-15 degrees
  - Cottle test
    - Lateral traction on cheek
    - Diagnostic of collapse of internal nasal valve
    - Indicates need for spreader grafts
- External Nasal Valve
  - Caudal to internal nasal valve
  - Tx for obstruction:
    - Alar batten grafts
    - Lateral crural strut grafts
    - Lysis of adhesions

- Scar revision
- Mucosal grafts
- Skin grafts
- Composite grafts
        - Multiple surgical interventions available:
  - Open or closed rhinoplasty
  - Indications for Open:
    - Secondary rhinoplasty
    - Insufficient tip projection and columellar strut required
    - Spreader grafts easier to place (but can be done closed)
    - Disadvantage:
    - Loss of tip support
    - Increased and more prolonged post op edema
    - Anesthesia
      - Local
    - Pain control
    - Hemostasis
  - Major sensory nerves
    - Glabella (nasal branches supraorbital nerve V1)
    - Tip (external branch, anterior ethmoid V2 from ophthalmic nerve)
    - Alar base (infraorbital nerve V2)
    - Columella (nasal branches of infraorbital nerve V2)
    - Internal lateral mucosa (ant. ethmoid)
    - Internal medial mucosa (post. ethmoid)
  - Operative technique
    - 0.5% Lido with 1:200000 epi 3-5ml total
    - Oxymetazoline hydrochloride 0.05% (Afrin)
    - Toxic dose of Cocaine
    - IV antibiotics Ancef
    - General anesthetic
- COMMON ORDER OF RHINOPLASTY
  - Steps of open approach
    - Stair step incision at narrowest portion of columella
    - Lateral to medial along caudal border of lower lateral

- Medial to lateral transcolumellar incision to apex
- Double prong hooks and digital pressure to evert ala
- Skin envelope dissection
    - Meticulous
    - Supraperichondrial/submusculoaponeurotic plane
        - Avoid injuring arterial/venous/lymphatic blood supply to nose
    - Expose:
        - Dorsum
        - Upper lateral cartilage
        - Leave no soft tissue on lower laterals
        - On hump expose only areas that need to be addressed
- Dorsum
    - Address first if it requires lowering
    - Rasp or osteotome if greater reduction needed
    - Sequentially palpate to check for correct height
    - Err on undercorrection if necessary
    - Cartilaginous dorsum next
    - Septum reduced with paired lower lateral cartilages
        - Perform sequentially
- Septum
    - Address after dorsum reduced: Why?
        - If done first:
            - May leave insufficient dorsal cartilage for support
        - If dorsum rasped after septum it may dislocate the septal cartilage from the perpendicular plate resulting in loss of dorsal support
    - Long noses may require resection of caudal cartilage
    - Done prior to submucosal resection

- Need minimum of 1cm L strut for nasal support, more is preferable
- Part of vomer should be harvested to ensure optimum amount of cartilage is harvested
  - Dorsal augmentation
    - Septal cartilage is best
    - Crush edges with morselizer
    - Secondary cases use ear or rib cartilage
    - If dorsum is still deviated after submucosal resection
    - Then release caudal septum from maxilla and reposition with suture
  - Spreader grafts
    - Used to open up or preserve internal nasal valve
    - Fabricate from septal cartilage in the shape of a matchstick and suture into position
    - Can be used to give more pleasing dorsal aesthetic lines
    - Can camouflage nasal deviation
    - Can be placed asymmetrically if necessary to give straight appearance
  - Osteotomies
    - Three most common approaches:
      - Direct intranasal to piriform aperture
        - Simplest, no scar
        - Osteotome started on piriform aperture and directed cephalad
      - Gingivobuccal sulcus
      - Transcutaneous
    - In making osteotomy:
      - Feel nasal bones
      - Make osteotomy in a location where there will be a smooth transition from face of maxilla to nose
      - Gentle pressure to mobilize bone medially
    - Medial transverse osteotomies usually not needed
  - Manipulation of tip shape

- Goals refine and narrow external appearance
- Basic maneuvers:
  - Cephalic trim of lower laterals
  - Suture techniques for middle crura to help define nasal tip
- There is a learning curve
- Tip Projection
  - Columellar strut to increase
  - Placement w/i columella b/w lower laterals pushing on underlying maxilla
- Tip rotation
  - Increased by:
    - Columellar strut
    - Increased by resection of caudal septum
    - Resection of cephalic scrolls
    - Tip sutures
    - Resection of lateral crura
  - Decreased by:
    - Extended spreader grafts sutured to medial crura
    - Can deproject by dividing medial and lateral crura
- Ala
  - Change of position usually done to decrease circumference of nasal aperture
  - Must decide "What is the most objectionable portion of the nostril?"
    - Nasal sill
    - Ala
    - Internal nostril
    - External nostril
    - Combination
- POSTOP
  - Antibiotics
  - Analgesics
  - Nasal normal saline for postop congestion
  - Head of bed elevation
  - Drip pad
  - No nasal manipulation or sneezing through nose 3 weeks

- Splint 1 week
- No foods requiring excessive lip movements

3. Select appropriate options in diagnosis and management

- In this case I would select…?
- Tell why?
- Specify areas that should be addressed and how…
- What technique would be used…?
- Open or closed and sequence of operation
- Approach and plan should be based on anatomic findings in scenario photo.
- INCISIONAL APPROACHES AND OPERATIVE TECHNIQUE
    - Open vs. Closed
        - Open
            - Preference stair step incision
                - Why?
                - Facilitates reapproximation
                - Breaking up scar prevents contracture
            - Excellent exposure and control
            - Direct visualization
            - Minimal negative consequences
            - Predictable results and negligible external scar
            - Best approach for:
                - Secondary rhinoplasty
                - Posttraumatic deformity
                - Cleft lip nose deformity
                - Complex tip modification
        - Closed
            - Best for isolated deformity of dorsum or minor tip modification
    - Options
    - Delivery vs. Nondelivery
        - Delivery
            - Intercartilaginous incision
            - Marginal incision (1mm cephalad to caudal margin of lateral crus)
            - Transfixion/hemitransfixion incision

- - - Subsequent transposition of lower lateral cartilages outside skin envelope
  - Nondelivery
    - Transcartilaginous incision (several mm cephalad to caudal margin of lateral/medial crura) OR
    - Eversion (retrograde) incision with lower laterals in native position
    - Osseocartiaginous framework work carried out skin envelope not reflected as in open approach
  - Skin envelope elevation
- REDUCING OSTEOCARTILAGINOUS HUMP
  o Component fashion
  o Four steps:
    - Separation of upper lateral cartilage (ULC) from septum
      - Elevate mucoperichondrium from dorsal septum
      - Preserve mucosa
      - Spreader grafts can be placed if needed
    - Incremental reduction of septum proper
      - Trim septum by serial shave
      - Reduce upper laterals if needed
        o Minimal trim of ULC minimizes deformity
        o Overresection
          - Internal nasal collapse
          - Dorsal nasal deformity
    - Incremental dorsal bony reduction (using rasp)
      - Large hump >5mm power burr or guarded 8mm osteotome
      - Small hump <5mm down biting rasp
    - Three-point palpation test
      - Redrape skin

- Moisten fingers with saline
- Palpate, visualize, assess
- Performed repeatedly to assess dorsal aesthetic lines, detect irregularities or contour depression
- SEPTAL RECONSTRUCTION/CARTILAGE GRAFT HARVEST
    - For deformed septum or first choice cartilage harvest if available
    - Closed approach
        - Killian or hemitransfixition incision
        - Avoids decreased tip projection
    - Open approach
        - Separate middle crura and expose anterior septal angle
        - Incise perichondrium
        - Elevate mucosa in submucoperichondrial plane posterior to perpendicular plate to nasal floor
        - Caution at cartilaginous and bony septum junction
        - Same dissection on both sides
        - Swivel knife or 15 blade harvest cartilage
        - PRESERVE L-STRUT
            - DORSAL SEPTUM 10MM (Minimum)
            - CAUDAL SEPTUM 10MM (Minimum)
        - Preserve in saline
        - Rongeur or resect residual deformity
        - Repair mucosal perforations
- INFERIOR TURBINOPLASTY
    - Consider if hypertrophy present and airway obstruction refractory to medical management
    - Options:
        - Turbinate outfracture
        - Conservative composite tissue removal and cauterization
        - Submucous morselization of turbinate bone
        - Submucous resection anterior 1/3 to 1/2 inferior turbinate
            - Develop mucoperiosteal flaps

- Expose conchal bone
- CEPHALIC TRIM
    - If tip boxy or bulbous
        - Needs refinement and definition
        - Tip rotation needed
    - PRESERVE 6 mm strip
- SPREADER GRAFTS
    - Avoids inverted V deformity or saddle nose deformity
    - Stents internal nasal valve
    - Stabilizes septum
    - Preserves dorsal nasal lines
    - Size: 25-30mm by 3mm
    - Fit underneath bony dorsum
        - Place at septal angle if no lengthening needed
        - Extended spreader if lengthening desired
    - Secure with 5-0 PDS or other suture of choice
- TIP MODIFICATION
    - KEY ANATOMIC ELEMENTS
        - Supporting ligament between anterior septal angle and overlying dermis
        - Length and strength of lower lateral cartilage
        - Suspensory ligament bridging anterior septal angle
        - Fibrous connections between upper and lower lateral cartilages and septum
        - Abutment of cartilages with piriform aperture
        - Anterior septal angle
- INCREASED PROJECTION
    - Ideally- precise, incremental and nondestructive
    - Algorithm
        - Suture modification (increase projection 1-2mm)
            - Natural fibrotic reaction will solidify result
        - Open technique best exposure
    - Techniques
        - Medial crural sutures- unify medial crura of LLC

- Can be used with columellar strut
- Option to straighten out flaring of medial/middle crura
- Medial crural septal sutures
    - Anchor crura to septum, alters projection
- Interdomal sutures
    - Placed in medial walls of domes in mattress
    - Narrow interdomal distance
    - Increases tip refinement and projection
- Transdomal sutures
    - Placed across dome of middle crura, mattress
    - Corrects anatomic asymmetries
    - Place on each LLC then tied to each other
    - Can narrow tip defining points
- Columellar struts
    - Septal or other cartilage can be used
    - Size: 25mmx4mm
    - Fixed (secured to anterior maxilla)
    - OR
    - Floating (not secured)
    - Bolsters tip
    - Placement via pocket between medial crura
    - Secure with 25 gauge wire until suture placement
    - Horizontal mattress
- Tip grafts
    - Use if prior more predictable methods do not result in satisfactory tip projection
        o Onlay tip graft (shield or umbrella graft)
        o Infratip lobular graft
        o Columellar tip graft
        o Combination graft

- DECREASED PROJECTION
  - Primary means:
    - Alter LLC via open approach
    - Transection, setback and resuturing medial or lateral crura
  - Avoid or correct resulting alar flare or columellar bowing

- ALTERING TIP ROTATION
  - Evaluate using nasolabial angle
    - Line through most anterior to posterior edges of nostril and plumb line from natural horizontal facial plane
    - 95-100 women and 90-95 men
  - Techniques:
    - Cephalic trim- separation of ULC from LLC
    - Caudal septal resection- Release fibrous attachments of medial crura and caudal septum
    - Adjunct- limited nasal mucosal resection to maintain harmony
    - After rotation:
      - Maintain position with suture techniques
        - Medial crural septal sutures and/or
        - Columellar strut or septal extension graft

- NOSTRIL SHOW
- ALAR-COLUMELLAR RELATIONSHIP
  - Think about BC AC relationship (line on long axis of nostril, and line from alar rim to columellar rim)
  - Class I- Hanging Columella >2mm from long axis
    - Resect caudal septum
    - Resect portion of medial crus
    - Resect caudal portion of middle crus
    - Combination
  - Class II- Retracted ala > 2mm from long axis
    - Insert elliptically shaped composite graft from vestibular skin access incision
    - Mild with no tissue deficiency- release lateral crura from accessory chain

- Alar contour graft
- o Class III- hanging columella and retracted ala
  - Use combo of above techniques
- o Class IV- hanging ala <1mm from long axis
  - Elliptical excision of vestibular skin AVOID overresection
- o Class V- retracted columella <1mm from long axis
  - Columellar strut
- o Class VI- Combination
  - Combination of above
- OSTEOTOMY TECHNIQUES
  - o INDICATIONS
    - To narrow lateral walls of nose
    - Close open roof deformity (after dorsal hump resection)
    - Create symmetry by straightening nasal bony framework
  - o CONTRAINDICATIONS
    - Short nasal bones
    - Elderly with thin, fragile nasal bones
    - Heavy eyeglasses
  - o TECHNIQUES
    - Medial
    - Lateral
      - Low to high
      - Low to low
      - Double level
    - Transverse
    - Approach (internal or external)
  - o ALWAYS PRESERVE Webster's Triangle
    - Triangular area on caudal aspect of frontal maxillary segment near internal valve
    - It supports valve and prevents nasal obstruction from collapse
  - o Goals
    - Smooth fracture line without step off
    - Cephalic margin not higher than intercanthal line (medial canthal ligament)
    - Avoid iatrogenic injury to lacrimal system
  - o Lateral Osteotomy
    - Low to high Osteotomy
      - Corrects small open roof deformity

- Mobilizes medium-wide nasal base
- Starts at piriform aperture and ends on dorsum
- Low to low Osteotomy
  - Large open roof deformity
  - Correct wide bony base
  - Starts low and stays low
  - Often may need medial Osteotomy to mobilize better
- Medial Osteotomy
  - Facilitates medial positioning
  - Indicated in thick nasal bones or wide bony base
  - Usually performed before lateral osteotomy
  - AVOID placing too central
  - Cephalic margin should not cross intercanthal line

- CLOSURE
  - Skin 5-0 nylon
  - Vestibular incisions 5-0 chromic
  - Intranasal splint to prevent synechiae
  - Dorsal splint (plaster or technique of choice)
  - Tape
  - Drip pad
- ALAR BASE SURGERY
  - Performed after closure prior to splint placement
  - Corrects:
    - Wide or excessive nostril sills
    - Wide alar base
    - Asymmetric or malpositioned alar bases
  - Wide nostril sills (alar flaring)
    - Small crescentic resection of alar base
    - Avoid extension into sill
    - Incision 1-2mm above base to avoid notching
  - Wide alar base
    - Crescentic excision, wedge like includes small portion of sill

4. Understand risks and benefits of various approaches

- Have familiarity with risks and benefits of various techniques

- o Scarring
- o Effect on airway
- o Potential residual deformity
- o Mobidity of donor sites
- o Other
   - When would you use one technique over another? Why?
   - Describe interventions available to minimize the risk of complications

5. Address complications and unexpected problems adequately

   - Overresection of dorsum
     - o Possibly secondary to edema formation during procedure
     - o Secondary cartilage graft required to augment
   - Crooked dorsum
     - o Inaccurate judgment during procedure
     - o To minimize chance of shifting
       - Pack 1 to 2 days
       - Splint 1 or 2 weeks
     - o If deviated require repeat osteotomy
   - Collapse of external valve
     - o Occurs on inspiration due to insufficient support of nasal rim
     - o Overresection of lower lateral cartilage
     - o Cartilage graft needed to correct to provide support
   - Obstruction of airflow through internal nasal angle
     - o Secondary to scarring at the angle
     - o Correct with spreader grafts either at primary surgery or secondary surgery
   - Rhinoplasty revision rate: 1 in 30
     - o Reasons
       - Further tip refinement or tip asymmetry
       - Parrot beak or pinched supratip deformity
       - Excessive dorsal reduction or dorsal irregularities
   - Infection rare
     - o Toxic shock syndrome
       - Management
       - Use antibiotics
       - Early packing removal
   - Hematoma

- Temporary/permanent numbness
- Rare
    - Anosmia
    - Lacrimal duct injury

6. Demonstrate ability to structure alternative plan

    - Be prepared to manage complications
    - Inadequate correction- did you miss something?
    - Unsatisfied, belligerent or litigious patient
    - Patient doesn't agree with your proposed operative plan
    - Preferred donor site for cartilage grafts if septum not available
    - Roll for alloplastic materials in rhinoplasty?

Chapter Forty

Genioplasty

40
Genioplasty

1. Identify General Problem/Diagnosis/Planning
   (Describe photo, give working diagnosis, key problems, evaluates patient)

   - Analyze photo and describe all findings as in cosmetic face patients
   - PRINCIPLES
     - Labiomental groove
       - 4mm in women
       - 6mm in men
     - Riedel's plane
       - Line drawn by connecting most projecting portion of upper and lower lips
       - Should touch most projected portion of chin
     - Anatomy
       - Canine tooth longest tooth (25.5mm in length)
       - Horizontal osteotomies 5mm caudal to canine to avoid injury (30.5mm)
       - Osteotomy location 5mm caudal to mental foramen to reduce risk of injury to mental nerve.
       - Mental foramen located in a plane between 1st and 2nd premolar
       - Deep labiomental groove and Class II Occlusion
         - Benefit most from Orthognathic surgery compared to genioplasty
       - Intraoral incisions
         - 1cm anterior (labial) to gingivolabial sulcus to maintain soft tissue for closure (important to leave a good cuff for closure)
     - Genioplasty
       - Implant preferred in older patients
       - Genioplasty preferred in younger patients
     - Angle II or III malocclusion

- Orthognathic surgery in addition to or instead of genioplasty
    - Augmentation genioplasty
        - Use submental incision reduces risk of:
            - Infection
            - Cephalic migration
            - Wound dehiscence
    - Complications treated with implant removal
    - Chin affects lower third of face:
        - May be vertically deficient or excessive OR
        - Horizontally deficient or excessive
- MOST IMPORTANT IN RELATION TO THE NOSE
    - Large nose frequently has deficient chin
    - Improvements are via implants, grafts for augmentation OR
    - Osseous procedures
        - Burr reduction
        - Osteotomy with caudal segment repositioning
        - Osteotomy with grafting
        - Osteotomy with segmental sectioning
    - Problems with alloplastic augmentation
        - Limited correction in large augmentation without lip retraction
        - Lower success in symmetry
        - Limited in vertical dimensional correction
- ANATOMY
    - In horizontal osteotomy
        - Blood supply maintained by terminal lingual artery periosteal perforating branches that travel through musculature on lingual side.
    - Mental Nerve
        - Sensation to anterior mandibular gingival, mucosa and lower lip
- PE
    - As in cosmetic patient
    - Focus on:
        - Cardinal determinants
            - Projection symmetry and vertical length
        - Chin symmetry

- (vertical line from midglabella, tip of nose, philtral dimple)
- Midpoint of chin should fall on this line
      - Maxillary vs. mandibular disharmony or chin itself
      - In pure genial asymmetry- genioplasty will address this
    - Check vertical dimension in frontal view analysis
    - Check horizontal excess or deficiency in profile view
    - Use Riedel's line for ideal chin projection
    - Labiomental groove
      - 4mm women
      - 6mm men
    - Deep groove generally not amenable to augmentation alone
  - MUST CHECK INTRAORAL EXAM FOR OCCLUSION
    - What is maxillary/mandibular occlusal relationship?
    - Periodontal disease?
  - Life-size photo with soft tissue cephalometric analysis

2. Consider reasonable goals in diagnosis and management *(Management and treatment, surgical indications, operative procedures and anesthesia)*

   - INDICATIONS AND CONTRAINDICATIONS
     - Genioplasty addresses chin disharmony does not replace orthognathic surgery
     - Augmentation genioplasty
       - Best serves
         - Older pt (>60) with mild to moderate horizontal defect
         - Osseous procedures can be used
       - Must be conservative in long face deformities who do not want maxillary intrusion
       - Contraindicated in poor surgical candidates
         - (Diabetes, immunodeficiency)
       - Avoid if it will not sufficiently correct dysmorphology
       - Avoid implants in smokers

- Most other patients should have osseous genioplasty
- Classification of chin deformity (Types I-VII)
- Type dictates procedure
- Group I- Macrogenia
  - Horizontal/Vertical/Combo
    - Tx:
    - Mild to moderate burr
    - Moderate to severe- setback
    - Pure vertical- horizontal block or wedge
    - Combo
- Group II- Microgenia
  - Horizontal/Vertical/Combo Tx:
    - Mild to moderate horizontal augmentation
    - Horizontal osteotomy with advancement of caudal segment
    - Pure vertical- horizontal osteotomy and caudal repositioning
- Group III- Combined Macro/microgenia
  - Combination
  - Horizontal excess/vert deficiency- horizontal osteo caudal and posterior repositioning
  - Vertical excess/Horizontal deficit- two osteotomies remove anterior wedge caudal segment advanced cephalically, graft gap
- Group IV- asymmetric chin
  - Avoid alloplast
  - Wedge osteotomies
- Group V- pseudomacrogenia
  - Excess soft tissue gives appearance
  - Reduce via submental incision
- Group VI- pseudomicrogenia
  - From vertical maxillary excess and clockwise rotation of mandible
  - Orthognathic surgery
- Group VII- Witch's chin soft tissue ptosis
  - Excise soft tissue via submental incision
- Postop

- o Antibiotics
- o Avoid heavy exercise 3 weeks
- o Foam type compressive tape dressing removed in 2-3 days

3. Select appropriate options in diagnosis and management
Operative technique

- Ostectomy- reduction genioplasty
    - Excess horizontal dimension
    - Local or general
    - 4cm submental incision or intra oral incision
    - Leave 1cm cuff of mucosa
    - Visualize mental nerve and protect
    - Burr incrementally ½ at a time
    - Use irrigation to avoid thermal damage to bone
    - Bone excised primarily in central region and tapered laterally
    - Repair mentalis during closure
  - o Osteotomy with caudal segment repositioning
    - Intraoral approach
    - Osteotomy 5mm caudal to projected canine roots, 5mm caudal to mental foramen
    - Wide blade centrally, narrow laterally
    - Prefabricated step plate contour
    - 2 screws on each side of osteotomy
    - Can use wire
  - o Augmentation
    - Implant silicone and porous polyethylene
    - Place subperiosteally in all cases
      - Prevents
        - o Soft tissue injury
        - o Dimpling and migration
    - Place over denser portion of bone to minimize erosion
    - Soft tissue response 0.8 to 1.0
    - Submental incision preferred
      - 0.5cm anterior to submental crease
      - Local
      - Pocket made just large enough to accommodate implant

4. Understand risks and benefits of various approaches

    - Be able to compare risks benefits of various approaches based on presented deformity.

5. Address complications and unexpected problems adequately

    - Genioplasty Complications rare
    - Wound dehiscence and infection
        - Tx:
        - Usually will close spontaneously if no loose or exposed hardware
        - Debride oral antibiotics
    - Hematoma
        - Drain to prevent abscess
        - Infection increases risk of resorption
        - Antibiotics used postop
    - Tooth devitalization
        - Take precautions
    - Dental root exposure
        - Manifests as caudal retraction of gingival, painful exposure of sensitive portion of teeth
        - May require gingival grafting
    - Neurosensory loss
        - Temporary in most cases
        - Permanent loss no recovery after 1 year
        - Exploration and neurorrhaphy
    - Soft tissue ptosis
        - Excise excess tissue via submental incision
    - Asymmetry
        - Most commonly missed preop asymmetry
        - Mild observe
        - More severe consider correction
        - If significant correct prior to osseous union
    - Over- or Under-correction
        - Faulty planning
        - Imprecise surgical enactment
        - Revision osteotomy
    - Irregularities and step-type deformities
        - Revise as appropriate

- Lower lip retraction
    - Loss of lower lip support
    - Improper mentalis repair
    - Resuspend through intraoral incision
- Augmentation complications
- Dehiscence
    - Leads to exposed implant
    - Remove implant
    - Oral antibiotics 5-7 days
- Extrusion
    - Remove implant
    - Antibiotics
    - Residual deformity treat with osteoplastic genioplasty
- Infection
    - Rare in absence of exposure
- Malposition/dislodgement
    - Remove and osseous genioplasty
- Bone resorption
    - More common with nonporous implants
    - Avoid or minimize by caudal placement of implant
- Capsular contracture
    - Almost exclusively in smooth implants
    - Remove implant, capsulectomy, osseous genioplasty
- Lower Lip Retraction
- Inadequate soft tissue closure and coverage following intraoral incision
- Common error inadequate tissue left at sulcus for closure

6. Demonstrate ability to structure alternative plan

- Have multiple options of treatment. Back-up plan for failure or complications.

Chapter Forty-One

Secondary Rhinoplasty

41
Secondary Rhinoplasty

- COMMON DEFORMITIES TO ADDRESS
  - Supra-tip deformity
    - Under-resected or over-resected caudal dorsum with resultant scar tissue
    - Postop loss of tip projection
  - Inverted V deformity
  - Inadequate tip projection
  - Alar rim retraction
- CONSIDERATIONS
  - Patient concerns
    - Aesthetic
    - Functional
  - Require longer consultation time
  - Refer to previous surgeon?
  - Check operative records
    - Septal availability
    - Turbinectomy performed?
  - Is facial disharmony contributing to problems?
    - Forehead prominence
    - Chin deformities
    - Hypoplasia malar bones
    - Dysmorphic maxilla, mandible
  - Focused Physical Exam
    - Skin quality
    - Previous incisions (generally can ignore)
    - Telangiectasia will be more pronounced
    - Note all deformities present
- INDICATIONS AND CONTRAINDICATIONS
  - Wait one year in general before reoperating
  - May always be unpredictable factors that can affect result
  - Informed consent
  - Potential graft use
  - Recognize and identify imperfections
- TECHNIQUES
  - Revision generally requires open rhino approach except for minor revision

- - - Skin usually safe to re-elevate, slight delay phenomenon
  - ALTERATION OF RADIX
    - Under-corrected radix
      - Remove bone with guarded burr
      - Incrementally lower radix
  - DORSAL HUMP
    - Residual hump
      - Easily removed with rasp
      - Osteotome more likely to cause problems in re-do nose
      - If too wide after removal
        - May need unplanned osteotomy
    - Septal harvest after hump reduction to preserve dorsal strut
  - NASAL BONE OSTEOTOMY
    - Lateral depressions
    - Camouflage with cartilage or fat graft
    - In cases of difficulty breathing may need to out-fracture nasal bones
  - DORSAL DEFICIENCY
    - Depression from over resection common in secondary rhino of midvault
      - Correct with cartilage graft
        - Septum first choice
        - Conchal cartilage second choice
      - Suture to dorsum
  - CARTILAGE HARVEST
    - Conchal cartilage graft harvest
      - Tattoo
      - Posterior incision
      - Leave support for frame
    - Costal cartilage harvest
      - Submammary or anterior chest incision
      - Split rectus muscle
      - Expose 5th or 6th rib
      - Avoid pleural tear
      - Valsalva maneuver after harvest
      - Take 6cm segment
      - Avoid warping
  - CORRECTION INVERTED V-DEFORMITY AND NASAL COLLAPSE

- Collapse of ULC causes inverted V-deformity
  - Nasal function affected
  - Aesthetic deformity
- Mild deformity
  - Correct with spreader graft
  - Thickness dependent on internal valve collapse
- Moderate deformity requires splay graft
  - Splay graft spans the anterior septum from posterior extent of one ULC to the opposite side
- ADJUSTMENT CAUDAL DORSUM
- SUPRA-TIP DEFOMITY
  - Caudal dorsum appears over-projected from inadequate resection
    - Recontour while maintaining mucoperichondrium over caudal nasal vault intact
  - Avoid dead space for hematoma collection which can cause recurrent deformity
    - Supra-tip suture prevents
    - Over-resection increases risk of recurrence (Increased dead space)
- TIP REFINEMENT
  - Use standard techniques
- LATERAL CRURA STRUT
  - Can correct collapse of lower lateral cartilage
  - Placed under surface of existing LLC from maxilla to ipsilateral dome
- PROTRUDING COLUMELLA
  - Rectangular caudal resection
- COLUMELLAR STRUT
  - Corrects short columella 2cm long 3mm wide
  - Causes cephalic rotation of tip
  - Caudal projection of subnasale
  - Increase in tip projection
- TIP GRAFT
  - For deficient lobule or inadequate tip projection
  - Onlay or shield type tip graft are used
  - Can give nasal elongation for over-shortened nose
- FOOTPLATES
  - Widened displaced or asymmetric

- o Under-projected-tip and splayed footplates
  - ▪ Approximation of foot plates will strengthen the tip support and narrow base of columella
- ▪ RETRACTED ALAR RIM
  - o If minimal
- ▪ Alar rim graft (3mm wide, 1mm or less thick, 8-10mm long) Placed in pocket along alar rim
  - o V-Y flap may be needed in severe cases
  - o Two stents to hold in place
- ▪ ALAR BASE ABNORMALITIES
  - o Use standard techniques
- ▪ SHORT NOSTRIL
  - o Increased by alar rim graft
  - o Columellar strut
  - o Narrowing footplate
  - o If no osteotomy splint not needed
  - o Stents used in extensive secondary or primary septoplasty with secondary rhinoplasty

EXTREMETIES

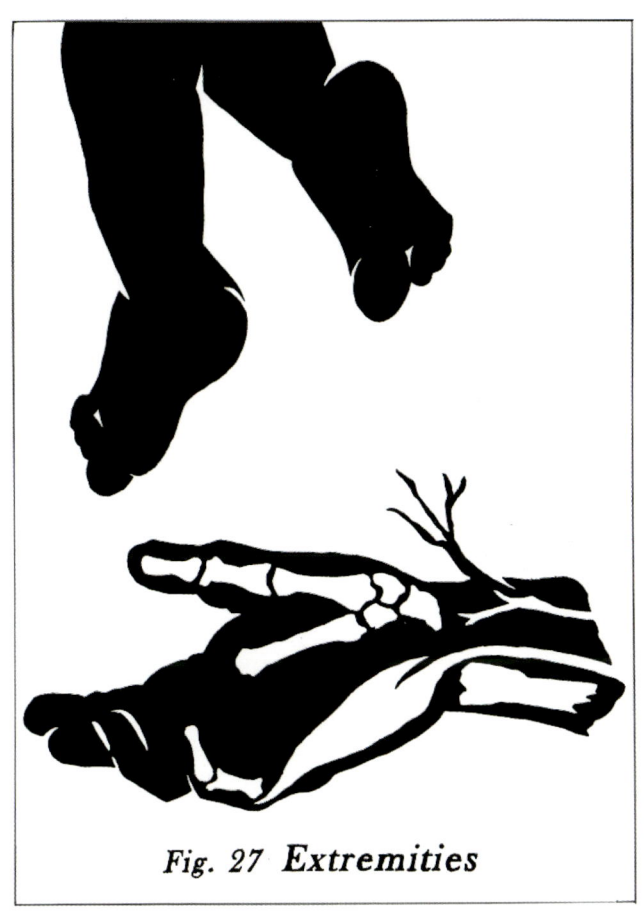

Fig. 27 *Extremities*

Section Nine
Lower Extremity

Chapter Forty-Two

Lower Extremity Overview

42
Lower Extremity Overview

1. Identify General Problem

   - Describe photo
   - Give working diagnosis
   - Key problems
   - Evaluate patient
   - Diagnosis/Planning
   - Classify defect
     - Upper leg, Middle leg, Lower leg, Ankle, Heel, Foot
   - Determine etiology of wound
     - Trauma, Tumor, Chronic, Diabetes, Infection
   - What is missing?
   - Length of time present
     - Acute, Subacute, Chronic wound
   - Note patient age and medical status
     - PVD, DM, Anticoagulants, Steroids
   - In trauma cases:
     - Go through ABC's of trauma management
     - Brief relevant medical and surgical history
     - Control airway, bleeding, resuscitation
     - Fracture type (Gustilo classification)
   - Need for additional work-up
     - Consultants, Imaging studies, Angiography

2. Consider reasonable goals in diagnosis and management

   - Management and treatment
   - Surgical indications
   - Operative procedures and anesthesia
   - Surgical goals
     - Preservation of length
     - Preservation of function
     - Optimal ambulation
   - Amputation last resort unless:
     - Gross contamination, Farm injury, Severe crush injury
   - Timing of intervention

- What type of coverage is needed?
- Can hardware be removed at this time?

3. Select appropriate options in diagnosis and management

    - Surgical options
    - Give your surgical choice and treatment plan and why?
    - Post-op management
    - Drains
    - PT/OT
    - Anticipated time to full weight bearing
    - What are you trying to achieve?
    - Goal of therapy?
    - How is procedure performed?
    - Key steps of surgery
    - Markings and relevant anatomy

4. Understand risks and benefits of various approaches

    - Discuss risks, benefits in regard to:
        - Choice of operation, timing, donor site choice
    - Your anticipated outcome?

5. Address complications and unexpected problems adequately

    - Be prepared to manage:
        - Failing free flap
        - Flap loss
        - Local wound complications
        - Osteomyelitis
        - Intra-op problems
    - Explain why any complication may have occurred
        - Eg. inadequate debridement, anastomosis in zone of injury

6. Demonstrate ability to structure alternative plan

    - Lifeboat or back-up plan for failed flap
    - Timing of next intervention
    - Cross-leg flap is your friend
    - Amputation intervention of last resort except for grossly contaminated wound

Chapter Forty-Three

Lower Extremity Trauma and Reconstruction

43
Lower Extremity Trauma and Reconstruction

1. Identify General Problem Diagnosis/Planning
   (Describe photo, give working diagnosis, key problems, evaluates patient)

   - In trauma: number one priority:
     Salvage the patient not necessarily the limb
   - ATLS protocol
   - ABC's
   - Rule out life threatening injuries to head/chest/abd
   - History:
   - Age- No absolute criteria for intervention
     o Children better nerve injury recovery
     o Elderly may not tolerate extensive procedures
   - Time of injury
     o Lengthy time (>4-6 hours)
     o Consider:
       - Tissue damage and wound colonization
       - Muscle ischemia
       - Fasciotomy may be needed
   - Mechanism
     o Crush vs. laceration
     o May affect surgical options
   - Compartment syndrome
     o High suspicion in closed injuries
     o Need for fasciotomies
     o Classic Signs
       - Pain out of proportion to exam
       - Pain on passive flexion or extension
       - Palpably swollen or tense compartment
       - Poikylothermia
       - Absence of pulses (late sign)
       - Paresthesia's (late sign)
     o Check compartment pressures
       - Stryker or zeroed central venous pressure-line set up

- Pressure 12-20mmHg can observe and repeat
- Pressure >20mmHg consider fasciotomy
- Pressure >30mmHg emergent fasciotomy
- COMPARTMENTS OF THE LEG
  - Anterior
  - Lateral
  - Superficial posterior
  - Deep posterior
  - Be able to draw compartments of the leg
- Medical hx
  - Preexisting peripheral vascular disease
  - Diabetes
    - Higher morbidity
    - Equal mortality
    - Free flap results equivalent to nondiabetics
  - Smoking
    - Adverse effect on outcomes
- PE
- Wound location
  - Thigh easier to manage than distal leg
  - Distal leg has a paucity of muscle and soft tissue
- Extent of soft tissue injury
  - Amount of necrotic tissue
  - Free tissue transfer in larger defects >25cm^2
- Gustilo Classification of Wound (Type I-IIIC)
  - I- open fx wound <1cm
  - II- open fx wound >1cm
  - III- open fx + extensive soft tissue injury
    - III A- Open fx with adequate soft tissue coverage
    - III B- Open fx with tissue loss, periosteal stripping or bone exposure
    - III C- Open fx with arterial injury requiring repair
- Classify traumatic lower extremity injury
- Amount of dead space
- What is exposed in the wound? What is missing?
  - Hardware
  - Bone

- o Tendon
- o Vessels
- o Skin
- o Muscle
- Will need reliable coverage to achieve healing and prevent infection.
- Distal pulses palpable?
  - o Vessels may be in spasm or kinked secondary to injury
    - Reduce fracture, check for return of pulses
    - **Rule out posterior knee dislocation**
      - Prone to disruption of popliteal vessels
      - Vascular emergency
  - o Check with doppler
  - o Angiogram may be needed:
    - Severely mangled extremity
    - Free flap needed for reconstruction
- DISTAL SENSATION CRITICAL
  - o **Loss of posterior tibial nerve function**
    - Absent sensation plantar aspect of foot
    - RELATIVE CONTRAINDICATION FOR LOWER EXTREMITY SALVAGE
  - o Posterior tibial nerve disruption
    - Loss of plantar flexion of foot, facilitates step-off during ambulation
    - Devastating loss is plantar sensation, results in:
      - Loss of position sense
      - Risk of chronic injury/wounds
  - o Peroneal nerve disruption
    - Foot drop
    - Loss of sensation dorsum of foot- minimal morbidity
    - Not crippling but morbid
    - Management:
      - Lifelong foot splinting
      - Tendon transfers
- NERVE GRAFT IN LOWER EXTREMITY RESULTS GENERALLY POOR
  - o Long distance spinal cord to motor end plate, end organ atrophy

- Work-up
  - Plain x-rays for bony injury pattern
  - Angiography indications:
    - If suspected disruption of blood supply or
    - Free flap anticipated
  - Can consider noninvasive angiography
    - MR or CT angiogram- may not be available emergently
  - On the table angio acceptable in trauma scenario
- Consults
  - Trauma for management of concomitant injuries
  - Ortho for stabilization of fracture
  - Vascular for major arterial injury
  - Other as appropriate
    - Polytrauma
    - Other medical conditions?

2. Consider reasonable goals in diagnosis and management *(Management and treatment, surgical indications, operative procedures and anesthesia)*

- Indications for coverage with vascularized soft tissue
  - Extensive periosteal stripping
  - Comminution
  - Marrow obliteration
- ACUTE INJURY MANAGEMENT
- Stabilize fracture, may require external fixation (ex fix)
- Restore inflow if required
- Four compartment fasciotomy
  - Incisions ankle to knee
  - Medial and lateral
  - Release all compartments
- Debridement washout (all devitalized tissue must go!)
  - Vascular exposure immediate coverage
  - No vascular exposure repeat debridement
  - Inadequate debridement can lead to infection
- Goals of treatment:
- Preserve a limb that will be more functional than an amputation.
- If salvage not possible optimize length especially in regard to knee joint

- Below knee amputation (BKA) if knee salvageable
  - Ideal BKA 6cm stump of tibia, but any length acceptable to make BKA possible.
  - BKA decreased work of ambulation
    - 25% increased energy and O2 consumption vs. 65% in above knee amputation (AKA)
- Severe mangled extremity will require multiple operative procedures, months to years before weight bearing attained.
- INDICATIONS FOR SALVAGE
  - Pediatric patients
  - Adult with preserved plantar sensation
  - Reasonable hope of ambulation within 1 year
- ABSOLUTE INDICATION FOR PRIMARY AMPUTATION
  - Crush injury with warm ischemia time >6 hours
  - Severe, gross contamination, eg. Farm injury
- RELATIVE INDICATIONS FOR PRIMARY AMPUTATION
  - Serious associated polytrauma
  - Unstable patient cannot tolerate prolonged salvage operations
  - Severe ipsilateral foot trauma
  - Anticipated protracted course to obtain soft tissue coverage and tibial reconstruction
  - Segmental tibial fractures
  - Multiple zones of injury
  - Transection of posterior tibial nerve
- Consider AMPUTATION if two or more present:
  - 3 or more fascial compartments involved
  - Two or more injured tibial vessels
  - Failed vascular reconstruction
  - Cadaveric foot at initial examination
  - Severe muscle crush injury or muscle tissue loss
- Initial treatment (tx):
  - Antibiotics
    - Pseudomonas and Klebsiella most common pathogens
  - Tetanus
  - Debridement with pulse lavage
  - Skeletal stabilization ASAP
- If other life threatening injuries:

- o Limit extremity management to:
  - Stabilization of extremity
  - Control of bleeding
  - Consider amputation in unstable patient
- Orthopaedic Tx
- Closed treatment
  - o For low-energy, closed wounds
- Ex Fix
  - o Ideal for severely traumatized lower extremity with massive soft tissue and bone injury
  - o Gives rigid fixation without additional soft tissue injury, minimal bone devascularization
  - o Ilizarov technique may be used for bone gaps >6cm or
  - o Left in place after cancellous or vascularized bone grafting
- Internal fixation
  - o Faster union time
  - o Lower malunion rate
  - o Intramedullary nailing
    - Useful only for minimally comminuted fractures without significant bone loss
    - Reamed nails obliterate entire endosteal blood supply by stripping out medullary canal
    - Not indicated in massive trauma
    - Risk of progressive infection
- Options for bone gap
  - o Nonvascularized cancellous bone graft defects up to 10cm under vascularized muscle flaps
  - o Intact fibula facilitates bone grafting of long defects
  - o Free fibula, iliac crest, scapula for longer defects
  - o Vascularized bone graft for defects 6cm or greater
    - Up to 15 months for stable union
  - o Ilizarov (Distraction osteogenesis) may be used in defects >10cm
- TIMING OF SOFT TISSUE COVERAGE
  - o Determined by need to cover vital structures
  - o Early coverage lower complication rate (within 5-6 days)
  - o More complications in open tibial fractures allowed to progress to subacute phase (1-6weeks post injury)

- Options
  - Serial debridements may be necessary
  - Control of wound colonization or infection
    - Antibiotic coverage based on cultures
  - Flap donor sites outside zone of injury
  - Vacuum assisted closure devices uses:
    - Temporize wound until definitive coverage
    - Salvage flap loss
    - Treatment for patients in whom free flap contraindicated
  - Tissue expansion
    - High failure rate in lower extremity
    - Generally not indicated in acute injuries
    - May be useful in non-acute reconstruction
    - Not an ideal choice in the lower extremity
- MANAGEMENT BY ANATOMIC REGION
  - Thigh
  - Local tissue advancement usually available
    - Large anterior thigh muscles may fill defects
    - Rectus femoris flap
    - Tensor fascia lata
  - Proximal third of leg
    - Medial gastrocnemius flap frequently best option
      - Proximal pedicle and broad muscle belly, larger than lateral
      - Originates on tibia inserts into calcaneus via Achilles tendon
      - Increase reach by release from origin on tibia
      - No functional deficit
    - Lateral gastrocnemius flap
      - Useful for lateral knee defects
      - AVOID injury to peroneal nerve during harvest
      - No functional deficit
  - Middle third of leg
    - Soleus flap frequently best option
      - Arises from tibia, inserts in calcaneus as part of Achilles tendon
    - Medial or lateral gastroc flap may be an option

- Small defects
  - Flexor digitorum longus flap
  - Extensor digiti longus flap
  - Extensor hallucis longus flap
  - Flexor hallucis longus DO NOT sacrifice needed for push off for ambulation
- Fasciocutaneous flaps
- Distal Third of Leg
  - Free tissue transfer best option
    - Recipient vessels
      - Anterior tibial artery and vein outside of zone of injury
        - Located between tibialis anterior and extensor digitorum longus
      - Posterior tibial artery and vein
        - Approached medially above the soleus
    - Use vein grafts if necessary to have anastomosis outside zone of injury
  - Common flaps
    - Latissimus dorsi based on thoracodorsal vessels
      - Long pedicle, bulky
      - Avoid if long term crutch walking anticipated
    - Rectus abdominis- myocutaneous or muscle only
      - Long pedicle, reliable
    - Serratus muscle flap
    - Gracilis- smaller muscle, shorter pedicle
    - Anterolateral thigh flap
      - Good for weight bearing areas
    - Vastus lateralis

- Cross leg flap
  - Life boat flap if free flap not an option or fails
  - High morbidity
    - Local flap necrosis 40%
    - Infection 28%
  - Fasciocutaneous units ratio 3:1 or 4:1
- Reverse turndown sural artery flap
  - Include sural nerve and lesser saphenous vein

o Heel
- Free flaps often required in trauma
- Local flaps more useful in chronic wounds
- Instep fasciocutaneous (medial plantar) flap
  - Perforator between abductor hallucis and flexor digiti brevis
  - Based on medial or lateral plantar artery
  - Skin graft donor site
- Lateral plantar flap
  - Medially based durable rotation flap
- Retrograde sural nerve flap (retrograde sural artery flap) useful for heel and ankle defects

o Forefoot
- Avoid incisions on weight-bearing surfaces
- Instep fasciocutaneous flap
- Toe fillet flap
- Free flap

3. Select appropriate options in diagnosis and management

- Make your plan and choose your operative intervention based on the presented clinical scenario and the available clinical options.
- Location of wound and extent of tissue loss primary considerations.
- You must decide on your plan and be prepared to defend it.
- Postop care
  o Monitoring
    - Gold standard for free flaps- clinical exam

- Doppler examination early postop period 2-3 days
- Temperature probe is an option
- Other
    o Anticoagulation
        - Heparinization prior to cross clamp, 3000-5000 units heparin
        - Postop heparinization generally reserved for patients with:
            - Intimal damage
            - Crush injury
            - Wide zone of injury
        - Dextran 40 after test dose
            - Risk of pulmonary edema, anaphylactic reaction
            - Often used for 24-72 hours in initial postop period
        - Aspirin 325mg/day for one month
        - No anticoagulation in the postop period is an acceptable option.
        - Be familiar with anticoagulation protocols, use the one you are comfortable with.
        - Be prepared to defend it and discuss risks and benefits of different protocols.
        - No consensus on this aspect of microsurgery, yet.
    o Subq heparin for deep vein thrombosis (DVT) prevention
    o Bed rest first 2 days
    o Progressive regimen of sitting and standing
    o Extremity elevation
    o After 10-14 days limited dangling (5 min at a time)
    o Ace wrap for edema control started 3 weeks post op

4. Understand risks and benefits of various approaches

- Consider extent of injury, anatomic location and what is missing for flap choice/reconstructive options
- What is your prognosis for the extremity based on the clinical presentation?
- Consider potential for ambulation long term

- Understand risks and benefits of various reconstructive options
- How do you manage these patients post-op?

5. Address complications and unexpected problems adequately

    - Bleeding- related to anticoagulation
    - Infection related to traumatic insult, inadequate debridement
    - DVT- prophylaxis critical
        - How do you manage DVT or PE?
    - Ischemic flap
    - Chronic pain
    - Flap loss
        - 8% failure rate for free flaps
        - Doubled with vascular trauma
        - Tripled with large bony defects
        - Quintupled if vein grafts needed
    - Thorough work-up to evaluate reasons for free-flap failure:
        - Anastomosis in zone of injury
        - Venous or arterial thrombosis
        - Underlying clotting disorder
        - Other
    - May require repeat free flap or leave in place until full demarcation with hope skin graft may salvage reconstruction.
    - Cross-leg flap lifeboat
    - Integra in vascularized wound bed, can be used for salvage even in extensive soft tissue injuries.

6. Demonstrate ability to structure alternative plan

    - Have alternative flap options
    - Know when to stop, temporize and come back to fight another day

Chapter Forty-Four

Special Lower Extremity Topics:
Diabetic and Chronic Wound Care

44
Special Lower Extremity Topics:
Diabetic and Chronic Wound Care

- Diabetic peripheral polyneuropathy major cause of morbidity
    - Secondary to chronically elevated blood glucose
    - Nerve swelling and tight compartment double crush injury
    - Concurrent macrovascular disease
- Ischemia work-up
    - Palpable pulses
    - Ankle Brachial Index
    - Doppler
    - MRA vs. Angio
    - Vascular surgery consultation
- In your wound evaluation specifically note:
    - Size, Depth, Area
    - What is exposed, i.e. Affected structures
    - Culture results
    - MRI for osteomyelitis (osteo) in diabetic foot ulcer
    - Don't do MRI if operative debridement planned, do bone biopsy
- Labs
    - CBC (WBC with diff, Hb/Hct check for anemia)
    - Iron, Transferrin levels
    - Glucose + Hgb A1C
    - Albumin >3.0 ideal
    - Pre-albumin (16-35 normal range)
    - ESR, C-reactive protein
    - Culture and sensitivities
    - Wound or Bone Biopsy
- Imaging
    - X-ray- minimum, Other as indicated
- Infection may track along tendon sheath
- Check sensation and motor function of foot
- Lack of protective sensation may warrant other interventions

- Infection work-up
    - X-ray- check for gas (clostridia perf.)
    - Compartment pressures
    - US or CT to check for deep abscess
- Debridement
    - Four odor is an indication for debridement
    - Avoid amputation if possible
- Hyperbaric O2 good adjuvant treatment
- Aerobic and anaerobic cultures from deep tissue
- Broad-spectrum antibiotics
    - Multiple organisms often present in diabetic wounds
    - Suspected osteo treat with antibiotics for 6 weeks based on deep wound culture.
- Reconstruction options
- Single stage vs. Two stage
    - Two stage reconstruction preferred: Less morbidity
- Goal of wound treatment
    - Promote healing within timely fashion
    - Establish clean, healthy wound bed
    - Debridement and immediate reconstruction OR
    - Debridement and temporization with wound VAC
    - Followed by reconstruction
- CHRONIC WOUNDS
    - Chronic wounds are arrested in inflammatory stage of wound healing and cannot progress
    - Wounds of long duration (years) consider diagnosis of Marjolin's Ulcer
    - Chronic wounds are colonized by bacteria in a protective bio-film.
    - In chronic wound one must:
        - Correct medical abnormalities
        - Correct coagulopathy
        - Restore adequate blood flow
        - Administer antibiotics
        - Decolonize the wound
    - Delayed closure after debridement of chronic wound is critical.
        - Single stage closure complication is high because of bacterial burden, adequate clearance not achieved.
        - Single stage vs. Two stage amputation
        - Complication rate (21% vs. 0%)

- o Debridement
  - ▪ Use atraumatic technique
  - ▪ Sharp dissection
  - ▪ Skin hooks
  - ▪ Bipolar cautery
- ▪ AVOID DAMAGE TO UNDERLYING TISSUE
- ▪ Excise wound until only normal vascularized tissue remains
- ▪ Use tissue color as guide
  - o Beefy red is the end point
  - o Yellow or white- more debridement will be needed
- ▪ Methylene blue useful in guiding level and adequacy of debridement
- ▪ Excise hard indurated tissue
- ▪ Debridement can be done serially
- ▪ Collagenase may be used as an adjunct for debridement
- ▪ Tendon
  - o Soft and liquefied- Excise
  - o Hard and shiny- Preserve
- ▪ General Debridement Instruments
  - o Forceps
  - o Scalpel
  - o Scissors
  - o Curettes
  - o Rongeurs
  - o Cobb elevator
  - o Pulse lavage
  - o Versajet (works by Venturi effect)- vacuum around high-pressure stream of water
    - ▪ Hydro-surgical water knife
    - ▪ Forces narrow stream of water across a small gap (8-14mm) at speeds of 15K miles/hour
    - ▪ Stream sucks in surrounding tissue and pulverizes
- ▪ Once wound bed vascularized may use VAC
- ▪ Closure when all paranormal parameters corrected
- ▪ Choice of reconstruction based on reconstructive ladder
  - o Primary considerations
    - ▪ What is missing?
    - ▪ Size of defect
    - ▪ What is exposed?

Section Ten
Hand

Chapter Forty-Five

Hand Overview

45
Hand Overview

1. Identify General Problem

   - Describe photo
   - Give working diagnosis
   - Key problems
   - Evaluate patient
   - Diagnosis/Planning
   - Determine etiology of problem
     - Trauma, Chronic wound, Tumor, Infection
   - Give specifics of injury and defect
   - Classify problem
   - Describe what is missing and functional implications
   - Go through ABC's of trauma management
   - Open fractures?
   - Need for escharotomy, fasciotomy, compartment syndrome?
   - Relevant medical history (smoking, DM, CAD, HTN, steroids)
   - Pertinent positives and negatives in history (drug abuse)
   - Nutritional status and work-up (pre-albumin, anemia)
   - Previous surgeries
   - Relevant medications especially anticoagulants
   - Right or left handed?
   - Occupation
   - Age of patient
   - Every Hand Trauma Case:
     - Give IV antibiotics, Tetanus, X-rays
   - Need for further work-up or consultations?
     - Imaging studies, labs, consultants

2. Consider reasonable goals in diagnosis and management

   - Management and treatment
   - Surgical indications
   - Operative procedures and anesthesia
   - Indications for replantation/revascularization
     o Consent for blood transfusion
     o Consent for vein grafts, skin grafts, tendon grafts

- Inform patient of the need for the extension of wounds or additional incisions for exposure or graft harvest
  - What are the surgical goals?
  - What are your surgical options?
  - Timing for soft tissue, tendon, bone, nerve reconstruction
  - Amputation last resort unless gross contamination, farm injury, severe crush, other.

3. Select appropriate options in diagnosis and management

   - What is your choice for proceeding and why?
   - Surgical sequence
   - Timing of intervention
   - Post-op management
   - Splinting/casting/rehab
   - Anticipated functional outcome
   - Familiarity with common tendon transfers
   - How is procedure performed?
   - Key steps of surgery
   - Markings and relevant anatomy

4. Understand risks and benefits of various approaches

   - Discuss risks, benefits of various approaches
   - May relate to:
     - Handedness of patient
     - Age or occupation (especially in less extreme scenarios)
     - Timing of intervention
     - Need or benefits of staged reconstruction?

5. Address complications and unexpected problems adequately

   - Note potential immediate post-surgical and long-term complications
     - Osteomyelitis
     - Malrotation
     - Flap loss with exposed bone
     - Compromised replant
     - Indications for tendon transfer
   - Noncompliant patient

- No insurance coverage for therapy
- Indications for non-operative vs. operative management of postop or other problems
- Use of occupational therapy
- Splinting- how do you do it
- Tenolysis and indications

6. Demonstrate ability to structure alternative plan

    - Have lifeboat and back-up plans in mind for failed reconstruction (groin flap)
    - Why did reconstruction fail?
    - What if patient will have poor compliance post-op?
        - Drug-abuse
        - Psychiatric patient
        - Children
        - Will this change your management plan?

Chapter Forty-Six

Flexor Tendon Injury

46
Flexor Tendon Injury

1. Identify General Problem/Diagnosis/Planning
   (Describe photo, give working diagnosis, key problems, evaluates patient)

   - This patient has an injury consistent with flexor tendon injury, why?:
     o Describe photo
     o Explain key problems
     o Give working diagnosis
     o Based on history given and absence of natural flexion cascade
   - History
     o Determine mechanism of injury
       - Sharp vs. crush
     o Are nerve, bone, vessels involved?
     o Contaminated vs. uncontaminated
       - Delay tendon repair in grossly contaminated wounds
       - Clean laceration tendon may be repaired anatomically and early
     o Timing of injury (when did it occur)
       - Acceptable to repair within first 10 days which is ideal (up to 3-4 weeks)
     o Position of finger at time of injury
       - Digit in flexion, anticipate greater retraction of tendon ends
     o Plan for appropriate exposure, note this in consent form
     o Hand dominance
       - Dominant hand injury greater dysfunction but rehab the same
     o Occupation
       - FDS- associated PIP joint dysfunction
       - FDP- associated DIP joint dysfunction
       - Different occupations different needs of fingers
         • Primary repair in all if possible

- Staged reconstruction of DIP if a musician
- Arthrodesis of DIP joint, tenodesis or simple observation may be more appropriate in a laborer, quicker return to work
    - PE
        o Resting cascade
            - Loss of cascade may indicate transection
        o Ischemia
            - Devascularized digit needs immediate revascularization
        o Sensation of digit
            - Gross sensation and two-point discrimination
        o Individual tendon function
            - FDS- Inserts middle portion, middle phalanx
            - FDP- Inserts distal phalanx
            - Passive tenodesis test useful in extensive trauma to fingers
        o Joint stability
            - Is a dislocation present?
        o Adequate overlying soft tissue to allow repair and subsequent rehab?
        o Get plan x-ray to rule out bone injury if necessary

2. Consider reasonable goals in diagnosis and management *(Management and treatment, surgical indications, operative procedures and anesthesia)*

    - Loupe magnification and tourniquet
    - Debride contaminated tissue thoroughly, irrigate
    - Early repair < 1 week if possible
    - Late repair results in:
        o Greater inflammatory phase, worse outcome- adhesions
        o Late repair may mandate staged recon if fibro-osseous canal collapsed
        o Delayed repair results in tendon retraction
            - More difficult to advance
            - Increased tension on repair may require staged repair

- Absolute contraindications to flexor tendon repair:
    - Gross infection
    - Human Bite injuries
    - Cellulitis
- Ideal tendon repair:
    - Easy suture placement
    - Secure knots
    - Anatomic approximation with minimal interference with blood supply
    - Strength to permit early motion protocol (minimum 4 strands)
- Exposure:
    - Zigzag Brunner type incision or
    - Longitudinal incisions along midaxial line of digit
- Technique:
    - Loupe Magnification
    - Tourniquet control
    - Atraumatic
        - Handle only severed ends
    - Suture material
        - Nonreactive
        - Small caliber
        - Excellent knot handling
        - 3-0 for core sutures if possible better than 4-0
        - Epitendinous sutures 6-0 nylon
        - Prolene or nylon preferred
    - Number of strands
        - The greater the number of strands, the greater the strength
        - 4 strands or more, minimum for active motion protocols
    - Suture bites minimum of 7-10mm
    - Leaving part of the sheath open no effect on healing and may be beneficial in healing and glide by decreasing constriction
- Tendon retrieval:
    - Finger held in flexion
    - 25-gauge needle may be used to hold tendon in position for suturing

- Informed consent critical!
    - Make patient aware of functional goals
    - Stress importance of rehabilitation and therapy
    - Expected time off
    - Possible complications
        - Stiffness
        - Staged repair
        - Need for revision surgery
        - Tendon rupture
        - Infection
- Delay reconstruction if:
    - Severe wound contamination
    - Bony injuries involving joint components
    - Extensive soft tissue loss
    - Destruction of a series of annular pulleys and lengthy tendon defects
- PARTIAL TENDON REPAIRS
    - 60% or less no repair needed- trim or epitendinous sutures to decrease risk of entrapment and friction
    - 60-80% minimum of epitendinous repair
    - 80-90% treat like complete laceration

3. Select appropriate options in diagnosis and management

- Make diagnosis, explore wound, identify injured structures
- Treatment by Zone of injury
    - Zone I- distal to FDS insertion
    - Zone II- distal palmar crease to FDS insertion
    - Zone III- distal edge of carpal tunnel to distal palmar crease
    - Zone IV- carpal tunnel
    - Zone V- proximal to carpal tunnel
- Zone I- distal to FDS insertion
    - Primary repair by advancement if gap <1cm
    - Tendon graft if gap >1cm
    - May need periosteal elevation and suture passage through nail with button
    - Tenodesis
    - DIP arthrodesis
- Zone II- distal palmar crease to FDS insertion
    - "No man's land"
    - Most challenging flexor tendon injuries

- o Variables for optimal range of motion:
  - Active range of motion protocol
  - Age
  - Edema formation
  - Presence of composite tissue injury
  - Associated fractures
  - Zone of injury
  - Adequate repair of A-2 and A-4 pulleys
  - Epitendinous suture
  - Avoidance of gap formation
- o Maintain FDS to preserve blood supply to FDP
- o Reconstructive choices:
  - Primary repair whenever possible, within 7 days if possible
    - 4-core suture technique, 3-0 sutures if possible
  - Delayed primary- grossly contaminated wounds, second or third look surgeries, repair after adequate debridement
  - Secondary repair weeks after initial injury- usually unsuccessful
  - Profundus advancement- used distal to FDS insertion if >1cm of tendon lost
    - Excess shortening of tendon flexes repaired digit with limited flexion in remaining digits (quadriga effect)
  - Tendon grafting- shown to grow with patient, but, not advocated in children if noncompliant with therapy
  - Tendon transfer FDS to ring finger most frequently used
  - Arthrodesis of DIP joint loss of 15% of total arc of rotation of digit
  - Dynamic tenodesis- looping proximal cut end of FDP around FDS insertion
  - Pulley reconstruction via slip of FDS tendon or wrist extensor retinaculum
- o Attempt to preserve pulleys if necessary
  - If necessary in primary repair try to limit sheath incisions to 2cm, but, entire A4 pulley and up to 2/3 length of A2 can be surgically released if it improves access

- Zone III- Distal palmar crease to carpal tunnel
    - Primary repair
    - Lumbricals originate from FDP tendon
    - Functional result more dependent on nerve repair than tendon repair
- Zone IV- Carpal tunnel
    - Primary repair
    - Functional result dependent on median nerve repair
- Zone V- Proximal to carpal tunnel
    - Primary repair
    - Results similar to zone IV usually excellent
    - If median nerve or ulnar nerve injury need to maintain PIP joint extension in postop period
    - Tenolysis needed in 15%
- FPL tends to have more primary contraction
- POSTOPERATIVE REHABILITATION
    - Early controlled mobilization improves repair process and decreases adhesion formation
    - Immobilization reserved for noncompliant cases, small children, mentally incapable of following therapy
    - Early controlled passive motion Duran or Kleinert
    - 0-4 weeks
        - Passive flexion/active extension with therapist
        - Dorsal blocking splint
            - Wrist flexed 20-30 degrees
            - MP 40-60 flexion
            - IP straight
    - 4-6 weeks
        - Active ROM 4 to 6 times/day
        - Scar massage within splint
    - 6-8 weeks
        - Active and passive ROM with removal of blocking splint
    - 8-12 weeks
        - Resisted flexion
    - 12 weeks full use
        - Active mobilization protocol (with dorsal blocking splint with a wrist tenodesis splint)

- o Passive flexion within splint must have 4 strand or greater repair to prevent early rupture.
- o Edema control important
- o 4 weeks active exercise without tenodesis splint
- o 6 weeks remove dorsal blocking splint
- o 8 weeks add light resistance

4. Understand risks and benefits of various approaches

  - Early repair if possible
  - Debride all devitalized tissue
  - Antibiotics
  - Atraumatic technique
  - Minimum 4 strand repair for active motion protocols
  - AVOID
    - o Tendon bunching
    - o Exposure of suture knots
    - o Trauma to uninjured portions
    - o Gap formation
  - Active motion protocols better outcomes
  - Reconstruction approach based on clinical presentation: contamination, tendon loss, soft tissue coverage, age of patient, time of injury and presentation

5. Address complications and unexpected problems adequately

  - Infection
  - Bleeding
  - Hematoma
  - Stiffness
  - Tendon Rupture
    - o Confirm by clinical exam, U/S or MRI
    - o 5% incidence (higher with FPL)
    - o Treat by prompt re-exploration and repair
  - Skin loss
  - Need for revision surgery
  - Need for staged reconstruction
  - Limited postop function
  - Quadriga effect- tight tendon repair or graft
  - Lumbrical plus deformity- loose tendon repair or graft
  - Adhesions
    - o Common Causes

- Tendon and composite tissue damage
- Loss of tendon sheath
- Gap formation
- Ischemia
- Immobilization
- Persistent inflammation
- Secondary trauma
  - Treatment Options:
    - Tenolysis
      - Indicated if passive range of motion exceeds active range of motion despite aggressive hand therapy
      - Timing- 3 or more months after initial repair if therapy has plateaued with no gains
    - One-stage reconstruction
      - Pulp to palm graft in digit with minimal scarring
      - Supple joints
      - Adequate pulley system
    - Staged reconstruction
      - Salvage procedure following attempt at one or more other reconstructive options
      - Silicone rod sutured or screwed to distal phalanx A2 and A4 pulleys reconstructed on top
      - Period of therapy and scar massage to maintain maximal passive range of motion
      - Second stage at 2-3 months
      - Graft distally attached into hollow in distal phalanx with pull out suture
      - Proximal end secured with Pulvertaft weave
    - Arthrodesis
    - Amputation

6. Demonstrate ability to structure alternative plan

   - Know when to do primary vs. delayed primary vs. secondary reconstruction. Management of failed tendon repair.

- Graft options
- Palmaris longus absent in 15-25% (13cm)
- Plantaris tendon absent in 10-20% (31cm)
- Long extensors or central three toes (30cm of length)
- EIP 10cm
- EDM 11cm

Chapter Forty-Seven

Extensor Tendon Injury

47
Extensor Tendon Injury

1. Identify General Problem/Diagnosis/Planning
   (Describe photo, give working diagnosis, key problems, evaluates patient)

   - In this injury I suspect that the patient may have:
   - Describe all findings in photo include suspicion of nerve injury
   - Radial Nerve- innervation to extensor tendons
   - Extensor muscles of wrist, thumb, fingers all radial nerve innervated
   - Understand anatomy of extensor tendon, be able to draw it
   - Radial nerve
     - Direct branches to:
       - Brachioradialis (BR)
       - Extensor carpi radialis longus (ECRL)
     - Posterior interosseous nerve (branch of radial) does the rest:
       - Order of innervation proximal to distal:
       - ECRB>Supinator (S)> EDC> EDM> ECU> APL> EPB> EPL> EIP
     - Recovery of radial nerve predictable by this sequence:
       - Wrist extension, finger extension, thumb extension
   - Extensor Tendon
     - Paratenon
     - At wrist extensor retinaculum
       - 6 distinct anatomic compartments
       - Lister's tubercle- bony prominence
         - EPL (3rd compartment) courses radially
     - Distal to retinaculum juncturae tendinum (junc. tend.) connect index, middle, ring and small fingers
       - Consistent ring to middle and small
       - Variable index and middle

- Index and small have separate extensors EIP and EDM
  - ALWAYS **ULNAR** TO EDC TENDON
  - Spare part for tendon reconstruction (EIP and EDM)
  - Communis to small absent in up to 80%
  - Replaced by substantial junc. tend. from ring finger.
- At level of MCP joint
  - Tendon stabilized by sagittal bands
    - Prevents ulnar or radial subluxation
- More distally
  - Oblique and transverse fibers
  - Tendinous contributions from intrinsic muscles through lateral bands
- Lumbrical muscles
  - Pass volar to MCP joint
  - Dorsal to PIP
  - Through lateral bands
  - ALLOW simultaneous MCP flexion and PIP extension
- At level of PIP joint
  - Extensor tendon becomes central slip and attaches to dorsal base of middle finger
  - ALLOWS extension of PIP joint along with oblique fibers from lateral bands
  - Over the middle phalanx controlling position of the lateral bands
  - Triangular ligament- stabilizes lateral bands dorsally
    - Prevents volar sublux-Boutonniere Deformity
  - Transverse retinacular ligament- stabilizes volarly
    - Prevents dorsal sublux- swan-neck deformity
- Further distally
  - Lateral bands join to insert onto base of distal phalanx for DIP joint extension

- Extensor Compartments (Six) Radial to Ulnar

- Abductor pollicis longus/Extensor pollicis brevis APL/EPB

- Extensor carpi radialis longus/Extensor carpi radialis brevis (ECRL/ECRB)
- Extensor pollicis longus (EPL)
- Extensor digitorum communis, extensor indicis proprius (EDC/EIP)
- Extensor digitorum minimi (EDM)
- Extensor carpi ulnaris (ECU)

- 1st dorsal compartment- likely to have subcompartments
  - Abductor pollicis longus (APL)
  - Extensor pollicis brevis (EPB)
- EPL- no attachments (junctura connection) to other extensor tendons
  - Laceration of EPL may result in full retraction of proximal end, prevents easy repair
- Juncturae tendinae prevent retraction of EDC tendons

- ACUTE INJURIES
- Note Zone of injury (Nine zones)
  - Zone 1- DIP joint
  - Zone 2- Middle phalanx
  - Zone 3- PIP joint
  - Zone 4- Proximal phalanx
  - Zone 5- MCP joint
  - Zone 6- Metacarpal (dorsum of hand)
  - Zone 7- Extensor retinaculum (wrist)
  - Zone 8- Distal forearm
  - Zone 9- Mid/prox forearm
- DIFFERENTIATE INTRINSIC AND EXTRINSIC TIGHTNESS WITHIN EXTENSOR SYSTEM
  - Complex balance between extrinsic and intrinsic tendons and ligamentous support
  - Normally intrinsic muscles:
    - Tightened with MCP joint extension
    - Loosened with MCP joint flexion
- INTRINSIC TIGHTNESS
  - Less passive flexion of PIP jt. When MCP jt. Extended than when MCP jt. Flexed
- EXTRINSIC TIGHTNESS
  - Extrinsic extensor tendon limits the ability of finger to achieve combined flexion of MCP joint and the PIP joint.

- o Less passive flexion of PIP jt. When MCP jt. is flexed than when MCP jt. Extended
- o This guides treatment
  - Causes of rupture
  - Attrition after prolonged abrasion against bony surfaces
  - Chronic inflammation (rheumatoid disease)

  - PE
    - Passively extend finger to 0 degrees
      - o Proximal tendon injury
    - Cannot maintain full MCP joint extension
      - o Radial nerve palsy
    - No active extension possible
      - o Sagittal band rupture
    - Passive extension returns extensor tendon to apex of metacarpal head, can actively maintain position
    - Test for Boutonniere deformity
    - Place finger in 90-degree flexion at PIP
    - Test ability to actively extend PIP joint against resistance
    - If extension possible, central slip is in continuity.
  - COMMON EXTENSOR PROBLEMS
    - o Extensor tendon rupture
    - o Sagittal band injury
      - Frequently diagnosed 2-3 wks after injury
      - Associated with open injury Zone V
    - o Swan neck deformity
      - DIP flexion/PIP hyperextension
      - Intrinsic muscle tightness- lateral bands sublux dorsal to axis of PIP rotation
      - Causes
      - Chronic mallet finger
      - Volar plate laxity of PIP joint (congenital or traumatic)
      - Dynamic imbalance normal joint
    - o Boutonniere deformity
      - DIP hyperextension/PIP flexion
      - Causes
      - Disruption of central slip from middle phalanx
      - Trauma or attrition from underlying arthritis
      - May not respond to splinting

- Mallet Finger
  - Disruption of terminal slip from base of distal phalanx
  - Can be closed or open
  - DIP joint flexed at rest
  - Inability to actively extend the distal phalanx
- Classification Four Types
  - Type I: Closed with attenuation or disruption within substance of tendon, may be associated with small bone fragment
  - Type II: Open, post direct laceration of distal extensor tendon
  - Type III: Open with loss of soft tissue overlying extensor tendon and requires soft tissue coverage of tendon
  - Type IV: Includes distal phalanx fracture
- Degloving injuries (See Mutilating Hand, Chapter 58)
  - Is there exposure of and/or damage to extensor tendons?
  - Principles
    - Debridement of all nonviable tissues
    - Definitive repair of fractures
    - Coverage with durable tissue
    - Tendon reconstruction

2. Consider reasonable goals in diagnosis and management *(Management and treatment, surgical indications, operative procedures and anesthesia)*

- Zone of tendon injury dictates management.
- Extensor tendon rupture
  - Commonly seen in rheumatoid and osteoarthritis
  - Caused by attrition
  - Presents with extensor lag with no history of trauma or excessive force
- Sagittal band injuries
  - As tendon passes over metacarpal head
  - At level of MCP joint
    - Tendon stabilized by sagittal bands
      - Prevents ulnar or radial subluxation
    - Centralizes extensor tendon

- With lac or rupture extensor tendon slips off apex of metacarpal head
- Zone V injury treatment
  - Open injury repair immediately if no contraindication
  - Closed injury-spontaneous rupture rheumatoid
    - Ulnar subluxation, radial side rupture
    - (power grip stronger on ulnar side)
  - Presentation
    - Pain, swelling over MCP jt.
    - Snapping or locking with active extension
    - Normal flexion
  - X-ray
    - R/O arthritic changes
    - R/O trigger finger
- Inspect sagittal bands in ZONE V injuries
  - If not repaired
    - Subluxation of tendon over MCP joint
    - Loss of normal joint excursion
    - Late diagnosis direct suture will not be possible
- Late repair of sagittal band
  - Use tendon tissue around region of extensor hood/sagittal band
    - Juncturae tendinae or proximally or distally based portion of extensor tendon itself may be used
  - Sutured to remaining extensor hood or passed around lumbrical tendon
  - Tension set to ensure centralization with flexion and extension of finger

- Swan neck deformity
  - DIP joint flexion
  - PIP joint hyperextension
  - Intrinsic muscle tightness as lateral bands sublux dorsal to axis of PIP joint rotation
  - Associated ligamentous abnormalities:
    - Tightening of triangular ligament

- Laxity of the transverse retinacular ligament
- Chronic mallet finger
  o Volar plate laxity (congenital or traumatic)
  o May have dynamic deformity that manifests during attempted maximum extension or fixed deformity with underlying contracture and joint changes.
  o Generally refractory to conservative treatment (splinting or exercises)
  o Operative Management
  o Reserved for:
    - Dynamic imbalance but normal underlying joint architecture
    - Severe contracture or PIP joint arthritis- arthrodesis
    - Imbalance secondary to mallet deformity
    - Correction of DIP joint may restore normal length tension relationships around PIP joint
    - Primary volar plate laxity- tenodesis
- PIP JOINT VOLAR PLATE LAXITY
  o Treat by tenodesis procedures
    - Common principle
      • Tendon graft use or tendon re-routing to prevent PIP joint hyperextension.
    - Spiral oblique retinacular ligament reconstruction
      • Free tendon graft for tenodesis (palmaris longus)
    - Superficialis tenodesis technique
      • Slip of FDS used for tenodesis at PIP joint
  o Postop Care (same for both):
    - Continuous splinting for 4 weeks
    - Then dorsal blocking splint that maintains the PIP joint flexed at 20 degrees and DIP joint neutral
    - Active joint flexion and extension exercises splint prevents extension beyond 20 degrees
    - After 10 weeks splint adjusted to allow PIP joint to straighten another 10 degrees
  o Boutonniere deformity
    - DIP hyperextension

- PIP joint flexion
- Disruption of central slip from middle phalanx
  - Traumatic
  - Attenuation, arthritis
- Causes subluxation of lateral bands volar to PIP joint axis of rotation
- Associated ligamentous abnormalities opposite of swan neck:
  - Laxity of triangular ligament
  - Transverse retinacular ligament contracture
- Initial treatment
  - Static extension splinting of PIP joint/active flexion DIP joint
  - Early injury may respond
- Late cases
  - Treat with splinting and exercise prior to surgical release
  - Serial splinting of PIP into greater degrees of extension gradually alleviate any flexion contracture of PIP joint
- GOALS OF SURGICAL INTERVENTION
  - Attempt to divert increased tone at DIP joint toward PIP joint
  - Fowler procedure
  - Transversely divides extensor mechanism at junction of middle and proximal thirds of middle phalanx
  - Allows lateral bands to slide proximally increasing tone over PIP joint
  - Post op splint in full extension, DIP free
  - After several weeks dynamic splinting protocol
  - Correction very difficult recommended only for patients unresponsive to splinting
  - Acute traumatic injuries
  - Principles
    - Debridement of all nonviable tissues
    - Definitive repair of fractures
    - Coverage with durable tissue
    - Tendon reconstruction
- ZONE I INJURIES

- Mallet Finger
- Disruption of terminal slip from base of distal phalanx
- Can be closed or open
- Clinically DIP joint flexed at rest/inability to actively extend the distal phalanx
- Treatment
  - Type I:
    - Treated with closed reduction extension splinting 6 to 8 weeks
    - Protocol- Strict continuous extension 6-8 weeks/When splint removed rest finger in extension/Proper fit DIP slight hyperextension/PIP free
    - Remove after 6-8 weeks in no lag then nighttime splinting additional 2 weeks. If lag then splint 6 more weeks or until lag resolved
    - Controlled active flexion exercises are required to regain DIP flexion
  - Type II:
    - Direct repair of skin laceration with 4-0 or 5-0 suture
    - Deep passage of suture allows simultaneous tendon and skin approximation (tenodermodesis)
    - Splinted as in type I
  - Type III:
    - Reconstruction facilitated by K wire pinning across DIP
    - Local flap- reverse cross finger/homodigital island flap
  - Type IV:
    - Reduction of distal phalanx fx
    - May sublux overtime if inadequate reduction
    - K-wire or screw fixation
    - Edge of tendon then advanced onto distal phalanx and affixed with a suture anchor or tie-over button

- **ZONE II INJURIES- Central slip injuries**
    - Level of middle phalanx- central slip injuries
    - Level of proximal phalanx in thumb
    - Usually direct lacerations
    - <50%
        - Less than 50% of tendon injured- NO REPAIR NEEDED
        - DIP splinted in extension 14 days until sutures removed
        - Then active, gentle ROM at DIP
    - >50%
        - Repair primarily- horizontal mattress
            - Bunching or shortening of tendon will cause incomplete DIP joint flexion after healing
            - Splinting as in mallet finger
                - Protocol- Strict continuous extension 6-8 weeks/When splint removed rest finger in extension/Proper fit DIP slight hyperextension/PIP free
                - Remove after 6-8 weeks if no lag then nighttime splinting additional 2 weeks. If lag then splint 6 more weeks or until lag resolved
                - Controlled active flexion exercises are required to regain DIP flexion
- **ZONE III INJURIES- Boutonniere deformity**
    - Injuries over PIP joint-
        - Disruption of central slip from base of middle phalanx
        - Can give rise to BOUTONNIERE DEFORMITY (PIP flex/DIP hyperex) due to volar migration of lateral bands
    - Causes
        - Direct laceration
        - Closed avulsion after hyperflexion or volar dislocation of PIP joint

- BOUTONNIERE DEFORMITY may present as late as 3 weeks after trauma.
- Treatment
  - Closed injury
    - Splinting
    - PIP joint in extension/DIP free
  - Treat operatively when x-ray shows small fragment of bone avulsed from middle phalanx and volar subluxation of joint.
  - Dorsal approach
    - Open injury with clear laceration repair
- POSTOP CARE
  - Splint all injuries postop
  - PIP joint extended DIP free
  - At 3 weeks spring-loaded splint
  - Allows active PIP flexion and passive extension
  - Worn at all times up to 8 weeks post injury
  - Night splinting and active and passive ROM instituted after 8 weeks.

- ZONE IV- Sagittal band injury
  - Level over proximal phalanx- broad tendon in this area
  - <50%- Treat conservatively, ROM beginning at 7-10 days/ after skin healed
  - >50%- Repair with mattress sutures
    - Early controlled ROM protocols to reduce need for tenolysis
- ZONE V-Human bites common here (clenched fist), sagittal band injuries
  - Over MCP joints
  - Clenched fist injuries often partial
  - Management
    - X-ray
    - Explore in all cases of clenched fist injuries- joint involvement common
      - Explore
      - Irrigate
      - Leave wound open in cases of human bite, contaminated

- Proximal tendon does not retract except EPL
- Antibiotics!
    - <50% no repair
    - >50% repair
  - Inspect sagittal bands- if not repaired
    - Subluxation of tendon over MCP joint
    - Loss of normal joint excursion
    - Late diagnosis direct suture will not be possible
  - Late repair of sagittal band
    - Use tendon tissue around region of extensor hood/sagittal band
      - Juncturae tendinae or proximally or distally based portion of extensor tendon itself may be used.
    - Sutured to remaining extensor hood or passed around lumbrical tendon
    - Tension set to ensure centralization with flexion and extension of finger
- ZONE VI INJURIES
  - Level over metacarpal bones
  - Tendon more cord-like
  - Injuries mostly lacerations fewer spontaneous ruptures
  - Operative technique
    - Use core sutures and epitenon sutures
    - Early ROM can be done- greater strength of repair
    - Retraction uncommon due to juncturae tendinae
    - Attention to correct reapproximation- abnormal tension may affect other fingers
- ZONE VII INJURIES
  - Level of extensor retinaculum
  - More frequently multiple tendons involved
  - Treat retinaculum by lengthening in step-cut fashion to avoid restriction in gliding while preventing bowstringing
- ZONE VIII INJURIES
  - Treat as in ZONE VII

- At level of musculotendinous junction isolate tendon fibers
- Repair core and figure of eight sutures
- ZONE IX INJURIES
    - Injury through extensor muscle substance with denervation of muscle distal to injury
    - Return of function may be limited due to denervation of muscle
    - Repair muscle fascia directly with figure-of-eight sutures
- EXTENSOR TENDON RUPTURE
    - Rheumatoid arthritis
    - Ruptures occur in ulnar to radial fashion
        - EDC and EDM first followed by EDC of ring finger
    - Distal radius fracture may cause extensor tendon rupture. Most commonly EPL.
    - Early diagnosis
        - Primary repair or short tendon graft
    - Multiple tendons or delayed diagnosis
        - Tendon transfer!
            - Rupture of EPL
                - EIP or palmaris longus transfer
            - Rupture of EDC
                - EIP or EDM transfer
                - Side to side tenodesis to adjacent intact communis tendon
            - Rupture of ECRL or ECRB
                - Pronator teres tendon transfer
- DORSAL HAND DEGLOVING INJURIES
    - Principles of management
        - Thorough debridement of all nonviable tissues
        - Definitive repair of fractures
        - Coverage with durable soft tissue
        - Tendon reconstruction
        - Ipsilateral reverse radial forearm workhorse flap
        - Allen's test prior to harvest

- Posterior interosseous artery flap
- Lifeboat distant flap- pedicled groin flap
- Fasciocutaneous coverage is the best option if available
              - If local/regional/distant flaps not available then free tissue transfer
                    - Ideally thin pliable flap (fasciocutaneous)
                        - Contralateral radial forearm flap
                        - Anterolateral thigh flap
                        - Temporoparietal fascia flap
                        - Lateral arm flap
              - Staged tendon reconstruction
                    - Segmental tendon losses
                        - Staged tendon recon
                        - First Stage
                              - Silicone rods placed at time of coverage.
                        - Second stage once flap healed and maximal passive flexion and extension achieved.
                              - Silicone rod removal and placement of free autologous tendon
                                    - Donor sites for graft
                                    - Palmaris
                                    - Plantaris
                                    - Toe extensors
                              - Bridge defects between proximal motor and distal tendons

3. Select appropriate options in diagnosis and management

   - Choose from above, diagnosis, intervention will be based on:
       - Presentation
       - Open or closed injury
       - Zone of Injury
       - Anatomy of tendon
       - Length of time of deformity (acute vs. chronic)
       - Disease process (trauma vs. rheumatoid)
   - POST OP CARE ZONE V-IX INJURIES
       - Immediate postop: Static volar splint

- Wrist 30 degrees extension
- (majority of unloading of tension of repair)
- MCP joints 0-15 degrees flexion
- IP full extension
- Worn at all times!
- No active or passive ROM allowed at fingers
- While in splint may start passive MCP hyperextension exercises

- 3-6 weeks postop: Dynamic splint
  - Wrist 30 degrees extension
  - MCP joints increasing flexion
  - IP joints full dynamic extension
  - Guarded active flexion at IP joints using volar guard
  - Static splint at night
- 6-8 weeks postop: Exercises out of splint
  - Active flexion with wrist in extension
  - Active finger extension
  - Wrist flexion and extension with fingers in relaxed, extended posture
- 8 weeks: Wean from splints
  - FROM allowed with avoidance of simultaneous finger and wrist flexion
  - Light grip strength exercises
- 12 weeks
  - Allowed to flex both fingers and wrist

4. Understand risks and benefits of various approaches

- Extensor tendon injury is generally a straightforward surgical question.
- Be able to discuss the risk and benefit of various approaches
  - Risk of no intervention based on presentation
  - Surgical options based on acuity of presentation
  - (acute vs. chronic, closed vs. open injury)
  - Choices of soft coverage based on presented defect
  - Anticipated outcome
  - Appropriate postop management

5. Address complications and unexpected problems adequately

- Wound infection
- Wound dehiscence
- Contracture
- PT non-compliance
- Failed tendon reconstruction
- Management of intrinsic or extrinsic tightness
- Uninsured patient

6. Demonstrate ability to structure alternative plan

- Failed flap or soft tissue coverage
- Alternate tendon donor sites
- Alternate flap sites

Chapter Forty-Eight

Boutonniere Deformity

48
Boutonniere Deformity

1. Identify General Problem/Diagnosis/Planning
   (Describe photo, give working diagnosis, key problems, evaluates patient)

   - Describe finding from photo in detail.
   - Note: Flexion at PIP + hyperextension DIP joint = Boutonniere deformity
   - Caused by disruption of central slip of extensor tendon.
   - Zone III- extensor tendon injury
   - Hx:
     - Trauma
       - Most commonly closed injury
       - Sudden forceful flexion of extended PIP
     - Direct blunt trauma
       - Open laceration
       - Burn injury
     - Other causes
       - Rheumatoid
       - Inflammatory arthropathies
       - Ligamentous laxity
       - Advanced Dupuytren's
   - Timing
     - In acute closed injury
       - Injury may not be immediately evident
       - Often manifests over time (10-14 days)
   - Pathology
     - After disruption, triangular ligament and transverse retinacular ligament stretches over time
     - Lateral bands sublux volar to axis of rotation of PIP joint- result PIP flexion
     - Lateral bands sublux dorsal to axis of rotation of DIP- extension
   - Stages
     - Acute 0-2 wks
     - Subacute 2-8 wks
     - Chronic >8 wks or fixed PIP joint flexion contracture

- Concomitant medical conditions
  - Inflammatory and connective tissue disorders (rheumatoid, lupus, other)
- Considerations
  - Age
  - Handedness
  - Occupation
- Impacts effect of deformity
  - 20 degree PIP joint flexion contracture tolerated well in most
- PE
  - Assess active and passive motion
  - Presence of fixed contracture
  - Extensor function
  - Signs of trauma
  - Swelling, ecchymosis, tenderness over middle phalanx
  - Mobility
  - Central slip evaluation:
    - Passively flex PIP 90 degrees
    - Hold pressure on middle phalanx
    - Ask patient to extend
    - If extension force present
    - Central slip likely intact
    - In this maneuver
      - Normally when central slip intact DIP will not be extended
      - In boutonnière deformity DIP will extend via lateral bands!
    - NEXT
    - Hold PIP in full extension
    - DIP passively flexed
    - In Boutonnière- there will be decreased passive DIP joint extension
  - Pseudo-boutonniere
    - Hyperextension injury to PIP joint
    - Contracture of volar structures but no effect on DIP joint
  - Look for stability of collateral ligaments of PIP; may indicate central slip injury may be from volar PIP joint dislocation
  - Zancolli stage of injury

- Stage I:
  - Weak PIP joint extension (lateral bands)
  - Resting flexion of PIP joint
  - Can be passively corrected to full extension
- Stage II:
  - Loss of active PIP joint extension
  - Secondary stretching of triangular ligament
  - Sublux of lateral bands volar to axis of PIP joint
- Stage III:
  - Progressive hyperextension of DIP joint via subluxed lateral bands
  - MCP joint may hyperextend
- Stage IV:
  - Fixed PIP joint contracture
  - Contracture of oblique retinacular ligaments and PIP joint volar plate
- Stage V:
  - Fixed deformity +
  - Secondary PIP joint arthritis on x-ray

- Plain x-ray:
  - AP, lateral, oblique views
  - Visualize MCP, PIP and DIP joints
- In acute injury:
  - R/O associated avulsion fracture off dorsal middle phalanx
  - Look for degenerative joint changes
- Consultations: Rheumatology

2. Consider reasonable goals in diagnosis and management *(Management and treatment, surgical indications, operative procedures and anesthesia)*

- Majority of Boutonnière deformities are treated nonoperatively with splinting:
  - Most common type:
    - Static extension splint- PIP in extension, MCP and DIP free, full time for 6 wks
  - Chronic cases with established PIP joint contracture:
  - First step:
    - Serial extension casts or dynamic extension splints to regain PIP extension

- Then:
  - PIP joint status splinting additional 6 wks
- INDICATIONS FOR SURGERY
  - Acute boutonnière
    - Displaced, nonreducible avulsion fracture of dorsal base of middle phalanx
    - Boutonnière secondary to laceration or open wound
    - Boutonnière associated with lateral and axial instability of PIP joint
    - Failure of splinting

3. Select appropriate options in diagnosis and management

- Surgical options in acute boutonnière deformity:
  - ORIF displaced avulsion fracture
  - Tendon repair
    - Non-absorbable suture
    - Avoid shortening
    - Can fix central slip to dorsal base of middle phalanx by anchoring suture
    - Lateral bands must be relocated and sutured to dorsal axis of PIP joint
  - Immobilize PIP joint for 4-6 weeks in full extension
  - Oblique K wire or static splint
  - DIP left free and active DIP flexion encouraged- to prevent adhesions
  - If central slip cannot be reconstructed
    - Lateral bands released, mobilized dorsally to reconstruct central slip and rebalance extensor tendon. (Salvi procedure)
- Surgical options chronic boutonnière:
  - First step:
    - Correct PIP joint flexion contracture
    - Serial casting or dynamic splinting
  - If full PIP extension not restored THEN:
    - Surgical joint release and secondary central slip reconstruction
  - Central slip reconstruction:
    - Excise distal scar tissue
    - Reattach central slip to insertion
    - Do not shorten (reduces PIP flexion)

- Immobilize 6wks in full extension with K wire
- Turndown procedure
  - V-Y advancement
- Joint arthritis- relative contraindication to soft tissue reconstructive procedures
- PIP joint arthrodesis viable option in laborers and degenerative PIP joint and unreconstructable tendon
- Rheumatoid patients may function quite well with a significant boutonnière deformity and require no other intervention

4. Understand risks and benefits of various approaches

   - Consider timing issues in reconstruction
   - Management of open vs. closed injuries
   - Indications for surgery
   - Surgery for chronic boutonnière high failure rate, high recurrence rate of PIP joint flexion contracture

5. Address complications and unexpected problems adequately

   - Complications
     - Failure to properly diagnose and treat before fixed PIP flexion contracture develops
     - Failure to fully correct PIP joint flexion contracture prior to extensor tendon reconstruction, result- persistent contracted boutonniere deformity
     - Skin necrosis
     - Limited PIP joint flexion due to tight central slip repair
     - K-wire related complications- pin tract and joint infections, bending or breakage of the wire
     - Nonunion of dorsal avulsion fractures

6. Demonstrate ability to structure alternative plan

   - Management plan for common complications
   - Local flaps for extensive soft-tissue loss
   - Cross finger flaps

Chapter Forty-Nine

Swan Neck Deformity

49
Swan Neck Deformity

1. Identify General Problem/Diagnosis/Planning
   (Describe photo, give working diagnosis, key problems, evaluates patient)

   - This patient appears to have a joint deformity characterized by **hyperextension at the PIP joint and flexion of the DIP joint- Swan neck deformity.**
   - Give working diagnosis of pathology:
     o Either DIP joint or PIP joint…
       - DIP joint
         - Inciting event disruption of terminal extensor mechanism
         - **Mallet Finger**
         - **Causes gradual hyperextension of PIP joint**
       - PIP joint
         - Primary pathologic structure
           o Incompetent volar plate as in rheumatoid arthritis
           o Volar plate laxity causes hyperextension and dorsal displacement of the lateral bands
           o Dorsal migration of lateral bands and volar plate laxity leads to PIP hyperextension.
           o Once lateral bands migrate dorsally they also cause DIP flexion
           o Intrinsic muscle tightness
     o Rare causes
       - Rupture of FDS tendon leading to hyperextension
   - Key points in hx:
     o Hx of finger fracture
       - Fracture of distal phalanx may cause mallet deformity

- Fracture of middle phalanx that heals in hyperextension may cause swan deformity
    - Length of time present
        - Acute- rare, indicates rupture of volar plate of PIP or traumatic mallet deformity
            - Tx: Splinting
    - Other medical conditions
        - Rheumatoid- may weaken volar plate of PIP and/or rupture of terminal extensor tendon- both may cause swan neck
        - Medical conditions that cause systemic ligamentous laxity will unbalance tendon forces and lead to dorsal displacement of lateral bands
    - Occupation- splinting in older patient vs. ligament recon in athlete
    - Handedness
    - Effect on daily routine
        - No interference may consider observing
- PE
    - Look for:
        - Which/how many digits affected?
            - More than one consider
                - Systemic pathology vs. one traumatic isolated injury
        - Is PIP joint flexible?
            - PIP joint used for classification:
                - Type I- flexible
                - Type II- PIP flexion dependent on position of MP joint (relaxation of intrinsic)
                - Type III- stiff PIP with joint preservation on x-ray
                - Type IV- stiff PIP, x-ray destruction
        - Is DIP joint flexible?
            - Important to ascertain prior to reconstruction
        - MP joint flexible? MP flexion (relaxation of intrinsic) gives more PIP laxity?

- o Important to ascertain intrinsic tightness as part of management strategy.
  - If not addressed tight intrinsic muscles prevent return of normal posture and function
- o Neurovascular status
  - Poor blood supply
  - Poor surgical candidate
- o Surgical scars on hands
  - Sign of prior surgical attempts
  - Incorporate into other attempts
- Work up
  - o Plain X-ray- 3 views to:
    - R/O fracture
    - Evaluate joint spaces- rheumatoid disease?
    - Visualize joint spaces preop
- Consultants:
  - o Rheumatology if rheumatoid disease present

2. Consider reasonable goals in diagnosis and management *(Management and treatment, surgical indications, operative procedures and anesthesia)*

   - Acute swan neck deformity treat by splinting!
   - In rheumatoid MCP joint must be addressed first
   - Consultant: rheumatology, esp. for immunosuppressant management
   - Functional deficit is primary indication for intervention!
   - Key to treatment- degree of passive flexibility of PIP joint

3. Select appropriate options in diagnosis and management

   - Options for management of swan neck deformity:
     - o Non-surgical
       - Splinting- will not permanently correct
         - Okay for supple deformities and minimal functional deficits
       - DIP splinting for primary mallet finger
       - Primary PIP pathology- figure-of-eight splinting- prevents hyperextension while allowing flexion
     - o Surgical intervention

- Type I
  - DIP joint
    - Repair of mallet deformity with subsequent maintenance of PIP in 20 degrees of flexion via splint or K-wire removed at 4 weeks
    - DIP joint fused and PIP splinted at 20 degrees
  - PIP joint
    - Figure-of-eight or "silver ring"
    - Volar plate repair- tighten capsule or volar plate
    - Sublimus tenodesis
    - PIP dermodesis
    - Surgical procedures build in flexion contracture to PIP joint
    - Oblique retinacular ligament reconstruction
- Type II
  - Requires release of intrinsic muscles and treatment of MP joint abnormalities
- Type III
  - Restore passive PIP motion via mobilization of lateral bands and physical manipulation of PIP joint
- Type IV
  - Requires arthroplasty or arthrodesis
- PIP JOINT VOLAR PLATE LAXITY
  - Treat by tenodesis procedures
    - Common principle
      - Tendon graft use or tendon re-routing to prevent PIP joint hyperextension.
    - Spiral oblique retinacular ligament reconstruction
      - Free tendon graft for tenodesis (palmaris longus)

- Superficialis tenodesis technique
  - Slip of FDS used for tenodesis at PIP joint
- Postop Care
  - Same for both:
    - Continuous splinting for 4 weeks
    - Then dorsal blocking splint that maintains the PIP joint flexed at 20 degrees and DIP joint neutral
    - Active joint flexion and extension exercises splint prevents extension beyond 20 degrees
    - After 10 weeks splint adjusted to allow PIP joint to straighten another 10 degrees

4. Understand risks and benefits of various approaches

- Intervention dependent upon:
  - Medical status
  - Status of digit:
    - Pliability of PIP and DIP joints
    - Pliability of MP joint
    - Assessment of intrinsic tightness
    - Previous surgery and perfusion
  - Occupation and functional needs of patient
  - Time of deformity
  - **Functional deficit**
- Based on classification and nature of pathology choose non-operative or operative therapy

5. Address complications and unexpected problems adequately

- Potential complications
  - Postop stiffness
    - Most common complication following ligamentous recon.
    - Prevented by early mobilization
    - Must balance risk of early disruption
    - Experienced hand therapist critical
  - Wound infection
  - Disruption
    - Early- re-repair

- Delayed- re-repair vs. other options (arthrodesis)
  - Nonunion- risk of arthrodesis

6. Demonstrate ability to structure alternative plan

    - Consider alternatives for failure of therapy or treatment plan altered by complications
    - What if patient not insured or will not comply with postoperative therapy?
    - How much time will you give for non-operative therapy?
    - What is your time frame for operative therapy?
    - Any benefits of staging surgery?

Chapter Fifty

Extensor Mechanism

50
Extensor Mechanism: Swan neck, Boutonniere, Sagittal Band

1. Extensor Mechanism

- Anatomy of extensor tendon
    - Extensor muscles of wrist, thumb, fingers all radial nerve innervated
- Radial nerve
    - Direct branches to:
        - Brachioradialis (BR)
        - Extensor carpi radialis longus (ECRL)
    - Posterior interosseous nerve (branch of radial) does the rest:
        - Order of innervation proximal to distal:
        - ECRB>Supinator (S)> EDC> EDM> ECU> APL> EPB> EPL> EIP
    - Recovery of radial nerve predictable by this sequence:
        - Wrist extension, finger extension, thumb extension
- Extensor Tendon Anatomy
    - Paratenon
    - At wrist extensor retinaculum
        - 6 distinct anatomic compartments
        - Lister's tubercle- bony prominence
            - EPL (3rd compartment) courses radially to this
    - Distal to retinaculum juncturae tendinum (junc. tend.) connect index, middle, ring and small fingers
        - Consistent ring to middle and small
        - Variable index and middle
    - Index and small have separate extensors EIP and EDM
        - ALWAYS **ULNAR** TO EDC TENDON

- Spare part for tendon reconstruction (EIP and EDM)
- Communis to small absent in up to 80%!
- Replaced by substantial junc. tend. from ring finger.
    - At level of MCP joint
        - Tendon stabilized by sagittal bands
            - Prevents ulnar or radial subluxation
    - More distally
        - Oblique and transverse fibers
        - Tendinous contributions from intrinsic muscles through lateral bands
- Lumbrical muscles
    - Pass volar to MCP joint
    - Dorsal to PIP
    - Through lateral bands
    - ALLOW simultaneous MCP flexion and PIP extension
- At level of PIP joint
    - Extensor tendon becomes central slip and attaches to dorsal base of middle finger
    - ALLOWS extension of PIP joint along with oblique fibers from lateral bands
    - Over the middle phalanx controlling position of the lateral bands
        - Triangular ligament- stabilizes lateral bands dorsally
            - Prevents volar sublux-Boutonniere Def.
        - Transverse retinacular ligament- stabilizes volarly
            - Prevents dorsal sublux- swan-neck
- Further distally
    - Lateral bands join to insert onto base of distal phalanx for DIP joint extension
- Extensor Compartments (Six) Radial to Ulnar
    - I - Abductor pollicis longus/Extensor pollicis brevis (APL/EPB)
    - II - Extensor carpi radialis longus/Extensor carpi radialis brevis (ECRL/ECRB)
    - III - Extensor pollicis longus (EPL)

- o IV - Extensor digitorum communis, extensor indicis proprius (EDC/EIP)
- o V - Extensor digitorum minimi (EDM)
- o VI - Extensor carpi ulnaris (ECU)
- 1st dorsal compartment- likely to have subcompartments
  - o Abductor pollicis longus (APL)
  - o Extensor pollicis brevis (EPB)
- EPL- no attachments (junctura connection) to other extensor tendons
  - o Laceration of EPL may result in full retraction of proximal end, prevents easy repair
- Juncturae tendinae prevent retraction of EDC tendons
- DIFFERENTIATE INTRINSIC AND EXTRINSIC TIGHTNESS WITHIN EXTENSOR SYSTEM
  - o Complex balance between extrinsic and intrinsic tendons and ligamentous support
  - o Normally intrinsic muscles:
    - Tightened with MCP joint extension
    - Loosened with MCP joint flexion
- INTRINSIC TIGHTNESS
  - o Less passive flexion of PIP jt. When MCP jt. extended than when MCP jt. Flexed
- EXTRINSIC TIGHTNESS
  - o Extrinsic extensor tendon limits the ability of finger to achieve combined flexion of MCP joint and the PIP joint.
  - o Less passive flexion of PIP jt. When MCP jt. is flexed than when MCP jt. Extended
- This guides treatment.

2. Swan Neck Deformity

- Hyperextension at the PIP joint and flexion of the DIP joint
  - o Working diagnosis of pathology:
    - Either DIP joint or PIP joint…
    - DIP joint
      - Inciting event disruption of terminal extensor mechanism- Mallet Finger
      - Causes gradual hyperextension of PIP joint
    - PIP joint
      - Primary pathologic structure-

- Incompetent volar plate as in rheumatoid arthritis
- Volar plate laxity causes hyperextension and dorsal displacement of the lateral bands
- Dorsal migration of lateral bands and volar plate laxity leads to PIP hyperextension.
- Once lateral bands migrate dorsally they also cause DIP flexion.
          - Rare causes
            - Rupture of FDS tendon leading to hyperextension
          - Key points in hx:
            - Hx of finger fracture
              - Fracture of distal phalanx may cause mallet deformity
              - Fracture of middle phalanx that heals in hyperextension may cause swan deformity
            - Length of time present
              - Acute- rare, indicates rupture of volar plate of PIP or traumatic mallet deformity
            - Tx: Splinting
          - Other medical conditions
            - Rheumatoid- may weaken volar plate of PIP and/or rupture of terminal extensor tendon- both may cause swan neck
            - Medical conditions that cause systemic ligamentous laxity will unbalance tendon forces and lead to dorsal displacement of lateral bands
          - PIP joint used for classification:
            - Type I- flexible
            - Type II- PIP flexion dependent on position of MP joint (relaxation of intrinsic)
            - Type III- stiff PIP with joint preservation on x-ray
            - Type IV- stiff PIP, x-ray destruction
          - DIP joint flexible

   3. Boutonnière Deformity

- Flexion at the PIP and hyperextension at DIP joint
- Caused by disruption of central slip of extensor tendon.
- In acute closed injury
    - Injury may not be immediately evident
    - May manifest over time (10-14 days)
    - After disruption, triangular ligament and transverse retinacular ligament stretches over time.
    - Lateral bands sublux volar to axis of rotation of PIP joint- result PIP flexion
    - Lateral bands sublux dorsal to axis of rotation of DIP- extension
- Central slip eval:
    - Passively flex PIP 90 degrees
    - Hold pressure on middle phalanx
    - Ask patient to extend if extension force present
    - Central slip likely intact.
    - In this maneuver
        - Normally when central slip intact DIP will not be extended,
        - In boutonnière deformity DIP will extend via lateral bands!
- NEXT
    - Hold PIP in full extension
    - DIP passively flexed
    - In Boutonnière- there will be decreased passive DIP joint extension
- Pseudo-boutonniere
    - Hyperextension injury to PIP joint
    - Contracture of volar structures but no effect on DIP joint
- Look for stability of collateral ligaments of PIP may indicate central slip injury may be from volar PIP joint dislocation

4. Zancolli stage of injury (Boutonnière Deformity)

- Stage I:
    - Weak PIP joint extension (lateral bands)
    - Resting flexion of PIP joint
    - Can be passively corrected to full extension
- Stage II:
    - Loss of active PIP joint extension
    - Secondary stretching of triangular ligament

- - o Sublux of lateral bands volar to axis of PIP joint
  - Stage III:
    - o Progressive hyperextension of DIP joint via subluxed lateral bands
    - o MCP joint may hyperextend
  - Stage IV:
    - o Fixed PIP joint contracture
    - o Contracture of oblique retinacular ligaments and PIP joint volar plate
  - Stage V:
    - o Fixed deformity +
    - o Secondary PIP joint arthritis on x-ray

Chapter Fifty-One

Tendon Reconstruction

51
Tendon Reconstruction

1. Absolute contraindications to primary flexor tendon repair:

   - Gross infection
   - Human bite injuries
   - Cellulitis

2. INDICATIONS FOR SECONDARY RECONSTRUCTION

   - Delay tendon reconstruction in cases not indicated for primary repair:
     o Contaminated fields
     o Hand injuries with extensive soft tissue loss
     o Infection
     o Destruction of pulleys
   - Rupture that cannot be re-repaired directly
   - Cases not treated during primary or delayed primary stage

3. Prior to tendon reconstruction

   - Stable soft tissue coverage
   - Supple joint prior to reconstruction of the pulley system
   - Tendon grafting can growth with patient
     o Not advocated in children if cannot comply with therapy.
   - Secondary tendon grafts
     o Indicated when:
       - Primary repair fails
       - Repair is delayed due to:
         • Contamination
         • Concomitant injuries preclude tendon repair

4. Post tendon grafting regimen

   - 3-4 weeks immobilization followed by unrestricted motion
   - Options for failed tendon repair or gross contamination:
     o 2-stage tendon graft

- o Tendon transfer
- o DIP arthrodesis for zone II failure
- Graft options
  - o Palmaris longus absent in 15-25% (13cm)
  - o Plantaris tendon absent in 10-20% (31cm)
  - o Long extensors or central three toes (30cm of length)
  - o EIP 10cm
  - o EDM 11cm

5. Adhesions

- Causes of Adhesions
  - o Tendon and composite tissue damage
  - o Loss of tendon sheath
  - o Gap formation
  - o Ischemia
  - o Immobilization
  - o Persistent inflammation
  - o Secondary trauma
- Treatment of adhesions
  - o Tenolysis
    - Indication
      - Passive range of motion exceeds active range of motion despite aggressive hand therapy
    - Timing
      - 3 or more months after repair
      - If therapy has plateaued with no gains
    - Prerequisites:
      - All fractures healed
      - Wounds and scars mature
      - Soft pliable skin, minimal reactions around scars
      - Joint contractures corrected, near normal ROM
    - Technique:
      - Wide surgical exposure, Brunner or midlateral
      - Preserve sheath as much as possible
      - Maintain major pulleys

- Some cases resection of FDS may be helpful
- Try to retain both FDS and FDP if possible
- Separate as needed
        - Postop
            - Move fingers immediately 1st post op day
            - Passive ROM decreases and prevents joint contractures
        - Good tendons
            - Aggressive protocol
        - Poor tendon
            - Gentle motion or delayed initiation of finger motion
    - One-stage pulp to palm graft, requires:
        - Minimal scarring
        - Supple joints
        - Adequate pulley system
    - Staged reconstruction- salvage procedure following attempt at one or more other reconstructive options
        - First Stage
            - Silicone rod sutured or screwed to distal phalanx A2 and A4 pulleys reconstructed on top
            - Period of therapy to maintain maximal passive range of motion
            - Scar massage
        - Second stage (at 2-3 months)
            - Graft distally attached into hollow in distal phalanx with pull out suture
            - Proximal end secured with Pulvertaft weave
        - Complications
            - Tight graft- quadriga effect
            - Too loose graft (lumbrical plus deformity)
            - Stiffness
            - Adhesions
            - Rupture, prompt re-exploration and repair

- o   Arthrodesis
- o   Amputation

6. Boyes classification

    - 1- Good- minimal scarring, mobile joints, no contracture
    - 2- Cicatrix- contractures from scar not joint damage, may need preliminary z-plasty or flap coverage
    - 3- Joint damage- restricted ROM, need improvement in joint ROM
    - 4 - Nerve damage- trophic skin, joint change, nerve injury
    - 5 - Multiple damage- multiple digits with tendon damage or scar, joint, nerve injury
    - Prognosis is worsened by additional hand conditions

7. EXTENSOR TENDON RECONSTRUCTION

    - If central slip cannot be reconstructed
        - o   Lateral bands released, mobilized dorsally to reconstruct central slip and rebalance extensor tendon. (Salvi procedure)
    - Central slip reconstruction:
        - o   Excise distal scar tissue
        - o   Reattach central slip to insertion
        - o   Do not shorten (reduces PIP flexion)
        - o   Immobilize 6wks in full extension with K wire
    - Joint arthritis- relative contraindication to soft tissue reconstructive procedures
    - PIP joint arthrodesis viable option in laborers and degenerative PIP joint and unreconstructable tendon

Chapter Fifty-Two

Tendon Transfers

52
Tendon Transfers

1. Identify General Problem/Diagnosis/Planning
   (Describe photo, give working diagnosis, key problems, evaluates patient)

   - Hx: Trauma or neurologic injury with loss of motion at joint and muscle imbalance
   - PE
     - Complete motor and sensory exam
     - Specify components of exam
     - Status of joints
     - Evaluate soft tissue and areas of scarring
   - Tendon transfers
     - Restore motion and balance
     - Functioning muscle-tendon unit preserved, distal tendon transferred to tendon of non-functional motor unit
     - Function does not return to normal
   - Tendon graft
     - Non-vascularized graft acts as interposition replacement of injured tendon
     - Motor function from original muscle
   - INDICATIONS
     - Muscle-tendon loss
     - Nerve injury
   - CONTRAINDICATIONS
     - Stiff joints
     - Poor soft-tissue equilibrium
     - Functional loss of donor tendon/muscle unit is unacceptable
   - CONDITIONS IT TREATS
     - CNS or PNS injuries
     - Closed or open tendon or muscle injury
     - Neurologic disease
   - Key points of tendon transfer:
     - Joints must be supple with maximal ROM prior to transfer
     - Capsulotomies pre-op if needed

- o Will not improve passive ROM
- o Soft-tissue coverage pliable, well vascularized, free of scar tissue
- o Prior to transfer fractures healed or rigidly fixed for post transfer therapy
- o If possibility of functional recovery, postpone until status known
- o Donor deficit of transferred tendon- gain outweigh loss
- o Excursion of donor unit adequate for intended function
- o One joint of action, one function
- o Line of pull as straight as possible
- o Pulvertaft technique, three weaves allows immediate active motion
- o Tension of repair replicates normal tension

2. Consider reasonable goals in diagnosis and management (Management and treatment, surgical indications, operative procedures and anesthesia)

   - During transfer some loss of excursion and strength will occur
   - Consider staging with silicone rods
   - Prepare wound bed
   - Silicone rods can create pseudosheath, facilitating glide
   - Correct skin contractures with z-plasty, local flaps or skin grafts
   - NEEDS
     - o Supple joints
     - o Good wound bed
     - o For optimized recovery
   - Surgical Considerations
     - o If possibility of functional recovery, postpone until status known
     - o Donor deficit of transferred tendon- gain outweigh loss
     - o Excursion of donor unit adequate for intended function
     - o **One joint of action, one function**
     - o **Line of pull as straight as possible**

- - -
    - - ○ Pulvertaft technique, three weaves allows immediate active motion
        - ○ Tension of repair replicates normal tension
    - Principles
        - ○ **Inventory injured and functional muscles**
        - ○ **Excursion**
        - ○ **Power**
        - ○ Length
        - ○ Expendability
        - ○ **Synergism of transfer**
        - ○ **Path of transfer**
        - ○ Condition of tissue
        - ○ Pulley for transfer
        - ○ Number of joints crossed
    - Timing
        - ○ Status of nerve and/or muscle unit
        - ○ Postpone until status known in low injuries
        - ○ If no motor function 3 months after expected time, proceed
        - ○ If no motor function anticipated, proceed as soon as soft tissue will allow
            - Immediate, time of nerve repair
            - Or later
        - ○ Early repair
            - High-level lesions of median, ulnar, radial nerves
            - Proximal injuries poor prognosis
                - Long innervation time
                - Poor function
            - Temporary substitute and later augments power or…
            - Permanent substitute
    - Technical Principles
        - ○ Release of contracted scars, joints
        - ○ Soft, supple tissue coverage
        - ○ Prevention of adhesions
        - ○ Pulvertaft weave- allows early active motion
        - ○ Appropriate postop therapy
        - ○ Tunnels for tendons must be straight line
        - ○ Fewer weaves or end-to-end repair
        - ○ Protect with dynamic splinting 4 weeks

- o Active motion for another 4 weeks allows progression to resistive exercises

3. Select appropriate options in diagnosis and management
    - MEDIAN NERVE PALSY
    - Low median nerve injury- distal to innervation of extrinsic finger and wrist flexors
        - o Thumb opposition- thumb pad to other finger pads
        - o Sensation thumb, index, middle, radial half of ring
    - Motor deficits
        - o Loss of Thumb CMC palmar abduction, pronation, flexion
        - o Thumb pronation
            - Lumbricals to index, middle, opponens pollicis, **abductor pollicis brevis**, flexor pollicis brevis
        - o Thumb MP abduction, flexion
            - FPB has dual innervation ulnar and median (70% retain adequate function)
        - o Sensory deficits
            - Thumb, index, middle, radial ring
    - TIMING LOW MEDIAN NERVE INJURY
        - o Nerve not far from muscle should allow time for recovery, good prognosis except in (i.e. consider early transfer):
            - Elderly patients
            - Poor prognostic signs:
                - Segmental nerve loss and nerve graft
                - Crush injury
                - Associated vascular, tendon or ulnar nerve injury
        - o Transfers for thumb opposition
            - EIP to APB (Burkhalter)
            - EDM to APB for palmar abduction
            - FDS of ring to APB (Bunnel)
            - Palmaris Longus to APB (Camitz)
            - Adductor digiti minimi to APB (Huber)
            - Extensor pollicis brevis transfer
    - PROCEDURES

- EIP or EDM- suitable for palmar abduction transfers (PREFERRED TRANSFER)
    - Sutured to adductor pollicis brevis
    - Short incision at MP joint
    - Ulnar tendon is harvested
    - Re-routed on dorsal ulnar side of wrist
        - (Pulley is ulnar side of forearm)
    - Tunnelled subcutaneously and sutured to adductor pollicis brevis muscle (APB)
    - Tension set with maximal tension on wrist and thumb in maximal palmar abduction
    - Neither EIP or EDM sacrifice significantly reduces hand function
    - Preferred because significant strength for opponensplasty not needed
- FDS of ring to APB
    - Strong tendon for opponensplasty, acceptable donor deficit
    - Distal tendon divided
    - Transverse incision at A1 and A2 pulleys
    - Incision made over pisiform and distal forearm
    - FDS is delivered into distal forearm
    - Distally based slip of FCU is sutured to main tendon creating loop to serve as pulley
        - Most effective pulley for this transfer
    - FDS passed through loop and sutured to APB
    - Tension set as in EIP and EDM transfer
- Palmaris Longus Opponensplasty
    - Palmaris longus tendon harvested with distal extension of palmar fascia through standard carpal tunnel incision
    - Fixed to distal palmar crease
    - Tunneled subcutaneously, superficial to thenar muscles
    - Inserted to Abductor pollicis brevis muscle on radial side of MP joint
    - Tension set with wrist neutral, thumb in maximal palmar abduction
    - Preferred in median nerve compression

- Hypothenar muscle opponensplasty (Huber)
  - Incision along ulnar aspect of hand
  - Muscle identified and transected as distal as possible
  - Id neurovascular bundle (on deep surface of muscle)
  - Free muscle proximally to pisiform
  - Pass subq over transverse carpal ligament
  - Insert into radial aspect of thumb metacarpal near MP joint, APB tendon
  - Allows abduction of thumb out of palm
    - Excellent flexion and pronation
    - Little palmar abduction
  - Useful in:
    - Combined median and ulnar nerve palsy
    - Congenital hypoplasia
- Extensor pollicis brevis transfer
  - EPB tendon transected at muscle tendon junction
  - Tendon brought out through incision at MP joint
  - Distally based tendon passed through subq tunnel to pisiform
  - ECU tendon divided at base of 5th metacarpal and passed around ulnar border of wrist
  - ECU is woven into EPB with thumb in palmar abduction
- High median nerve
- Low median nerve injury
  - Distal to innervation of extrinsic finger and wrist flexors
    - **Thumb opposition**
      - **Sensation thumb, index, middle, radial half of ring**
- Motor deficits
  - Loss of palmar abduction
    Thumb pronation (lumbricals to index, middle, opponens pollicis, **abductor pollicis brevis**, flexor pollicis brevis)
    PLUS

- Extrinsic flexor muscles
- Loss of:
- **Flexion index, middle at PIP and DIP**
- **Flexion of thumb at IP joint**
  - Deficit
    - All four FDS tendons
    - FDS to index and long ONLY
    - Pronator teres
    - Pronator quadratus
    - FPL
    - Thumb opposition
    - Sensation in median distribution
    - Long finger FDP may have cross innervation from ulnar nerve.
  - Goals of High Median nerve injury
    - Restoration of index and long finger flexion at PIP and DIP
    - Thumb flexion at IP joint
    - Focus on FDP function at expense of independent finger flexion
  - Operative Approach in High Median nerve
  - If ulnar nerve intact
    - Restore index and long finger by side to side suturing of FDP's of index and long to ring and small fingers- flexion but not independent
    - To increase power:
    - Consider ECRL tendon transfer to index and long FDP
    - ECRL transected at index metacarpal
    - Tunneled subq around radial border of wrist
    - Weave into FDP of index and long fingers
    - Tension- tips of index and long fingers approximate palm with wrist in 45 degrees dorsiflexion
    - Thumb flexion at IP
    - Restore by transferring brachioradialis to the FPL tendon
    - Brachioradialis transected at distal radius insertion
    - Interwoven with FPL tendon
    - Alternative

- If ECRL tendon not being used for index and long if may be transferred to FPL tendon
- Avoid over tightening
- LONGSTANDING MEDIAN NERVE PALSY
  - May cause adduction/supination contracture
  - May require release of web space
- ULNAR NERVE
  - Low ulnar nerve injury (distal to innervation of extrinsic finger flexors and ulnar wrist flexor)
  - Motor deficits
    - Hyperextension at MCP and hyperflexion at DIP of ring and small fingers
    - Claw deformity- lumbrical loss, unopposed extension at MCP by EDC and unopposed flexion at DIP by FDS
    - Common transfers to correct clawing
      - FDS of middle finger to radial lateral bands of middle, ring, small fingers (Stiles-Bunnell)
      - ECRB extended by grafts to radial lateral bands (Brand I)
      - ECRL extended by grafts to radial lateral bands (Brand II)
  - SEE ULNAR NERVE PALSY CHAPTER
- RADIAL NERVE
  - Motor deficits
    - Absent finger MP extension (EDC, EIP, EDQ)
    - Wrist extension (ECRB, ECRL, ECU)
    - Thumb abduction (APL)
    - Thumb MP extension (EPL, EPB)
  - Most disabling manifestation:
    - Diminished grasp and grip strength- inability to stabilize wrist
    - Other:
      - Inability to release an object
      - Sensory loss not that disabling compared to ulnar and median nerves
  - Low radial nerve injury (posterior interosseous nerve)

- Functional loss:
  - EDC
  - EDM
  - ECU
  - APL
  - EPL
  - EPB
  - EIP
- High radial nerve injury (radial nerve proper)
  - Functional loss: All of the above PLUS:
    - ECRL
    - ECRB
    - Brachioradialis
- Poorer prognosis
- Goals of transfer
  - Restoration of:
    - Finger extension at MP joint
    - Wrist extension
    - Thumb extension and abduction
- TIMING RADIAL NERVE, CONTROVERSIAL
  - Generally poorer prognosis
  - Indications for early repair:
    - Nerve repair not possible
    - Likely to have poor outcome
    - Transferred tendon acting as internal splint and substitute during nerve regeneration
    - Transferred tendon may act synergistically with reinnervated muscles
  - Delayed reconstruction:
    - Allow sufficient time for natural course of nerve regeneration and return of muscle function
    - No return of function in expected timeframe
    - Proceed with transfer
    - 3 month is timeframe for conservative observation

- Common transfer groups to restore finger and thumb extension:
  - FCU to EDC and palmaris to EPL (Jones)
  - FCR to EDC and palmaris to EPL (Starr)

- - - o FDS middle to EIP and EPL and FDS ring to EDC of middle, ring, small (Boyes)
  - Procedures: Three most widely used:
    - FCU transfer
    - FCR transfer
    - Boyes' superficialis transfer
  - o Standard flexor carpi ulnaris transfer
    - Triple transfer:
      - Pronator teres to ECRB
      - FCU to EDC
      - PL to EPL
  - o Flexor carpi radialis transfer- preferred in posterior interosseous nerve palsy
    - Triple transfer
      - PT to ECRB
      - FCR to EDC
      - PL to EPL
  - o Boyes superficialis transfer
    - PT to ECRB
    - FDS of long to EDC of long, ring and small
    - FDS of ring to EIP and EPL
    - FCR to abductor pollicis longus and EPB

4. Understand risks and benefits of various approaches

- Assess soft tissue and joints
- Assess likelihood of recovery
- High or low injury
- Limitations of FDS to APB tendon transfer
  - o Only ring finger can be used, FDS long unacceptable loss of strength
  - o Must leave 1cm of FDS attached to middle phalanx to prevent
  - o PIP hyperextension and swan neck deformity
  - o Cannot be used in high median nerve palsy or injury with forearm flexor muscle loss
  - o Cannot be used in combined low median nerve and high ulnar nerve injury
    - FDS only flexor in these patients
  - o Should not be used in combined low median and low ulnar injuries may be needed in anti-claw treatment

5. Address complications and unexpected problems adequately

    - Major problem inadequate tension or excessive tension
    - Inadequate contracture release prior to transfer
    - Recurrent scar tissue
    - Non-compliance with therapy

6. Demonstrate ability to structure alternative plan

    - Know available alternatives in different clinical scenarios for tendon transfer.

Chapter Fifty-Three

General Hand Fractures

53
General Hand Fractures

1. Identify General Problem/Diagnosis/Planning
   (Describe photo, give working diagnosis, key problems, evaluates patient)

   - Treat patient not x-ray
   - No degree of rotational deformity ever acceptable
     o 5 degrees rotation of metacarpal=1.5cm digital overlap
   - Consider:
     o Enveloping soft tissue
     o Tendons flexor and extensor
     o Intrinsic muscles
     o Neurovascular structures
   - May be involved due to force of injury
   - History:
     o Handedness
     o Occupation
     o Avocation
     o Mechanism of injury (Crush? Compartment syndrome?)
     o Time since injury ('golden period')
     o Place of injury (home, farm, industry)
   - PE:
     o Open fracture?
     o Localized tenderness, Swelling
     o Deformity (angulation, rotation, shortening)
     o Alignment (fingers gentle arc w/o overlap when partially flexed, all nail beds pointing toward scaphoid)
     o ROM (active/passive flexion and extension, intrinsic tightness)
     o Neurovascular status
   - X-rays are key
     o Three views (less than three can miss fracture)
       ▪ Anterior-posterior, Lateral, Oblique
     o Specify digit not general hand film (fingers are superimposed on each other)

- Post-reduction film at 5-7 days to check status of reduction
- Special views:
  - Brewerton view
    - For clarification of ligament-avulsion injuries of metacarpal head
  - Robert view
    - True AP view of thumb metacarpal with hand in maximal pronation
    - Shows thumb metacarpal-trapezium joint (Bennett or Rolando fx)
  - Reverse Robert view
    - 5th metacarpal-hamate joint

2. Consider reasonable goals in diagnosis and management *(Management and treatment, surgical indications, operative procedures and anesthesia)*

- Management
  - Attempt reduction
    - After accurate reduction immobilize and elevate
  - Immobilization
    - 'Intrinsic plus' or 'safe position'
      - MP joints in maximal or near maximal flexion
      - Prevents shortening of collateral ligament
      - Collaterals at maximal length
      - If Splinted in extension, collaterals shorten, lose flexion
    - IP joints splint in near maximal extension
      - Splinting in flexion causes development of checkrein ligaments, causes volar plate contraction, permanent loss of flexion at IP joint
  - Use internal fixation and early mobilization when appropriate
- Goals of management:
  - Not just bone healing in correct position
  - Minimization of soft tissue scarring

- 3R's: Reduction, Retention, Rehabilitation
    - Protective splinting and early mobilization
    - Avoid inappropriate or prolonged immobilization
- Majority of fractures treated non-operatively
    - Most are functionally stable before and or after closed reduction
- Indications for internal fixation:
    - Uncontrollable rotation
    - Angulation, Shortening
    - Displaced intra-articular fractures involving >15-20% of articular surface
    - Fracture dislocations of thumb and little finger CMC joint
    - Unstable fractures that failed closed manipulation
    - Metacarpal head fractures
    - Multiple digit fractures
    - Open fractures
- Bony union occurs quickly with simple splinting
- Unstable fractures
    - Cannot be reduced in closed position or…
    - If reduced, cannot be held in reduced position w/o supplemental fixation
    - Internal fixation needed
        - To provide stability
        - Allow early mobilization
    - Initial steps
        - Reduce convert to stable position by external immobilization
        - Closed reduction and K-wire or…
        - Open reduction and internal fixation (ORIF)
- Post-reduction management:
    - Immediate movement uninvolved fingers to prevent stiffness
    - Exercise program directed toward specific fracture or dislocation
    - Early mobilization of injured finger
- Non-displaced fracture treated by closed reduction:
    - Motion started within 3 weeks
- Mid-shaft proximal phalangeal fracture
    - 5-7 weeks immobilization for clinical stability
- Mid-shaft middle phalangeal fracture (>cortical to cancellous bone)

- - - o 10-14 weeks immobilization (same as scaphoid fx)
  - Comminuted fractures with disruption of periosteum
    - o 2x more time to bony union compared to simple, closed fractures
  - Failure of inadequate immobilization
    - o Loss of reduction with subsequent malunion
  - Radiologic union lags clinical, may not be seen for 3-5 months
  - Best criteria for initiation of mobilization- absence of pain at fracture site

3. Select appropriate options in diagnosis and management

  - Manage fracture according to guidelines in 2.
  - Management based on presented clinical scenario.

4. Understand risks and benefits of various approaches

  - Base treatment plan of type of fracture, location and digits involved
  - Note above mentioned risks and benefits based on type of fracture

5. Address complications and unexpected problems adequately

  - Complications may occur due to inappropriate management
  - Cosmetic deformity and/or functional loss
    - o Avoid by obeying basic principles
  - Inappropriate splinting can result in articular and extra-articular changes
    - o Stiffness
    - o Joint contracture
    - o Deformity
  - How do you manage malrotation, chronic pain, stiffness, joint contracture or residual deformity?

6. Demonstrate ability to structure alternative plan

  - Be familiar with common available treatment plans
  - When would you do open vs. closed reduction?
  - Backup plan for nonunion or malunion

Chapter Fifty-Four

Specifics of Hand Fractures

54
Specifics of Hand Fractures
Thumb, Metacarpal, and Phalanx Fractures

1. Identify General Problem/ Diagnosis/Planning
   (Describe photo, give working diagnosis, key problems, evaluates patient)

   - Treat patient not x-ray
   - No degree of rotational deformity ever acceptable
     - 5 degrees of rotation of metacarpal=1.5 cm digital overlap
   - Consider:
     - Enveloping soft tissue
     - Tendons flexor and extensor
     - Intrinsic muscles
     - Neurovascular structures
   - May be involved due to force of injury.
   - Hx:
     - Handedness
     - Occupation
     - Avocation
     - Mechanism of injury (Crush? Compartment syndrome?)
     - Time since injury ('golden period')
     - Place of injury (home, farm, industry)
   - PE:
     - Open fracture?
     - Localized tenderness
     - Swelling
     - Deformity (angulation, rotation, shortening)
     - Alignment (fingers gentle arc w/o overlap when partially flexed, all nail beds pointing toward scaphoid)
     - ROM (active/passive flexion and extension, intrinsic tightness)
     - Neurovascular status
   - X-rays are key

- o Three views (less than three can miss fracture)
  - ▪ Anterior-posterior, Lateral, Oblique
- o Specify digit not general hand film (fingers are superimposed on each other)
- o Post-reduction film at 5-7 days to check status of reduction
- o Special views:
  - ▪ Brewerton view
    - • For clarification of ligament-avulsion injuries of metacarpal head
  - ▪ Robert view
    - • True AP view of thumb metacarpal with hand in maximal pronation
    - • Shows thumb metacarpal-trapezium joint (Bennett or Rolando fx)
  - ▪ Reverse Robert view
    - • 5th metacarpal-hamate joint

2. Consider reasonable goals in diagnosis and management *(Management and treatment, surgical indications, operative procedures and anesthesia)*

- ▪ METACARPAL FRACTURES: HEAD
  - o Rare
  - o Intraarticular difficult to dx
    - ▪ Brewerton views
  - o Management
    - ▪ Nonoperative
      - • Indications
        - o Nondisplaced fx able to tolerate stress testing
        - o Small fragments <20% articular surface
        - o Less than 1mm articular step-off
        - o Comminuted fractures that are irreparable
      - • Immobilize in safe position (MP flex/IP extension) 2-3 weeks then
      - • Protected motion
    - ▪ Operative
      - • Goals of fixation

- Restoration of joint congruity
- Rigid internal fixation
  - To allow early active motion
  - To avoid scarring and contracture
- Indications
  - Non-comminuted fx >25% articular surface
  - >1-2mm articular step off
  - Unstable fx
  - Open fx
  - Comminuted or oblique fx with displacement requires ORIF
- Other treatment modalities
  - Skeletal traction
  - Silicone arthroplasty
  - Metacarpophalangeal joint arthrodesis
- **METACARPAL FRACTURES: NECK**
  - Most common
  - Boxer's fracture (little finger, 'real' boxers index and middle)
  - Secondary to direct blow axial load- Comminution of volar cortex
  - Intrinsic muscle flexes head of fragment
  - Apex dorsal angulation
  - MANAGEMENT
    - Non-op
      - Degree of acceptable angulation (CONTROVERSIAL)
        - Index and middle, fixed minimal compensatory motion CMCJ
          - 10-15 degrees of angulation tolerated
          - If greater then reduce fx
        - Ring and little finger

- 25-30 degrees of angulation tolerated (up to 40)
  - Controversial
  - Some say immediate mobilization irrespective of angulation
  - Minimal disability
  - Even 10-30 degrees in ring and little unacceptable if 'pseudoclawing' on active extension
  - Secondary to compensatory hyperextension of MP joint
  - Safe answer
    - Generally up to 40 degrees of angulation tolerated in ring and little
    - Attempt closed reduction if at least 15 degrees of angulation
  - In contrast
    - Index and middle no more than 15 degrees can be accepted
- ORIF required
  - <15 degrees
    - Ulnar splint 10-14 days
  - 15-40 degrees
    - Reduce
    - Ulnar gutter splint 3 weeks
- Surgery for:
  - >40 degrees
  - Volar Comminution
  - Extensor lag or unacceptable reduction
- Percutaneous pinning usually adequate
  - ORIF usually not necessary

- ANY ROTATIONAL DEFORMITY MUST BE CORRECTED!!!
  - Can be reduced up to 10-14 days post injury
  - Jahss "90-90" maneuver (MP and PIP in 90 degrees)
- Operative Treatment
  - Unstable fracture- re-angulation post reduction
  - Persistent pseudoclawing on active extension
  - Stabilize via:
    - K-wires
      - Longitudinal crossed
      - Transverse into adjacent metacarpal
  - ORIF any fracture that angulation and rotation cannot be achieved by closed means
- METACARPAL SHAFT
  - Transverse
  - Spiral
  - Oblique
  - Comminuted
  - Apex-dorsal angulation occurs
    - From interossei and flexor tendons
    - Causes
      - Pseudoclawing of MP
      - Pain with grip
      - Conspicuous dorsal prominence
    - More proximal fractures, less angulation can be tolerated
  - Comminuted fractures generally unstable require ORIF
    - Rotation never acceptable
    - Management
    - Non-op
      - Index and middle
        - 0-10 degrees on angulation acceptable
      - Ring and Little

- 20-30 degrees of angulation acceptable
- Compensatory mobility of CMCJ
- Shortening (controversial)
  - 2-5mm acceptable
- Treatment: Cast
  - Incorporate metacarpals
  - Digits free-wrist and IP joint immobilization does not add to stability only stiffness
  - 4 weeks gentle active, MP joint motion
    - Operative
      - Indications
        - Failure of closed reduction
        - Percutaneous K-wires usually adequate
          - Allows early motion
          - Not rigid fixation
      - Consider
        - Intramedullary pins
        - Transverse pins
          - Transfix distal fragment to adjacent intact metacarpal
      - ORIF
        - Malrotation
        - Irreducible fractures
        - Open fractures
        - Multiple fractures
        - Segmental bone loss
      - K-wire alone or in combo with:
        - Wiring
        - Screw
        - Plate
    - METACARPAL FRACTURE OF THUMB
      - Extra-articular
        - Fx at base of thumb metacarpal common

- Transverse or slightly oblique fractures
  - Angulate dorsally due to
    - Extension pull of proximal frag by APL
    - Flexion of distal frag by FPB
- Splinting alone cannot control muscle forces
- Progressive angulation results in malunion
- Intra-articular
  - Bennett's fracture
    - Intra-articular fracture-subluxation
    - Base of thumb metacarpal
      - Oblique ligament (volar beak ligament)
        - Stabilizes ulnovolar frag in anatomic position
      - Metacarpal shaft frag subluxates radially, proximally and dorsally
    - Tx:
      - Anatomic reduction
      - Any incongruity of articular surface unacceptable
      - Degenerative arthritis results in:
        - Pain, weakness, loss of motion
      - Reduction 'easy'
      - Retention 'difficult'
      - Reduction requires: Closed reduction and percutaneous pin fixation (CRPP) or ORIF (with K-wire or screw)
  - Rolando's fracture
    - Intra-articular fx of base of thumb metacarpal in T, Y or comminuted form
    - Tx:

- o Closed or open reduction and K-wire or screw placement
- Comminuted fx options:
  - o Thumb spica cast
  - o Oblique skeletal traction
  - o Limited open reduction and internal fixation or external fixation
- PHALANGEAL FRACTURES
  - o Goals
    - Anatomic reduction
    - Bony healing
    - Functional recovery
    - Correction of rotational deformity
    - Stability for bone healing
  - o Stable fractures
    - Undisplaced or stable following reduction
    - Brace, splint or cast
  - o Displaced or unstable fx
    - If reduction cannot be maintained
    - Percutaneous K-wire or screw fixation
  - o Typically angulate volarly
    - Imbalance of intrinsic tendons
  - o Post reduction
    - Must restore muscle balance- intrinsic plus position
  - o Poor prognostic factors
    - Intra-articular fx
    - Comminuted
    - Bone loss
- BASE FX PROXIMAL PHALANX
  - o Displaced split fractures
    - Reduce, tenacular clamp if necessary
    - Crossed K-wire
    - Attempt articular congruity
  - o Irreducible fx by closed means
    - Minicondylar plate application
  - o Can use CRPP with K-wire
    - Volar angulation of 25 degrees causes loss of motion necessitating corrective osteotomy
  - o Immobilize

- MP 70 degrees of flexion
- IP extended
- 3-4 weeks
- SHAFT FX PROXIMAL PHALANX
  - Transverse
  - Oblique (short)
  - Spiral (long)
  - Proximal phalanx angulates volar
  - Middle phalanx fx angulate depending on site of fx
    - Distal to FDS volar
    - Proximal to FDS dorsal
  - Long healing times
    - Mid-proximal phalanx 5-7 weeks
    - Middle phalanx 10-14 weeks-> cortical bone content
  - Long spiral, oblique fracture
    - Undisplaced spiral oblique of prox phalanx
      - If periosteum intact may be stable
      - Splint in functional position
      - Weekly x-ray 4 weeks- check for displacement
    - Displaced
      - Unstable
      - Static functional splinting in functional position combined with traction or…
      - ORIF K-wires or lag screw (2-3) perpendicular to plane of fx
  - Short oblique diaphyseal fx
    - Unstable fx except
      - Undisplaced fx may be stable if periosteum intact
      - Reduce plate reduction
      - Transverse K-wire or screws alone not adequate
  - Transverse diaphyseal fx
    - Unicondylar
      - Non-displaced and displaced are unstable fx
      - Preferred fixation
        - Two K-wires

- One or two miniscrews or Combo
  - Displaced best treated by ORIF
  - Often complicated by 20-30 degrees proximal IP flexion contracture or extensor lag
- Bicondylar
  - Small fragments more difficult to fix
  - Usually comminuted, intraarticular, unstable
- Options
  - Minicondylar plate
  - Dynamic traction
  - Primary joint arthrodesis

3. Select appropriate options in diagnosis and management

- See above in management
- Select management plan based on nature of fracture

4. Understand risks and benefits of various approaches

- Review above.
- Be aware of potential complications
  - Malunion
  - Nonunion
  - Malrotation

5. Address complications and unexpected problems adequately

- Malunions
  - Most common complication, more easily prevented than corrected
  - Rotational deformity
  - Overlap or scissoring during flexion
  - Diminishes grip strength and dexterity
  - Most frequently after
    - Spiral or oblique fx
  - Clinical diagnosis, x-ray hard to appreciate
  - Immobilization with adjacent normal finger may minimize this complication

- CRPP or ORIF low threshold in spiral or oblique fx
- Tx:
  - Osteotomy
    - Previous fx or base of metacarpal
    - Transverse osteotomy simplest approach
- Lateral angulation deformities
  - Cause displacement of condyle or bone loss at time of fx
  - Condyle hard to correct other types correctable
  - Tx:
    - Corrective Osteotomy- old fx or proximal to level of deformity
    - Fix with K-wire or interosseous wires
    - Arthroplasty in damaged joint surfaces
    - Arthrodesis
- Dorsal-volar angulation deformities
  - Typically secondary to transverse fx of metacarpal and phalangeal shafts
  - Muscle-tendon imbalance
  - Tx: Corrective osteotomy or refracture
- Shortening
  - Tx: Corrective osteotomy
- Nonunion
  - Uncommon
  - Occurs with:
    - Open fx with segmental bone loss
    - Soft-tissue interposition
    - Distraction at fracture site
    - Premature removal of internal fixation (shaft fx middle or proximal phalanx)
    - Loss of reduction
    - Inadequate immobilization
  - Greatest propensity in:
    - Middle phalanx
    - Proximal phalanx of thumb
  - Delayed union seen frequently-
    - X-ray union lags clinical union
    - May take 3-5 months
    - Undertake re-op at 4 months or later to avoid stiffness due to additional immobilization

- o Tx of nonunion:
  - Bone graft and rigid plate fixation
  - Frequently complicated by stiff finger
  - If adjacent to joint:
    - Bone excision
    - Arthroplasty
    - Arthrodesis
- Restricted Digital Motion
  - o Tendon adherence at fx site (extensor or flexor)
  - o Capsular contracture (Especially: PIP)
  - o Joint stiffness
  - o Must differentiate tendon adhesion from joint stiffness
    - Tendon adherence
      - Passive motion > active motion
    - Joint stiffness
      - Passive and active motion equally restricted
  - o Tendon adherence
    - Most frequent after crush injury
    - Prevention
      - Early active ROM
    - Surgical intervention ONLY after
      - Maximum passive ROM restored with aggressive OT
    - Extensor adherence
      - Significant active extensor lag of PIP w/o fixed contracture
    - Difficult to correct- extreme scarring
  - o Joint Stiffness
    - Improper immobilization (90-90 position)
    - Prolonged immobilization
    - Soft tissue capsular contracture
    - Intra-articular incongruity
    - Joint fibrosis
    - Inadequate rehab
  - o Tx:
    - May be correctable with aggressive OT
      - Active and passive ROM
      - Dynamic splinting
      - Serial casting

- **DO NOT OPERATE UNTIL ADEQUATE TRIAL OF THERAPY**
    - Operative Tx:
        - MP joint extension contracture
            - Dorsal capsulectomy
        - PIP flexion contracture
            - Checkrein release
        - Arthrodesis in functional position
        - Amputation
- Most common complication of ORIF- stiffness
- Infection
    - Rare
    - Antibiotics in open fx controversial
        - Often used but irrigation and debridement are primary treatment
    - Osteomyelitis
    - Infected non-union
        - Tx:
            - Stabilize fx
            - Debride infected, non-viable tissue
            - Antibiotics
    - If joint involved:
        - Fusion

6. Demonstrate ability to structure alternative plan

- Be familiar with different open operative approaches
- Plan if patient is not insured and cannot undergo therapy
- Patient refuses to comply with therapy

Chapter Fifty-Five

Thumb Amputation and Reconstruction

55
Thumb Amputation and Reconstruction

1. Identify General Problem/Diagnosis/Planning
   (Describe photo, give working diagnosis, key problems, evaluates patient)

   - Describe photo
   - It appears that this patient has a complete or partial amputation of the thumb.
   - Specify parts present and level of amputation.
   - Ask to review x-ray of hand and parts.
   - Thorough, expeditious history to determine if patient is a candidate for surgery:
   - Thumb indispensable
     - Loss of thumb = 40% impairment of the hand
   - Function prehensile- power grip, precision grip
   - Tactile gnosis (pulp sensation)
   - Position (length and web span)
   - Mobility (muscle and joint)
   - Hx:
     - Mechanism:
       - Sharp
         - Favorable for replant
       - Crush
         - Less favorable for replant
         - Greater areas of damage
         - Adverse effects on vessel and nerve
         - Wide zone of injury proximal or distal to amp site
       - Avulsion
         - Less favorable
         - Detaches tendons from musculotendinous junction
         - Devascularizes long segments of nerve important to functional reconstruction
         - Tendon detachment more proximal

- Limit of tolerable cold and warm ischemia
  - 12 hours warm
  - 24 hours cold
  - 1 hour of warm ischemia=6 hours cold ischemia
- Cooling extends window of opportunity:
  - Part wrapped in saline soaked gauze inside plastic bag on ice
- Site of injury
- Farm or garden increased risk of infection, less favorable
- Hand dominance- be more aggressive with dominant hand injuries
- Consider occupation
- Coexisting medical morbidities
  - CAD
  - PVD
  - DM
  - Kidney disease
  - DRUG ABUSE- cocaine
  - Other
- **Tetanus status**
  - Booster every 10yrs
  - Booster if >5yrs since last dose

- PE
  - ATLS
  - ABC's
  - R/O life threatening injuries (intracranial, intrathoracic, intraabdominal)
  - Which digits involved?
  - Radial digits- important in fine motor control
  - Ulnar digits- important in gross motor strength
  - Level of amputation:
  - Surgical options dependent on level of amputation
  - Plain x-ray assists in determination:
    - Bone- distal or proximal phalanx, metacarpal
    - Joint- interphalangeal, metacarpophalangeal
  - All hand trauma patients x-ray of hand and amputated parts
    - Three views (AP, lateral, oblique)
  - Looking for:

- Level of injury
- Comminution
- Joint involvement
  - Consultation- OT early
  - Labs in all replant patients:
    - CBC (Hb, Hct, Platelet count)
    - PT/PTT
    - Type and cross match 2-4 units, why? Transplant patients frequently require transfusion
    - EKG if hx of cardiac disease
    - CXR in some
  - Critical anatomic elements
    - Thumb pulp
    - Length of thumb
    - Span of first web- contracture or loss of web span equivalent to amputation of thumb. Loses its working ability
    - Thenar muscles
      - Extrinsic (FPL, Abductor pollicis longus, EPB, EPL)
      - Intrinsic (Abductor pollicis brevis, opponens pollicis, flexor pollicis, adductor pollicis)- stronger
    - First CMC joint
    - Classify by which elements are lost:
      - Type A- skin loss
      - Type B- loss of length
      - Type C- inadequate first web space
      - Type D- inadequate function of muscles
      - Type E- CMCJ
  - May be a combination of injuries, more than one option

2. Consider reasonable goals in diagnosis and management *(Management and treatment, surgical indications, operative procedures and anesthesia)*

   - Surgical candidate?
   - Determine level of amputation

- Type of injury- vein grafts more likely to be needed in crush or avulsion
- Stabilize life-threatening injuries prior to reconstruction
- Goals of reconstruction:
    - Good position relative to other digits
    - Stable joints
    - Painless skin, attempt to cover with protective sensation
    - Optimal length
    - Capacity for growth (children)
        - Type A injury- loss of skin
            - <1cm^2 and no exposed bone
                - Secondary intention
            - 1-1.5cm^2 Small palmar defects
                - Local flaps, Moberg flap
            - >1.5cm^2 Larger defects
                - Neurovascular island flap
                    - Cross finger
                    - Free toe pulp transfer
                    - Kite flap for dorsal skin loss
        - Type B- loss of length
            - Amputation distal to proximal phalanx
                - Do not need additional length for adequate return of function
            - Toe transfer needed for aesthetic thumb
            - More proximal injuries, multiple options:
                - Metacarpal lengthening
                - Toe transfer
                - Osteoplastic reconstruction
                - Pollicization
        - Type C- inadequate web space
            - Z-plasty or flaps
            - Posterior interosseous flap
        - Type D- inadequate function of thenar muscles
            - Associated with type B injury

- Toe transfer ideal for muscle loss amputations but need intact CMC joint
- Osteoplastic recon is an option, less ideal, but less OR time
  - Type E-Loss of CMC
    - Necessitates pollicization
    - Only finger metacarpophlangeal joint can approximate the CMC joint

3. Select appropriate options in diagnosis and management

   - Surgical options (depend on level of injury):
   - Replantation (completely severed) vs. revascularization (incomplete amp that requires vessel recon to maintain viability)
   - Simplest option (not always best): Shortening remaining bone and primary closure of skin
     o Type A Small soft tissue defects
       - Moberg Flap
         - Hypersupinated hand position
         - Must be no injury to dorsum of thumb or
         - Injury to dorsal branch of radial artery
         - Incision at midaxial line- to prevent contracture
         - Bilateral midaxial incisions
         - Plane of dissection
           o Deep to neurovascular bundles
           o Superficial to tendon sheath
         - Advance flap by flexing IP joint
         - Best for defects <2cm
         - Results in IP flexion deformity
         - Dorsal extension blocking splint 3 weeks
       - Littler Neurovascular Island Flap
         - Defects >2cm^2

- Sensate, well vascularized glabrous skin taken from ulnar side of middle or ring finger
- Digital Allen's test
- Distally leave 1cm pulp on donor finger
- Zigzag incision on palm
- Tunnel flap subcutaneously
- Critical to leave as much adipose around neurovasc. bundle as possible
- Inset flap with thumb in full abduction
- Primarily ulnar aspect of thumb pulp needs sensate cover, decreases flap requirement for tissue
- Post op
  - ROM donor digit POD 1
  - Graft donor site bolter for 7-10 days
  - Splint thumb one week then AROM
- Injury at or distal to IP (interphalangeal) joint:
  - Replant or revasc
    - Tourniquet
    - Bone shortening in most cases
    - Osteosynthesis with:
      - K-wire
      - 90-90 interosseous wire
      - Interosseous wire with k-wire (Lister technique)
    - Tendon
    - Artery
      - Anastomosis outside zone of injury
      - Microscope
      - Vein graft if needed

- - - Vein
    - Nerve
    - Skin closure
      - Loose
      - Unmeshed partial thickness skin grafts or allografts to avoid tension
    - Pulse ox to monitor perfusion
  - Metacarpal lengthening
    - Distraction osteogenesis- 2-3cm can be achieved
    - Requires:
      - K-wiring joint to prevent flexion deformity
      - Postop intensive therapy
      - May require secondary bone grafting
  - Deepening first web space
    - Four flap z-plasty
  - No reconstruction
  - Free pulp transfer
    - Advantages- better 2 point sensation
    - No need for cortical reorientation
    - Acceptable donor defect
    - Blood supply first plantar metatarsal artery
    - Great toe pulp preferred
    - Anastomosis to ulnar digital artery or radial artery in anatomic snuff box
    - Start AROM in thumb at 1 week, immobilize donor site 2-3 weeks
- Type B Injury- length deficiency
  - Injury within proximal phalanx:

- Great toe transfer (Ideal)
  - Indicated in any amputation from proximal phalanx proximally
  - Must have intact CMC joint
  - Flap based on first dorsal metatarsal
    - May be based on larger first plantar metatarsal a. (absent in 1/3)
  - Requires:
    - Intact thenar muscles
  - Advantage:
    - Single stage
    - Retention of growth potential
    - Motion at IP and MP level
    - Potential for sensibility
  - Disadvantages:
    - Large digit
    - Long OR time
    - Donor site morbidity
- Wrap around procedure
  - Best appearance
  - Free soft tissue and distal portion of distal phalanx flap
    - From first or second digit, toe
  - Placed around free bone graft (usually iliac crest)
  - Advantages
    - Single operation
    - Good strength
    - Less donor site morbidity
    - Better aesthetics
  - Disadvantages
    - Absence of growth potential
    - Potential for graft loss
- Second toe transfer (can be used in lieu of great toe)
  - Least satisfactory appearance, IP joint function weak

- Blood supply- first dorsal metatarsal a.
- Advantages
  - Single stage
  - Retention of growth potential
  - Adequate mobility
- Disadvantages
  - Small appearance
  - Long OR Time
  - Donor site morbidity
- WHAT IF PATIENT DOES NOT WANT TOE TRANSFER?
  - Web deepening- z-plasty with repositioning of the adductor insertion proximally
  - Distraction lengthening of first metacarpal and web deepening
  - Injury at MCP Joint level:
    - Distraction
    - Web space deepening
    - Wrap around
    - Toe transfers
    - Osteoplastic reconstruction
  - Injury at Metacarpal:
    - Toe- to thumb
    - Osteoplastic thumb reconstruction
    - (osteocutaneous reversed radial forearm flap)
  - Injury at carpal metacarpal joint (CMC) level or Type E Injury (CMCJ deficiency):
  - **POLLICIZATION ONLY OPTION**, due to absence of thenar musculature
  - Indications for pollicization:
    - Total or subtotal defects of thumb.
    - Narrows palm, less effective in adults
    - Type C injury (1st web deficiency)
    - Transverse or near transverse incisions will cause web contracture
    - Web contracture may involve skin as well as deeper structures like muscle and ligaments. CMC joint may require release
  - Treatment

- ▪ Skin only
  - • Z-plasty (jumping man flap or four limb z-plasty)
  - • Unaesthetic in dark skin patients
- ▪ Skin, muscle or joint
  - • Adductor release
  - • CMC joint capsulotomy
  - • Flap coverage
- ▪ Post op prolonged splinting
- o Type D injury (Motor deficiency)
- o Amputation or crush injury
- o Treatment:
- o Radical debridement of severely contused muscle
  - ▪ Inadequate debridement results in adduction contracture
- o Extrinsics provide adequate motion at MCP and CMC joints
- o Motor reconstruction
- o Goal
  - ▪ Restore opposition
  - ▪ Via tendon transfers
- o If length required:
  - ▪ Pollicization
  - ▪ Toe transfers
- o Toe Transfer Procedure
  - ▪ Identify arterial system
  - ▪ Preserve tendons
  - ▪ Osteotomy
  - ▪ Identify digital nerves
  - ▪ Ready the flexor tendons
  - ▪ Transfer and anastomose in snuff box
- o Post op
  - ▪ Hydrate
  - ▪ Warm
  - ▪ Anticoagulation
  - ▪ AROM after 1 week
  - ▪ Elevate foot, non-weight bearing for 3 weeks
- o Osteoplastic reconstruction
  - ▪ Iliac crest bone graft
  - ▪ Groin or forearm flaps

- Key points keep seam of flap used on palmar side
  - Allows placement of bone graft and inset of neurovascular island flap without making additional incisions
  - Harvest corticocancellous bone graft with some periosteum for suturing
  - Anticipate 30-50% resorption of iliac crest bone graft
- POLLICIZATION
  - Advantages over toe transfer:
    - Three functional joints
    - Arc of motion fully oriented into palm
    - Better option when basal joint is lost
    - Simultaneous web space deepening
  - Operation
    - Position
      - Supine
      - Upper limb abducted
      - Hand in mid-prone position
  - Preop
    - Is there adequate skin to reconstruct web?
      - Flaps may be needed
  - Two critical factors:
    - Safeguarding draining veins on dorsum
    - Position of new thumb
  - Procedure
    - Incision racquet-shaped with dorsal V top be placed in cleft made over thumb stump
    - Dorsal and palmar skin flaps
    - Expose second ray from PIPJ to base of metacarpal
    - Preserve dorsal veins
    - Severe juncturae tendinae
    - Intermetacarpal ligament divided
    - Radially, 1st dorsal interosseous sectioned
    - Two neurovasc. bundles released to palmar arch
    - Ulnar pedicle separated from middle
    - Osteotomy of 2nd at base
    - Include MCPJ depending on if CMCJ absent or present:

- CMCJ Present
  - Fix in position with K wire
  - Fine tune position
  - Transferred digit should not extend beyond PIPJ of middle finger (0.5 to 1.0cm proximal)
  - Position
    - Index pronated 90-100 degrees (tip-tip pinch with middle)
    - Four transferred tendons
      - EDC and FDP shortened sutured to EPL and FPL Pulvertaft weave
      - EIP ulnar side and FDS used to stabilize PIPJ, new CMCJ
- CMCJ absent
  - MCPJ acts as new CMCJ
  - Metacarpal fixed to trapezium or saphead using 90-90 wiring technique in 120 degrees of pronation
  - 1st dorsal interosseous sutured to radial aspect of proximal phalanx
    - Restores adduction and pronation
  - FDS released from insertion rerouted around pisiform inserted into radial aspect of PIPJ capsule
- Post op
  - Thumb splinted until bony union
  - Early ROM started, if rigid fixation achieved

4. Understand risks and benefits of various approaches

- See notes in 3.
- Be able to discuss risks and benefits of various approaches based on level of amputation.

- Understand risks and benefits of individual procedures
- What is the success rate of toe-to-thumb transfers?
- Risk of digital ischemia in pollicization

5. Address complications and unexpected problems adequately

- Moberg flap complications
    - IP joint flexion
    - First web space contracture
- Littler flap complications
    - Hematoma
    - Flap loss from kinking or vessel injury
- Post replant
    - Pulse ox to monitor perfusion
    - Management of failing free flap
    - Venous congestion management
    - Management of leeches
    - Hb/Hct monitoring, your protocol
- Complications
    - Infection- prophylactic antibiotics
    - Malunion or nonunion
        - Possible at site of reattachment
        - Tx: Secondary bone grafting across defect
    - Neuroma
        - Tx: Secondary excision and burying proximal stump
    - Chronic pain
        - May not have specific cause
        - Difficult to manage
        - Consult- Pain Management
    - Stiffness
        - Scarring of skin, tendon and/or joint capsule
        - Secondary tenolysis may be needed
    - Digit loss
        - Early ischemia post-op- re-explore
            - Inspect arterial and venous anastomosis
            - Check for technical problems
                - Anastomosis
                - Kinking of vessel
                - Compression
        - Anticoagulation

- Second toe transfer
    - DIP joint flexion deformity common
    - Pin for 3-4 weeks
- Pollicization
    - Avoid kinking of pedicle
    - Secondary procedures
    - May be needed
        - Shorten flexors
        - Extensor tenolysis
        - Opponensplasty

6. Demonstrate ability to structure alternative plan

- Have alternate plan based on failure of initial management
- What if patient does not agree with suggested operative plan?

Chapter Fifty-Six

Fingertip Injuries

56
Fingertip Injuries

1. Identify General Problem/Diagnosis/Planning
   (Describe photo, give working diagnosis, key problems, evaluates patient)

   - This patient appears to have:
     - Subungal hematoma
     - Loss or disruption of nail
     - Describe anatomic deformity in detail
   - Anatomy of fingertip
     - Hyponychium
     - Paronychium
     - Eponychium- epidermal shelf at base of nail
     - Fingernail
       - Proximal 1/3- germinal matrix
       - Two components, dorsal and intermediate
       - Distal 2/3- sterile matrix, distal to lunula
     - Fingernail production
       - Three areas
         - Dorsal nail
         - Intermediate nail of germinal matrix (90% of nail volume)
         - Ventral nail of sterile matrix
   - R/O other injuries- neurovasc, tendons, bone distal phalanx fracture

2. Consider reasonable goals in diagnosis and management
   (Management and treatment, surgical indications, operative procedures and anesthesia)

   - Tourniquet and Loupes
   - Indications
   - Based on:
     - Age
     - Hand dominance
     - Digit involvement
     - Gender
     - Pre-existing medical conditions

- o Mechanism of injury
- o Occupation
- o Anatomy of fingertip defect
- Operative Tx:
    - o Large wound >1cm or…
    - o Need for rapid healing
- Contraindications
    - o Advanced age for two stage or complex reconstructions
    - o Small wounds that will heal by secondary intention
- Large nail bed lacs involving germinal matrix heal poorly, nail plate abnormalities
- Association with large subungal hematomas
    - o Previous recommendation
        - Nail removal and nail bed repair every case
        - Study showed no deformity with drainage only, regardless of size of hematoma
    - o New recommendation
        - Drainage only for subungal hematomas
        - Reserve nail removal and nail bed repair for injury with disrupted nail edges or when nail is broken
- Associated distal phalanx fx
    - o Reduce and splint with nail
    - o If fx unstable or nail plate unusable, fixation of distal phalanx may be required

3. Select appropriate options in diagnosis and management

- Fingertip Injuries
    - o Operative goal:
        - Durable coverage
        - Restore protective sensation
    - o Small defects heal without significant loss of sensitivity
    - o Skin graft
        - Worse recovery of sensitivity
        - FT better than ST
        - Reinnervation >1yr
    - o Local sensory flap
        - Atasoy volar V-Y
        - Kutler bilateral V-Y

- - - Limited to small defects
  - Moberg for 1.5cm thumb defects
    - Not used in other digits because of:
    - High risk of dorsal skin necrosis
    - Flexion contracture deformities
  - Littler's neurovascular island flap
  - First dorsal metacarpal artery flap
  - Cross finger flap
  - Reverse homodigital artery flap
  - Larger defects

- Fingernail injuries
  - Intact nail/subungal hematoma
    - Drainage with battery-powered micro-cautery device
  - Nail edges disrupted or nail plate torn explore nail bed
  - Can preserve nail
  - Repair 7-0 chromic
  - Small defects of nail bed ST graft from sterile matrix of same injured nail bed or adjacent uninjured finger or great toe using 15 blade, thin
  - Large defects require entire sterile and germinal matrix from great toes complete loss of nail plate from donor

4. Understand risks and benefits of various approaches

- Be able to discuss options based on anatomic defect

5. Address complications and unexpected problems adequately

- Hypersensitivity
- Cold intolerance
  - In 50%
  - Tx:
    - Usually self-limited 1-2 yrs
  - Initial tx:
    - Scar massage
    - Desensitization
    - Edema control

- Hook nail deformity- secondary to loss of bony support for nail growth
- Postop complications
    - Nail growth or non-adherence abnormalities
    - Sterile matrix scar- causes split nail
    - Nail non-adherence- distal transverse or diagonally oriented nail-bed scars
    - Bone irregularities
    - Cornified nail ridge from scar within germinal matrix
    - Acute repair may prevent these complications

6. Demonstrate ability to structure alternative plan

- Be aware of various treatment options
- Management of complications tissue loss, non-viable fingertip repair, management of wound infection

Chapter Fifty-Seven

Compartment Syndrome Of the Hand

57
Compartment Syndrome Of the Hand

1. Identify General Problem/Diagnosis/Planning
   (Describe photo, give working diagnosis, key problems, evaluates patient)

   - This patient has an extensive injury of the upper extremity. Compartment syndrome should be considered in the work-up to prevent additional morbidity.
   - Suspicious history:
     - Fracture
     - Temporary vascular occlusion
     - Drug overdose
     - Intraosseous fluid replacement in infants
     - Gunshot wounds
     - Arterial Injury
     - Leakage from intravenous or arterial access
     - Contusions in hemophiliacs
   - R/O COMPARTMENT SYNDROME
     - Especially in crush injury, prolonged presentation
     - If clinically suspect
       - Can measure pressures with Stryker vs. 18 gauge on a-line or cvp line
       - Operative exploration justified on clinical suspicion alone
     - Indication for OR:
       - >30mmHg or in hypotensive patients less than 20mmHg difference between diastolic P and compartment pressure
     - Compartment syndrome requires urgent decompression.
   - Etiology
     - Decreased compartment size
       - Closure of fascial defects
       - Constrictive dressings or casts
       - Localized external pressure
       - Circumferential burn

- o Increased compartment content
  - Bleeding
  - Increased capillary permeability
  - Infusion infiltration
- Pathophysiology
  - o Increased capillary pressure
  - o Progressive muscle and nerve ischemia
- PE
  - o Pain on passive stretch
  - o Stryker measurements
  - o A-line transducer
- 5 P's
  - o Pain out of proportion to exam
  - o Paresthesia's
  - o Pulselessness
  - o Poikylothermia
  - o Pallor
  - o Paralysis 6th P- very late sign

2. Consider reasonable goals in diagnosis and management *(Management and treatment, surgical indications, operative procedures and anesthesia)*

- Indication for OR:
  - o >30mmHg or in hypotensive patients less than 20mmHg difference between diastolic pressure and compartment pressure
- Fasciotomy:
  - o Forearm 3 compartments:
    - Anterior
      - Flexors FDS, FDP, FPL, FCR, FCU, palmaris longus, pronators
    - Posterior
      - Extensors EDC, EIP, EDQ, EPL, EPB, ECU, APL, wrist supinator
    - Mobile wad
      - Brachioradialis, ECRL, ECRB
  - o Hand 10 compartments:
    - 4 Dorsal interossei
    - 3 palmar interossei
    - 1 thenar
    - 1 adductor pollicis

- 1 hypothenar

3. Select appropriate options in diagnosis and management

    - Operative approach
        - GOALS
            - Restore perfusion to affected region by:
                - Releasing confines of compartment via fasciotomy
                - Treating the source of pressure (Fracture reduction, hematoma evacuation, release of dressings/casts)
            - If pressure persists go to OR for urgent decompression by fasciotomy
    - Forearm and wrist
        - Forearm 3 compartments
            - Anterior (volar)
            - Posterior (dorsal)
            - Lateral
        - Wrist
            - Carpal tunnel
            - Closed space
            - Median nerve compression
        - Method
            - Ulnar based incision travels proximal on ulnar arm zigzags at antecubital fossa
            - or
            - S-shaped incision starting ulnar curves radial at midforearm and zigzags at antecubital fossa
            - Tourniquet without exsanguination, help visualize crossing veins
            - Extended carpal tunnel release
            - Travel proximally
            - Explore ulnar nerve
            - Volar forearm release usually adequate BUT
            - If mobile wad and extensor compartments still tense perform dorsal fasciotomies
                - Through longitudinal incision
            - IF still tense (electrical injuries)

- Deep forearm musculature mandates exploration and epimysotomies.
  - Hand fasciotomy
    - Hand 10 compartments:
      - 4 dorsal interossei
      - 3 palmar interossei
      - 1 thenar
      - 1 adductor pollicis
      - 1 hypothenar
    - Carpal tunnel must also be released each compartment must be individually released
    - Technique:
      - Two dorsal longitudinal incisions over index and ring finger metacarpals
      - Bridging veins, sensory nerves, extensor tendons preserved
      - Metacarpal spaces released for release of the dorsal and volar interossei
      - Incision over radial thumb metacarpal decompresses thenar musculature
      - Hypothenar region released with linear incision placed at junction of the glabrous skin

4. Understand risks and benefits of various approaches

   - Why is fasciotomy performed? What is the morbidity of the procedure?
   - Forearm: 3 compartments
   - Wrist: carpal tunnel
   - Hand: 10 compartments

5. Address complications and unexpected problems adequately

   - End state of untreated compartment syndrome
     - Volkmann's ischemic contracture
       - Muscle shortening and fibrosis
       - Joint contractures
       - Nerve dysfunction
       - Growth arrest
   - Wound infection
   - Unfavorable scarring

- Iatrogenic damage to neurovascular structures
- Persistent edema
- Chronic pain
- Tendon adhesions
- Claw deformity
- Nerve dysfunction

6. Demonstrate ability to structure alternative plan

- Post op
    - Carpal tunnel overlying skin closed
    - Other incisions left open
    - VAC therapy
        - Decreases edema
        - Maintains tension at wound edges
        - Protects vital structures from desiccation
- Elevate
    - Immobilize in intrinsic plus position
- Return to OR as needed for debridement
- Wound closure when wound controlled
    - Primary closure
    - STSG
    - Secondary intention
- Early initiation of therapy
    - Joint mobilization
    - Active and passive range of motion until function maximized

Chapter Fifty-Eight

Mutilating Hand Trauma

58
Mutilating Hand Trauma

1. Identify General Problem/Diagnosis/Planning
   (Describe photo, give working diagnosis, key problems, evaluates patient)

   - Describe photo in detail:
     o It appears that this patient has sustained significant injury to the right hand as a result of suspected type of trauma.
     o Specify digits and structures involved in injury
       - Status of skin
       - Extent of soft tissue loss
       - Tendon involvement
       - Joint involvement
       - Bones
       - Nerve
       - Vessels
   - Based on your best guess of what you see
     o Number one priority is to rule out life threatening injuries.
     o Initiate ATLS protocol, ABC's.
     o Limb salvage secondary priority.
   - Hx:
     o Mechanism of trauma:
       - Crush- bone, soft tissue, vessels, less likely tendon injury
       - Avulsion- tendons will be injured in addition to vessels
       - Laceration- better prognosis, expect vascular and tendon involvement, less likely bone
     o Timing
       - Prolonged time more colonization
       - Less likely primary closure will be an option
     o Hand dominance
       - Be more aggressive in dominant hand injuries
     o Occupation
       - Dictates needs of patient

- Laborer- quick return to work needed
- Musician- needs fine motor skills, more tolerant of long rehab
  - Smoking
  - Alcohol and drug use
  - DM
  - Tetanus status
  - Risk of infection
- PE:
  - Based on clinical presentation and what you want to know
  - First priority
    - **Compromised vascularity, warrants emergent surgery**
  - Vascularity Assessment
    - Specify
      - Color
      - Capillary refill
      - Digital pulp turgor
      - Temperature
    - Distal pulses
      - Spasm
      - Kinking secondary to injury?
      - Reduction of fracture, return of pulses?
      - Doppler if necessary
  - Pattern of distal sensation
    - Two-point discrimination
    - Gross sensation
      - Median- volar thumb
      - Ulnar- fifth digit
      - Radial- dorsal first web space
  - Motor function- flexors and extensors
    - Active ROM
    - Forearm squeeze test
    - Tenodesis effect- passive flexion and extension
  - Function of all joints proximal and distal to injury:
    - Start at neck end at DIP
  - Observe bulk, contour general posture
  - Digital cascade
- **R/O COMPARTMENT SYNDROME**

- - - Especially in crush injury, prolonged presentation
      - 6 P's
        - Pain out of proportion to exam
        - Pallor
        - Paresthesias
        - Pulselessness
        - Poikylothermia
        - Paralysis (late sign)
    - If suspected clinically: OR exploration is justified
    - Can measure pressures with Stryker vs. 18 gauge on a-line or cvp line
    - Indication for OR:
      - >30mmHg or in hypotensive patients less than 20mmHg difference between diastolic P and compartment pressure
    - **Note**
      - Extent of soft tissue injury
      - Size of wound
      - Consider free tissue transfer in defects >25cm^2
      - Exposure of hardware, bone or tendon
      - Consider solutions for coverage
  - Consider pre-op studies; for bony injuries or vascular injuries
    - X-ray
      - Degree of bone loss
      - Comminution
      - Intra-articular damage
      - X-rays can be prognostic
        - Intraop or preop angio
          - Reserved for distal extremity with suspected vascular disruption and in anticipation of free flap.
  - No preop studies needed for tendon or nerve injuries
    - Explore in OR
    - Exploration guided by clinical examination
  - Key Consults:
    - Trauma
    - Orthopedics
    - Vascular surgery, but you may be expected to manage vascular injuries

- OT post op for hand therapy

2. Consider reasonable goals in diagnosis and management *(Management and treatment, surgical indications, operative procedures and anesthesia)*

- INDICATIONS FOR INTERVENTION
    - Restore function and self-image
- Contraindications
    - Concomitant life-threatening injuries
    - Comorbid medical conditions
- Pre-op antibiotics key! Broad spectrum
- Bone injury with:
    - Extensive periosteal stripping
    - Comminution
    - Marrow obliteration
    - Require coverage with better-vascularized tissue
- Goals of treatment:
    - Preserve as much function as possible
    - If extremity not salvageable:
    - Maintain maximum functional length
- Initial treatment:
    - Antibiotics
        - First generation cephalosporin and gentamicin for farm, lawn, garden injuries
    - Tetanus prophylaxis
    - If life threatening injuries:
        - Initial treatment of the extremity should be:
            - Limited control of bleeding
            - Release of compartments
            - Stabilization of extremity
            - Operative debridement of nonviable tissue, pulse lavage
            - Repeated until soft tissue coverage completed
            - Preserve intact nerve, vessels, tendons
            - Free floating bone excised unless periosteal continuity or articular cartilage attached to achieve skeletal stability
    - TOURNIQUET CONTROL

- o LOUPE MAGNIFICATION
- If clinically unstable:
  - o Amputation may be more prudent than an extensive course of reconstruction
  - o Hemodynamic stability should be considered in the initial evaluation, stabilize prior to reconstruction
- Revascularization needed for arterial or venous injuries
- Re-innervation primary or delayed for major nerve injuries
  - o Note preop sensory and or motor deficits
- Skeletal stabilization
  - o May be temporary K-wire vs. ex fix
- Tendon and ligament repairs
  - o Primary or secondary
  - o Tendon transfer? (See Tendon Transfers chapter 52)
- Early soft tissue coverage
  - o Lower complication rate
  - o Timing- determined by need for coverage of vital structures
- Composite defect not amenable to skin graft requires vascularized coverage with local flaps, distant flaps or free tissue transfer.
- Compartment syndrome requires urgent decompression.
- SALVAGE VS. AMPUTATION
  - o Wants and needs of patient
  - o Age
  - o Medical comorbidities
  - o Smoking hx
  - o Decision frequently not clear-cut (No pun intended)
- GROSS CONTAMINATION
  - o Definitive osseous fixation delayed, return to OR Q24-48 hrs
  - o Temporary osseous fixation (ex fix vs. K wires)
  - o Cover with moist dressings, allograft, xenograft, or VAC
  - o Moist wound to prevent desiccation of the white structures
- KEY MANAGEMENT POINTS
  - o Splint and elevate, position of safety
  - o Ex Fix for exposed fractures with lack of soft tissue coverage (avoids infected internal hardware)
  - o Limit tourniquet use in presence of extensive devitalized tissue or ischemia

- o In degloving injury, tack skin flaps loosely in anticipation of edema and demarcating necrotic areas
- o Function takes precedence over aesthetics
- o Rehab and hand therapy from day 1 to minimize joint stiffness

3. Select appropriate options in diagnosis and management

- Sequence of reconstruction:
    - o After control of wound, same as replant!
    - o Osseous fixation
    - o Tendon
    - o Vessel (artery then vein)
    - o Nerve
    - o Soft tissue coverage
- Fracture management:
    - o Anatomic and stable fracture reduction
        - Earlier rehab
        - Decreased pain
        - Decreased infection rate
    - o Options
        - K wire, plates, screws, interosseous wires and ex fix
            - K wire
                - o Can be done percutaneously
                - o No compression of fracture
                - o Best option for temporary fixation until definitive fixation
            - Alternative
                - o Intraosseous wire with K wire
            - Screws and plates allow early active motion
            - Ex Fix good option for missing or comminuted bone
- Joint injury
    - o Significantly impairs function
    - o Can address with artificial joint replacement or vascularized autogenous joint transfers
- Tendon

- Primary tenorrhaphy if acceptable soft tissue coverage present
- Contaminated injury or extensive soft tissue injury stage reconstruction or perform tendon transfers in staged fashion
- Vessels
  - Specify repair under magnification (loupes vs. scope)
  - Section intima until healthy
  - Bone shortening, if anastomosis uner tension or not feasible
  - Vein graft if primary repair not possible
    - Prep lower extremity for vein graft harvest
    - Mark forearm veins after elevation of the tourniquet without exsanguination take down and re-elevate for surgery
    - Possibility of vein grafting important point in informed consent
- Nerves
  - Specify repair with loupes or microscope
  - Nerve graft if primary repair will be under tension
  - Nerve conduit okay in defects <3cm
  - Sources for nerve graft:
    - Sural nerve (large caliber nerves, medial, ulnar, radial)
    - Medial or lateral antebrachial cutaneous nerve
    - Posterior interosseous nerve (digital nerves, base of fourth extensor compartment)
    - Don't forget "spare parts"
  - Infection or soft tissue problems delay nerve recon, tag cut ends
- Soft Tissue Defects
  - Primary closure
  - Skin graft in superficial defects
  - Local flaps, regional or free flaps
  - Use simplest, fastest, safest and best functional outcome
- Considerations:
  - Defect size and volume
  - Amount of missing bone
  - Nerve gap

- - - o Tendon defect
    - o Requirement for vein graft
  - Regional flaps
    - o Reverse radial forearm (workhorse flap) if no vascular injury to hand
    - o Reversed posterior interosseous
    - o Ulnar artery perforator
    - o Reverse radial artery perforator
  - Distant flaps
    - o Ipsilateral groin flap (3 weeks to division)
  - Free tissue transfer
    - o Many choices (fasciocutaneous flaps ideal)
  - Replantation
    - o Indications
      - Importance of part
      - Level of injury
      - Mechanism of injury
      - Expected return of function
      - All thumb and multiple digit injuries
  - Amputation
    - o If cannot replant
    - o Use spare parts of needed
  - Fasciotomy:
    - o Forearm 3 compartments
      - Anterior
        - Flexors FDS, FDP, FPL, FCR, FCU, palmaris longus, pronators
      - Posterior
        - Extensors EDC, EIP, EDQ, EPL, EPB, ECU, APL, wrist supinator
      - Mobile wad
        - Brachioradialis, ECRL, ECRB
    - o Hand 10 compartments:
      - 4 Dorsal interossei
      - 3 palmar interossei
      - 1 thenar
      - 1 adductor pollicis
      - 1 hypothenar
  - Skeletal stabilization options:
    - o Nonoperative- splinting or casting
    - o External stabilization to internal fixation

- o Closed treatment acceptable for low-energy, closed wounds
- o Internal fixation faster time to union and lower malunion rate
  - Soft tissue coverage options:
    - o Skin graft- if viable wound bed, no bone stripping
    - o Local flaps (often not available, reverse radial forearm a workhouse flap)
    - o Regional flaps (groin flap)
    - o Fasciocutaneous free flap ideal (contralat radial forearm, parascapular, anterolateral thigh)

4. Understand risks and benefits of various approaches

   - Elaborate on why you would choose one procedure over another based on presented clinical scenario.
   - What would change or affect your management plan?
   - Be versatile and able to manage any proposed change in the clinical scenario.
   - Postop care
     - o Edema and stiffness common even in good reconstructions
     - o Early rehab during inpatient stay
       - Protective splint/gentle range of motion
     - o Intermediate rehab 6-8 wks postop
       - Wound care/scar management
       - Gentle controlled stress
         - To decrease adhesions
         - Increase tensile strength
         - Prevent contractures
     - o Late Rehab
       - Post 8 wks retraining and strengthening

5. Address complications and unexpected problems adequately

   - Wound infection
   - Soft tissue necrosis
   - Partial or complete flap loss
   - Persistent Chronic Pain
   - Postop ischemic flaps
     - o Release dressings and splint
     - o Doppler to confirm flow

- o Re-explore
- o Re-warm
- o Papaverin
- o Redo anastomoses
- Malunion or nonunion
  - o Debride and graft to stabilize bone
- Flap loss- life boats
  - o Can use second free flap but safer back up may be prudent (groin flap)
  - o Specify work-up of flap failure prior to attempting second free flap
  - o Complex regional pain syndrome (formerly reflex sympathetic dystrophy, RSD)
    - Three criteria for diagnosis:
      - Diffuse pain not related to distribution of peripheral nerve
      - Diminished function and stiff joints
      - Skin and soft tissue changes
      - Tx:
        - o Prevent stiffness
        - o Treat underlying nerve compression
        - o Sympathetic interruption with phenoxybenzamine or bretylium (no longer available)
- Long-term complications
  - o Stiffness
  - o Hypersensitivity
  - o Cold intolerance
  - o Neuromas
  - o Hyperesthesia
- Common secondary procedures
  - o Tenolysis
  - o Joint contracture release
  - o Release post-traumatic syndactyly, web space deepening
  - o Tendon transfers
  - o Thumb lengthening
  - o Toe-to-hand transfers

6. Demonstrate ability to structure alternative plan

    - Important to determine if life-threatening injuries are present
    - Determine if amputation is appropriate, may be difficult to determine
    - Err on the side of salvage and note possible downsides and potential late indications for amputation
    - Early vs. late reconstruction in tendon and nerve reconstruction

Chapter Fifty-Nine

Ulnar Collateral Ligament Injury

59
Ulnar Collateral Ligament Injury

1. Identify General Problem/Diagnosis/Planning
   (Describe photo, give working diagnosis, key problems, evaluates patient)

   - Diagnosis often made by history
   - Thumb MCP Joint
     - Ulnar collateral ligament injury of the thumb
     - Chronic Instability
     - Radial-sided injury
   - Anatomy
     - Little bony stability
     - Stabilizers:
       - Radial and ulnar collateral ligaments
       - Originate, metacarpal neck
       - Insert volar/lateral base proximal phalanx
     - Primary stabilizer against:
       - Varus instability-radial collateral
       - Valgus instability–ulnar collateral
     - Accessory collateral ligaments- primary stabilizer in extension
     - Volar plate- primary stabilizer in hyperextension, secondary stabilizer in varus/valgus instability
     - Classic 'gamekeeper's thumb'- chronic attenuation of ulnar collateral ligament
     - Acute injuries 'skiers thumb' more common
     - Secondary to forced hyperabduction/extension
   - Classified- complete or incomplete
     - X-ray
     - PE
     - X-ray performed before exam
       - To avoid displacing a nondisplaced fracture
   - Exam
     - Stress joint in full extension and maximum flexion to isolate ulnar collateral ligament
     - Compare to uninjured side

- o 30 degrees increased angulation in extension warrants operative repair
- o 15 degrees in flexion diagnostic of complete rupture
- o May require intra-articular local if exam not tolerated
- Stener lesion (14-83% of ulnar collateral injuries)
  - o Displacement of proximal ligament superficial to adductor aponeurosis
  - o Distal ligament deep to it.
  - o Prevents healing of ligament
- Other tests:
  - o Stress radiographs/arthrograms/arthroscopy/ MRI
- Chronic instability
  - o Presentation
    - Pain or instability and weakness
    - Degenerative changes on x-ray are contraindication to ligament reconstruction
  - o X-rays are mandatory
- WHAT ABOUT RADIAL SIDED INJURY?
  - o 1/10th as common as ulnar injuries
  - o Abductor aponeurosis prevents superficial displacement of ligament
  - o Broader than adductor aponeurosis

2. Consider reasonable goals in diagnosis and management *(Management and treatment, surgical indications, operative procedures and anesthesia)*

- Partial tear treat with immobilization in thumb spica cast or splint 4-6 weeks
- If Stener lesion present- surgical repair
  - o Midsubstance tear
    - Primary repair
  - o More commonly- there is little or no distal stump of ligament
    - Suture anchor or repair over button
  - o Must be precise, reattachment at site as little as 2mm from insertion alters MCP joint motion in vitro
  - o If fracture fragment:
    - Significant size
      - Internal fixation with k-wire, tension band or mini screws

- - Smaller fragments
    - Excised and ligament repaired
- Chronic instability
  - Surgical reconstruction
  - Static and dynamic techniques
  - Static
    - Free tendon graft (Palmaris longus)
    - Placed through drill holes to reconstruct the torn ligament
  - Dynamic
    - Tendon transfer or tendon advancement
    - Arthritic joints treat with arthrodesis
- Radial injuries usually treated with cast immobilization

3. Select appropriate options in diagnosis and management
   - Treatment dependent on extent of injury
   - Partial vs. complete
   - Goal of treatment

4. Understand risks and benefits of various approaches
   - Risk of stiffness
   - Due to Stener lesion ulnar collateral injuries unlikely to heal without surgical intervention

5. Address complications and unexpected problems adequately
   - Reconstruction may lead to stiffness of MCP joint

6. Demonstrate ability to structure alternative plan
   - If palmaris not available
   - Plantaris or toe extensors for graft material

Chapter Sixty

Ulnar Nerve Palsy

60
Ulnar Nerve Palsy

1. Identify General Problem/Diagnosis/Planning
   (Describe photo, give working diagnosis, key problems, evaluates patient)

   - This patient appears to have claw deformity of the ring and small fingers
   - Functional loss:
     - LOW ULNAR PALSY
       - Injury distal to innervation of FCU tendon and FDP tendons to ring and little fingers
         - I. Ring, little MP flexion (clawing)- intrinsic muscle paralysis
         - II. Ring, little coordinated MP, IP flexion- intrinsic muscle paralysis
         - III. Coordination for finger positioning
         - IV. Decreased strength tip pinch, - between thumb and index paralysis of adductor pollicis m. and first dorsal and second palmar interossei
         - V. Loss of lateral or key pinch- paralysis of adductor pollicis m.
         - VI. Flattening of metacarpal arch and hypothenar eminence
         - VII. Sensation in palmar little and ulnar ring
     - HIGH ULNAR PALSY
       - Injury proximal to innervation of ulnar FDP tendons and FCU tendon
         - Deficits of low ulnar palsy (Plus):
         - Loss of:
           - I. Ring, little DIP flexion- secondary to FDP paralysis
           - II. Decreases strength wrist flexion- FCU paralysis
           - III. Sensation dorsal little finger and dorsal ulnar hand

2. Consider reasonable goals in diagnosis and management *(Management and treatment, surgical indications, operative procedures and anesthesia)*

    - Operative Approach
        - Tendon transfers to correct clawing of the fingers
        - Static tenodesis
            - MP joint hypertext via extrinsic m. dominance
            - Contributes greatly to claw deformity.
        - Static procedures block MP joint hyperextension
            - Capsulodesis
                - Zancolli- advancement capsulodesis
                - Proximal edge MP volar plate pulled proximally and inserted into metacarpal neck, joint in 20 degrees of flexion
            - Tenodesis
                - Parkes- free tendon graft placed between radial lateral bands and dorsal
                - Carpal ligament with MP joint in 45 degrees of flexion
        - Tendon Transfers
            - Provide MP joint flexion alone or…
            - Combined MP joint flexion and IP joint extension

    - Exam Findings
        - Active extension of PIP and DIP with extrinsic extensors while MP joints in passive flexion
            - Then transfer should address MP joint flexion ONLY.
        - No active extension of PIP and DIP with extrinsic extensors while MP joints in passive flexion then
            - Transfer must include insertion on lateral bands of extensor apparatus

    - PROCEDURES
        - Tendon Transfer for MP flexion alone
            - Lasso Procedure (Zancolli)

- Divide FDS distal to A1 pulley
- Loop tendon around A1 and suture to itself with MP at 45 degrees of flexion
- Will provide MP flexion to ring and little fingers
  - In High Ulnar nerve palsy
    - FDS to long finger used
    - Divided into two slips and pulled around pulleys of ring and small
  - Tendon Transfer to provide simultaneous MP flexion and IP extension
    - Modified Stiles-Bunnell transfer
      - Radial mid-axial incision in long finger
      - Transverse palmar incision
      - FDS tendon exposed, transected and divided into two slips
      - Slips passed through lumbrical canals of ring and little fingers
      - Inserted on radial lateral band of extensor apparatus
      - IP joints in full extension
      - MP joints 80-90 degrees flexion
      - Wrist 30 degrees palmar flexion
    - Brand ECRL and ECRB transfers
      - ECRL or ECRB rerouted around radial forearm to palmar aspect of wrist and lengthened with four split free plantaris tendon grafts
      - Tendon Transfers to correct ulnar deviation of little finger
    - Modification of Fowler transfer
      - Ulnar portion of EDM detached and inserted on radial collateral ligament of MP joint of little finger
  - Tendon transfers to provide adduction of thumb
    - Provides power for thumb-index pinch, thumb adduction, index finger abduction
    - Ring finger FDS Transfer

- Partial division of FDS tendon distal to MP jt.
- Tunnel deep to index and long finger tendons in radial direction
- Insert on adductor pollicis tendon or ulnar prox phalanx thumb
- NOT EFFECTIVE IN HIGH ULNAR NERVE PALSY- NO FDP FUNCTION
  - Extensor carpi radialis brevis transfer
    - Restores thumb adduction ECRB transfer
    - Extend ECRB with plantaris or Palmaris tendon free graft
    - Passed through 2nd metacarpal space
    - Sutured to insertion of adductor pollicis longus tendon
  - Tendon transfer to provide index finger abduction
    - Key to thumb-index pinch, effective index finger abduction
    - Restored using abductor pollicis longus tendon
    - Accessory slips extended with free tendon graft
    - Tunneled subcutaneously and inserted at insertion of first dorsal interosseous muscle.

3. Select appropriate options in diagnosis and management

- Low ulnar nerve injury (distal to innervation of extrinsic finger flexors and ulnar wrist flexor)
  - Motor deficits
    - Hyperextension at MCP and hyperflexion at DIP of ring and small fingers
      - Claw deformity- lumbrical loss, unopposed extension at MCP by EDC and unopposed flexion at DIP by FDS
    - Common transfers to correct clawing
      - FDS of middle finger to radial lateral bands of middle, ring, small fingers (Stiles-Bunnell)

- ECRB extended by grafts to radial lateral bands (Brand I)
- ECRL extended by grafts to radial lateral bands (Brand II)

4. Understand risks and benefits of various approaches

    - Differentiate between low and high palsy
    - Determine what function needs to be restored
    - What is the morbidity of tendon transfer?

5. Address complications and unexpected problems adequately

    - Can patient comply with postop therapy
    - What is your post-op management? Splinting requirements?
    - Management of local complications
    - Complications of tendon transfer?

6. Demonstrate ability to structure alternative plan

    - Be familiar with available options and know how to perform one in detail.

Chapter Sixty-One

Finger Mass, Enchondroma, Giant Cell Tumor, Aneurysmal Bone Cyst

61
Finger Mass
Enchondroma, Giant Cell Tumor, Aneurysmal Bone Cyst

1. Identify General Problem/Diagnosis/Planning
   (Describe photo, give working diagnosis, key problems, evaluates patient)

   - Describe photo in detail
   - Give your differential diagnosis based on findings and clinical scenario.
   - **Must establish a diagnosis based on presentation and given information.**
     o Age of patient influences differential diagnosis
     o Skin cancer most common malignancy- risk factors?
     o History of trauma- infection? Felon, paronychiae
     o Chronic Candida Ablicans- recalcitrant cases require eponychial marsupialization
     o Recent fast growth
     o Pain involved?
     o Location
     o Handedness of patient
     o Scars on hand, note available flaps for closure
     o Nerve deficits
   - History for enchondroma most common bony tumor in hand 90%, most commonly proximal phalanx:
     o Slow-growing
     o Painless
     o Multiple lesions consider Ollier's disease (25% conversion to malignancy)
     o Multiple lesions and associated with hemangiomas Maffucci Syndrome (>25% conversion to malignancy)
   - History for aneurysmal bone cyst:
     o Pain and swelling months to years
   - PE
     o Check for mobility vs. fixation
     o Viability of digit

- Ulceration
- Lymphadenopathy of extremity
- Current level of function
- Further work-up with x-ray both hands!
  - X-ray findings for aneurysmal bone cyst:
    - Eccentric, lytic, ballooning expansion within metaphysis
    - Delicate rim of expanded cortical bone, best seen on CT scan
    - Fluid-fluid levels
  - X-ray findings for enchondroma:
    - Usually incidental finding or pathologic fracture
    - Most common in tubular bones of the hands, femur, humerus
    - Lesions show increase in calcification with stippled or 'popcorn' pattern
  - X-ray findings for Giant Cell tumor:
    - Lytic lesion
    - Cortical thinning and expansion
    - Rare pulmonary metastasis
- Consider need for:
  - MRI
  - CT Scan
  - Biopsy
    - Large lesions suspicious for skin cancer not amenable to simple excision
  - Consultations
    - Oncology
    - Ortho
    - OT
- Hand lesions are most frequently benign

2. Consider reasonable goals in diagnosis and management *(Management and treatment, surgical indications, operative procedures and anesthesia)*

- Treatment aneurysmal bone cyst:
  - Not all lesions require treatment if inactive state reached BUT no way to predict behavior
  - Treatment: curettage and bone graft
  - Local recurrence 25%

- Treatment of enchondroma:
  - Allow healing of pathologic fracture with immobilization
  - Then treat by curettage and bone graft for large echondromas or if cortical thinning present
  - Small enchondromas may be followed by serial x-ray
- Treatment giant cell tumor:
  - Curettage bone graft recurrence 50%
  - Curettage and adjuvant (phenol, hydrogen peroxide, liquid nitrogen) and pack with bone cement recurrence 6-25%
  - Close f/u for recurrent disease and pulmonary involvement

3. Select appropriate options in diagnosis and management

   - Establish diagnosis prior to surgical intervention
   - Plan extent of resection
   - Plan reconstruction
   - Need for on-going therapy or follow up?
   - Treatment based on pathology
   - Surgical options:
     - Skin grafts, local flaps, regional flaps
     - Free tissue transfer
     - In malignant lesions consider adjuvant therapy, chemo and/or radiation
   - Leave wound open if extent of lesion is unclear and…
   - Reconstruct later pending negative pathologic margins

4. Understand risks and benefits of various approaches

   - Risk of recurrence in aneurysmal bone and giant cell tumor
   - Risks and benefits of enchodroma treatment
   - Long-term follow up

5. Address complications and unexpected problems adequately

   - Decreased function, dependent on site of reconstruction, scarring. Plan for hand therapy in post-op period to restore function
   - Infection uncommon treat as appropriate

- Flap loss- too much tension, kinking of flap, poor design
- Recurrence plan for continued surveillance
- Wound breakdown with exposed bone graft or hardware

6. Demonstrate ability to structure alternative plan

- Know alternatives in management as mentioned above
- Small enchondroma, plan for recurrence

Chapter Sixty-Two

Dupuytren's Disease

———

62
Dupuytren's Disease

1. Identify General Problem/Diagnosis/Planning
   (Describe photo, give working diagnosis, key problems, evaluates patient)

   - Note position of fingers and which ones are involved
   - Nodes, cords?
   - Degrees of contracture: MCP, PIP and DIP (late)
   - State: I suspect this patient has Dupuytren's based on exam findings flexion contracture, nodes, cords, presented history of scenario.
   - Hx:
     o Any family history
     o Age (generally over age 40)
     o Involvement of:
       - Plantar fascia (Ledderhose's disease)
       - Penis (Peyronie's disease)
       - Dorsum PIP joint (Garrod's knuckle pads)
     o European descent?
     o Autosomal dominant with variable penetrance
     o R/O other disorders, how did problem begin?
     o Painful contracture more likely related to trauma
     o Occupation
     o Generally painless
   - PE
     o Flexion contracture
     o Nodes
     o Cords
     o Check the feet and penis (Peyronie disease)

   - Plain X-ray to rule out other problems
   - Benign fibroproliferative disease unknown etiology

2. Consider reasonable goals in diagnosis and management
   (Management and treatment, surgical indications, operative procedures and anesthesia)

   - Exam look for indications for surgical treatment:

- - - - - - o > 40 degree loss of extension MCP joint
        - o 20 degree loss of PIP extension
        - o Measure passive and active ROM
        - o Table top test (if cannot place hand flat on table top)
        - o Hand in pocket?
      - If less severe than above noted findings then monitor as surgery is not curative
        - o Pain not likely to respond to surgical therapy

3. Select appropriate options in diagnosis and management

    - Options for tx:
        - o Skeletal traction
        - o Percutaneous fasciotomy
        - o Collagenase therapy (enzymatic fasciotomy) not mainstream yet
        - o Fasciotomy- less advanced cases especially MCP only, elderly pts cannot tolerate more extensive surgery
        - o Partial (limited) fasciectomy- most common approach
        - o Dermofasciectomy- recurrent disease, young patients LOWER RECURRENCE RATE
        - o Amputation- severely flexed digits, after repeated failed surgery or elderly with severe disease
    - R/O concomitant carpal tunnel syndrome or ulnar nerve neuropathy, complicates recovery
    - POST OP CARE
        - o Plaster splint 1 week in extension including MCP joint (one of few hand cases in which this is done)
        - o Meticulous local hygiene
        - o Suture removal at 14 days
        - o MCP contracture no special therapy
        - o PIP contracture therapy with hand therapist
        - o Serial extension splinting may be needed at night 3 months

4. Understand risks and benefits of various approaches

    - PIP contractures more resistant to treatment
    - Primary risk neurovascular injury
    - Note risks and benefits of the above

- No benefit to more extensive surgery, do what is needed to get maximal extension
- Your f/u protocol?

5. Address complications and unexpected problems adequately

    - Surgery
        - Delay surgery if open wounds are present
        - Do not operate if patient will be noncompliant with therapy
        - H/O arthritis pain may worsen with surgery
        - Be sure to follow cords distal to joint and excise completely
            - Brunner zigzag- easier less tip necrosis (linear with z-plasty at closure acceptable) avoid scar contracture
        - Cause no harm, avoid injury to neurovascular bundles
            - Risk of ischemic digit with digit loss, permanent numbness, recurrent contracture.
        - If previous surgery check 2 point discrimination preop
        - General anesthesia
        - Tourniquet
        - Loupes
        - Zigzag incisions for exposure
        - Release proximal to distal
        - Spiral cords may displace neurovascular bundle more centrally
        - Identify neurovascular bundle in virgin territory proximal and distal to cord, complete dissection then excise cord.
        - In little finger check for abductor digiti minimi cord in addition to pretendinous cord.
        - Avoid exposure of flexor tendon, cover if exposed use cross finger flap in necessary
        - Compromised digit
            - Remove dressings
            - Still compromised re-explore
            - Consider vein graft
            - Rewarming
            - Papaverine

- **COMPLICATIONS**
    - Infection
    - Hematoma
    - Nerve or vessel damage
    - Skin necrosis
    - Complex regional pain syndrome, AKA RSD
    - Joint stiffness/loss of flexion
    - Pain cold intolerance

6. Demonstrate ability to structure an alternative plan

    - How do you manage ischemic digit after contracture release?
    - Still contracted after fasciectomy:
    - Sharp check rein ligament release until complete passive extension
    - K-wire 0.028 through PIP
    - Tight closure leave open heal by secondary intention
    - Recurrence 27-60%, common, your plan for recurrence

Chapter Sixty-Three

Syndactyly

63
Syndactyly

1. Identify General Problem/Diagnosis/Planning
   (Describe photo, give working diagnosis, key problems, evaluates patient)

   - This patient has complete/incomplete syndactyly involving specific digits.
   - X-ray will define simple or complex syndactyly by pattern of bone involvement.
   - Can cause functional impact primarily in 1st and 4th web space syndactyly. Functional impact usually mild.
   - More problems when growth compromised by fusion to a shorter digit (border digit syndactyly)
   - Cause: Failure of separation (apical ectodermal ridge)
   - In its management I would like to know:
     o Age of patient
     o If this is congenital or secondary to scarring (such as burn, other trauma)
     o Other congenital anomalies (syndactyly involving hand, foot or both)
       - Apert
       - Pfeiffer
       - Saethre-Chotzen
       - Poland
         - Check for pectoralis major
         - Hypoplasia chest wall development
         - Breast/nipple
       - Down Syndrome
     o Inherited (auto dom variable expressivity, incomplete penetrance), sporatic or syndromic
   - PE:
     o Describe digits involved, palpate for bony fusion (simple vs. complex)
     o Note complete vs. incomplete
     o Complicated (syndromic, mitten hand, seen in Apert Syndrome)
     o Look at entire body (face, trunk, extremities) clues to other anomalies

- o Most common digits 3rd > 4th > 2nd > 1st
- o Acrosyndactyly- fusion of distal parts as in Apert's
- o Symphalangism
- Work-up:
  - o Plain x-ray both hands only, defer until ready to reconstruct
  - o Other work up based on suspicion of other syndromes
- Consultations:
  - o Genetics
    - Determine risk of having other children with condition
    - Completion of syndromal work-up
  - o Hand therapist- to optimize surgical result

2. Consider reasonable goals in diagnosis and management *(Management and treatment, surgical indications, operative procedures and anesthesia)*

- Evaluate anomaly
  - o Rule out other syndromes and associations (uncommon in syndactyly)
- Timing for separation of digits (debated)
  - o Decide on your own preferred timing
  - o 1 year is a safe time (larger structures, safer surgery)
  - o Monitor for malrotation until surgery performed, move up intervention time if malrotation present
- Minimize impact on growth and post-op surgical scar
  - o Avoid growth restriction
  - o Optimize long-term function
  - o Separate digits allowing complete independent digital motion
- Management Principles
  - o Operate before development of prehension at age 2
  - o Earliest age 6 months.
  - o Expedite repair in cases of digital length discrepancy, earlier repair to avoid growth disturbance in longer digit.
  - o Border digits or significant length discrepancy operate in first several months of life
    - Prevents flexion, deviation, rotation of longer finger

- If equal length of digits, surgery at 18 months has lower incidence of web creep and other unsatisfactory outcomes
- Goal of surgery adequate skin cover and creation of web space with opposing skin flaps and full-thickness skin grafts
- Special Considerations In Complex Syndactyly
    - Optimal location of osseous separation (knife blade all that is needed)
    - Alignment of joints
    - Management of common nail
    - Ligation of artery to one side of digit
    - Mitten hand
        - Goal three digit hand
        - Avoidance of vascular compromise
            - Border digits first to allow unimpeded growth
            - Second stage index/middle
            - Third stage Middle ring
        - Alternative algorithm (Two stage):
            - Stage one- Thumb/index and middle/ring
            - Stage two- Index/middle and ring/small

3. Select appropriate options in diagnosis and management

- Cronin, mirror image zigzag incisions with full-thickness skin grafts in web spaces a classic approach.
- Be able to describe and mark your preferred operation.
- Planned surgical release
- Postop hand therapy
- Keys in surgery:
    - MARKINGS
        - Cronin- mirror-image zigzag incisions
        - Buck-Gramcko if shared nail
        - Proximally based dorsal flap
            - Trapezoidal, tapered
            - Distal transverse margin at junction of the middle and distal 1/3 of proximal phalanx
    - Skin grafts

- Optimal flap angle 60 degrees, minimum 45 degrees
- Place web space at distal 2/3 of proximal phalanx
  - Palmar surface
    - Web landmarks either slightly proximal to index-middle and ring-small or midway between distal palmar crease and the PIP joint flexion crease.
  - Base zigzag flaps over joints, tips should extend to midline of digits
- PROCEDURE
  - Identify and protect neurovascular bundles
  - Dissect distal to proximal
  - Intraneural separation of the nerve and possibly artery at the web space may be necessary
  - Stage separations of digits with bilateral syndactyly to reduce the risk of devascularizing the digit.
  - Skin flaps can be defatted by cautiously
  - Take down tourniquet prior to artery ligation to assess signs of ischemia
  - Must cast the patient with elbow in flexion postop for skin grafts Sugar-tong splint 10-14 days
  - Harvest graft from groin, lower abdomen, hypothenar eminence or instep (consider benefits and downsides of each)
  - If staging is necessary wait time is 4-6 months between surgeries
  - Use skin grafts in all cases of complete syndactyly as a general rule, although in recent years more congenital hand surgeons are avoiding grafts by aggressive defatting.
  - Aggressive defatting may not be a "safe" answer for boards.
- Postop dressing
  - Above-elbow splint or cast
  - Fingers in slight abduction
  - Bolster dressing of choice
  - Dressing 10-14 days up to 3 weeks

4. Understand risks and benefits of various approaches

- Generally one surgical approach:
    - Syndactyly release with flaps and skin graft closure
    - Reconstruction of nail bed if needed (Buck-Gramcko flaps)
- Note maneuvers to minimize risks of complications
- What are the consequences of no intervention?

5. Address complications and unexpected problems adequately

    - Separate one digit at a time/one side at a time in multiple digit syndactyly
    - Contracture, web space creep
        - Avoid by liberal use of skin grafts
    - Post op therapy
        - Expect 10% reop rate- web creep common culprit
    - Digital necrosis
        - If concerned about digit viability:
            - Take down cast
            - Return to OR and explore vessels
            - Vein graft if necessary
    - Skin graft loss
        - Most common complication, repeat if needed
        - Okay to defer repeat graft until wounds are healed
    - Shallow web space
        - Can deepen by:
            - 4 flap Z-plasty
            - Butterfly flap or dorsal proximal flap
    - Nail deformity
        - Fix by horizontal skin flap
    - Nighttime splint with scar mold pads may decrease hypertrophy
    - May need to revise web creep, scar contractures due to distal migration of web space (60% of pts)
    - Pubic hair growth on skin grafts in adolescence
        - Your management plan?
        - How do you avoid this?
            - Harvest groin skin from lateral 2/3 to flank region

6. Demonstrate ability to structure alternative plan

    - Be prepared for the need for revision

- Revascularize compromised digit
- Stage reconstruction if multiple digits
- Failed skin grafts
- Insurance refuses laser treatment for hair removal in case of pubic hair on skin graft

Chapter Sixty-Four

Thumb Hypoplasia

64
Thumb Hypoplasia

1. Identify General Problem/Diagnosis/Planning
   (Describe photo, give working diagnosis, key problems, evaluates patient)

   - This patient appears to have thumb hypoplasia.
   - Classify type:
     o Management is dependent on presence of stable CMC Joint.
     o Thumb hypoplasia (Blauth)
     o Type I- minor generalized hypoplasia
       - Tx- augmentation
     o Type II- absence of thenar muscles, narrowed 1st web space, insufficiency of ulnar collateral ligament
       - Tx- opponensplasty, release and Z-plasty, UCL reconstruction
     o Type III- all features of type II plus extrinsic muscle and tendon abnormalities.
       - Stable CMC joint- Reconstruction
       - Unstable CMC Joint- Ablation and Pollicization
     o Type IV- Pouce Flottant or floating thumb
       - Tx: Ablation and Pollicization
     o Type V Absence
       - Tx: Pollicization alone
   - Important to R/O radial deficiency
   - R/O syndromic associations, esp. Fanconi's Anemia, Holt Oram (cardiac), TAR, VACTERAL.
   - Radial deficiency requires full medical work up, pediatric subspecialists, hematology, cardiology, etc.
   - Note family history, etiology of deformity
   - PE
     o Length of extremities
     o Thenar muscles affected (helps differentiate type)
     o Web space open?
     o Stable CMC joint?
     o Observe how patient grasps objects, helps differentiate type and surgical needs

- - -
    - - Note is thumb used or not?
      - Other digits involved
  - Plain x-ray helpful three views
  - Tapered metacarpal without a base characteristic of type IIIB
  - Medically optimized plan for thumb reconstruction
  - Genetics evaluation for associated anomalies
  - A stable CMC joint can be incorporated into routine use.
  - An unstable CMC is ignored and prehension develops between index (pronates) and middle finger (pseudopollicization).

2. Consider reasonable goals in diagnosis and management *(Management and treatment, surgical indications, operative procedures and anesthesia)*

   - If radial deficiency is present this should be addressed surgically prior to thumb hypoplasia
   - Classify deformity
     - R/O Radial deficiency
     - Plan reconstruction based on CMC joint stability
     - Reconstruction requires addressing all hypoplastic structures
   - Indication for surgery
     - Improved function by making prehension, opposition of digits for pinch and grip possible
   - Surgical options as noted in 1.
     - Surgical goals
       - Widen first web/release adduction contracture
       - Increase bulk
       - Allow opposition or abduction of thumb
       - Transfer index finger to position of the thumb.
   - Timing
     - Ideal age between 1-5 years depending on procedure
     - Pollicization best at age 1-2 yrs, before the development of oppositional pinch

3. Select appropriate options in diagnosis and management

   - Type II and IIIA
     - Treatment

- Web space deepening and opponensplasty
- Four flap Z-plasty addresses adducted posture
  - If still adducted after skin release
  - First dorsal interosseous is released from index metacarpal
  - Anomalous connections b/w EPL and FPL may be present and require release along ulnar aspect of MP joint
  - Additional chondrodesis may be necessary
- Reconstruct ulnar collateral ligament via release and proximal advancement and insertion into metacarpal head
- After adduction contracture release:
  - Opponesplasty/abductorplasty performed
  - Abductor digiti minimi (Huber) transfer preferred
  - Second option ring FDS transfer
- Huber Opponensplasty
  - Incision along ulnar aspect of hand
  - Muscle identified and transected as distal as possible
  - ID neurovascular bundle, free muscle proximally to pisiform
  - Pass subq over transverse carpal ligament
  - Insert into radial aspect of thumb metacarpal near MP joint.
    - Allows abduction of thumb out of palm
- Type IIIA
  - May also require EIP transfer for EPL function and centralization of FPL tendon and pulley reconstruction
- Type IIIB, IV and V
  - Ablation and pollicization
  - Pollicization

- Skin incision on palmar side of index (must not cross 1st web space, avoid adduction contracture)
- Identify index radial and ulnar neurovasc bundles
- Create web space
- Common digital nerve to second web is dissected free to allow transposition without tethering
- Proper digital vessel to middle finger is ligated
  - Perfused by ulnar vessel
- A-1 pulley released
- Complete dorsal incision preserving dorsal veins
- Juncturae between index and middle fingers divided
- Interosseous muscles (first dorsal and palmar) elevated from index metacarpal protecting neurovasc bundles
- Metacarpal ostectomy with shortening
- Metacarpal head is new trapezium
- Index freely mobile and rotated 45 degrees abduction 100 degrees pronation for normal thumb posture
- Transferred index MP joint repositioned in hyperextension
- Stabilized with sutures then K wire
- First dorsal interosseous acts as abductor pollicis brevis
- EDC acts as abductor pollicis longus
- Adduction palmar interosseous acts as adductor pollicis
- Palmar skin closed
- Check for vasospasm
- Long arm splint with tip of thumb visible for monitoring

4. Understand risks and benefits of various approaches

- Surgical choice based on stability of CMC joint

- A stable CMC joint can be incorporated into routine use, unstable CMC is ignored and prehension develops between index (pronates) and middle finger (pseudopollicization)
        - Huber
            - Give muscle bulk to thenar eminence
            - Abducts thumb out of palm
        - Ring FDS
            - Abductorplasty, allows movement of thumb away from palm but no assistance in opposition
            - No bulk provided
        - Unstable CMC requires ablation and pollicization

5. Address complications and unexpected problems adequately

    - Postop care
    - Remove dressing at 2-3 weeks
    - Thumb spica splint fabricated to maintain first web space
    - Daytime thumb use nighttime splinting regimen
    - Complications
        - Malunion
        - Devascularization
        - MCP or CMC joint instability
        - First web space contracture
        - Weakness of thumb
        - Stiffness
        - Excessive length may require further shortening
        - Malrotation- secondary correction by repeat osteotomy and improved fixation

6. Demonstrate ability to structure alternative plan

    - 2nd choice to Huber
        - Ring ringer FDS transfer
            - Transect ring FDS at A1 pulley
            - Separate from FDP maximize length
            - Second incision in distal forearm
            - FDS pulled through FCU used as a pulley (longitudinal split in FCU or creating loop of FCU with radial half)

- FDS is tunneled above transverse carpal ligament passed to thumb and inserted into metacarpal at level of MP joint.
- Allows abduction of thumb away from palm (abductorplasty) does not assist in opposition of the thumb
- Free toe transfer not an option due to abnormal proximal structures present in thumb hypoplasia
- Management of ischemic pollicized index finger

Chapter Sixty-Five

Thumb Duplication

65
Thumb Duplication

1. Identify General Problem/ Diagnosis/Planning
   (Describe photo, give working diagnosis, key problems, evaluates patient)

   - Preaxial polydactyly
   - This patient has Wassel Classification deformity.
     - Indicate type based on x-ray
     - Types I-VII.
     - Type IV (Duplicated proximal phalanx) most common.
   - Types
     - I- Bifid distal phalanx
     - II- Duplicated distal phalanx
     - III- Bifid proximal phalanx
     - IV- Duplicated proximal phalanx
     - V- Bifid metacarpal
     - VI- Duplicated metacarpal
     - VII- Triphalangeal thumb.
   - Problem with split thumb, neither one complete.
   - X-ray of hand and forearm to r/o radial deficiency.
   - Primary problem poor thumb function, abnormal aesthetics.

2. Consider reasonable goals in diagnosis and management
   (Management and treatment, surgical indications, operative procedures and anesthesia)

   - Key points:
     - Thumb will not be same the normal thumb, but may function well.
     - Ulnar digit usually more developed
     - Augment with parts from radial digit
   - Reconstructed thumb
     - Smaller, more stiff than unaffected
     - Acceptable appearance
     - Good alignment

3. Select appropriate options in diagnosis and management

- R/O syndromic associations, esp. Fanconi's Anemia, Holt Oram (cardiac), TAR, VACTERAL.
- Consider if associated radial deficiency.
    - Radial deficiency full medical work up, pediatric subspecialists, hematology, cardiology, etc.
- Medically optimize then plan bifid thumb reconstruction:
    - General anesthesia
    - Loupes and tourniquet
    - Zigzag incision (Distal CMC along radial aspect of hand encircling more hypoplastic digit) to avoid longitudinal incision and potential progressive deformity
- Hypoplastic digit (Usually radial)
    - Identify extensor and flexor tendons
    - ID neurovascular structures
    - Cauterize digital artery
    - Transect digital nerve sharply and allow retraction to avoid neuroma
    - Perform distal tenotomy to preserve tendons for reconstruction if needed.
- Digit for preservation (Usually ulnar)
    - Key: visualize FPL and EPL insertions
        - If central and hearty, can excise ulnar tendons at bifurcation
        - If radially located or narrow at insertion, augment with ulnar tendons
        - Important to centralize tendon insertions to balance thumb.
    - Identify musculature on radial thumb
        - Radial collateral ligament is created from strip of periosteum from the base of the proximal phalanx including MCP joint capsule.
- If metacarpal head is bicondylar:
    - Narrowing osteotomy may be needed (performed with 15 blade)
- If metacarpal head angulated such that remaining thumb will be ulnarly deviated, closing wedge osteotomy needed
    - K-wire passed retrograde to align distal and proximal phalange, stabilizes and internally fixated.

- - - - -
            - Thenar musculature sutured into periosteum at the base of the proximal phalanx.
            - Confirm EPL and FPL centralization
            - Confirm vascularity at end of procedure
        - Postop Management
            - Thumb spica splint/cast 3 weeks
            - X ray if healing osteotomy remove pin
            - Splint or cast additional 3 weeks
            - Then second x-ray
            - Remove pin at 6 weeks if not removed already
            - Splint at night additional 3 months

4. Understand risks and benefits of various approaches
    - Surgical goals:
        - Preserve larger more complete digit
        - Centralize and balance tendons of remaining digit
        - Reconstruct radial collateral ligament
        - Proper alignment of metacarpal
        - EPL and FPL centralization
        - Confirm vascularity
    - Use parts of ablated digit to get optimal result, not simple ablation

5. Address complications and unexpected problems adequately
    - Potential problems
        - Wound healing
        - Devascularization
        - Malunion or nonunion

6. Demonstrate ability to structure alternative plan
    - Potential problems
        - Devascularization
        - Misalignment in adequate osteotomy or positioning
        - Malunion may require debridement and bone graft

PEDIATRIC PLASTIC SURGERY

Section Eleven
Congenital/Pediatric

Chapter Sixty-Six

Pediatric Plastic Surgery Overview

66
Pediatric Plastic Surgery Overview

1. Identify General Problem

   - Describe photo
   - Give working diagnosis
   - Key problems
   - Evaluate patient
   - Note pertinent positives and negative of history and physical exam. Findings that would influence your management
   - Consider if further work-up is necessary
   - Other interventions before surgery?
   - FOR CLEFT:
     - Note family history, prenatal exposures
     - Review transmission genetics, know numbers
     - R/O syndromic features other organ involvement prior to surgery
     - Classify cleft type, note severity
     - Be prepared for secondary revision cases
     - (Bilateral cleft-Abbe flap)
     - What are the problems caused by cleft lip/palate/congenital nevus/proposed extensive scar pattern or proposed excision?
   - GIANT NEVUS:
     - What is the risk for malignancy?
     - At what age does it occur?
   - Need for additional work-up for operative planning?
     - Speech and swallow
     - Orthodontics
     - Genetics
     - Neurology
     - Other
   - Be prepared for:
     - Facial reconstruction scenarios
     - Syndactyly
     - Burn
     - Trunk (meningomyelocele)

- o Facial paralysis
- o Poland
- o Prominent Ear deformity
- o Gynecomastia
- o Other
- o May qualify as a pediatric case

2. Consider reasonable goals in diagnosis and management

- Management and treatment options
- Specifically mention:
    - o Surgical indications
    - o Operative procedures and anesthesia
- Mention all options of management
    - o Even if they are things you are not going to choose
    - o Eg. Giant Congenital Nevus
        - Excision and closure
        - Serial excision
        - Excision and skin graft or integra
        - Tissue expanders
        - Expanded free flap
        - All options for management
    - o You choose what you think will be the best option
- For clefts describe your protocol
- Include timing of management of
    - o Presurgical orthodontics (all options)
    - o Lip
    - o Palate
    - o Alveolus
    - o VPI
    - o Rhinoplasty
    - o Midface deficiency
    - o Orthognathic surgery

- Stress importance of feeding and appropriate weight gain
- Cleft team
    - o Minimum team members according to American Cleft Palate Association (ACPA)
        - Speech and swallow therapist
        - Orthodontist
        - Cleft surgeon
    - o Can have other team members

- o Other important subspecialists
  - OMFS
  - ENT
  - Genetics
  - Ophthalmology
  - Social work
- Note potential effect of growth on long-term outcome in all pediatric patients.
- In giant congenital nevus or other wide lesions consider potential functional impact of resection and reconstruction.

3. Select appropriate options in diagnosis and management

   - How will you address the problem?
   - Commit to your choice of intervention
   - Justify decision
   - Discuss risks benefits vs. other options if relevant
   - Your preferred operation for lip and palate repair or other proposed problem and why?
   - Your post-op management
   - How is procedure performed?
   - Key steps of procedure
   - Markings and relevant anatomy
   - Your post-op management
   - Be familiar with tissue expanders all the in's and out's and your personal approach to their use.

4. Understand risks and benefits of various approaches

   - Expected outcomes
   - Need and timing for additional surgeries
   - Any additional interventions for wide lip/palate
   - Discuss risks benefits of various interventions
   - Include anticipated potential complications
   - What is your rationale for surgical intervention?

5. Address complications and unexpected problems adequately

   - In cleft be able to manage:
     - o Wound dehiscence
     - o Post-op bleeding
     - o Airway obstruction

- Abnormal scarring patterns
- Whistle deformity
- Notch in vermilion
- Malrotated lip
- Palatal fistula
- VPI
- Preventative measures
    - Palatal fistula repair reinforcement (alloderm)
    - Tongue stitch
    - Nasopharyngeal airway
- Common tissue expander complications
    - (exposure, infection)
- Ethical issues
- Family dissatisfaction
- Patient with no insurance coverage
- Parents want surgery but patient doesn't

6. Demonstrate ability to structure alternative plan

- Persistent VPI
- Palatal fistula
- Inadequate lip repair
- Early post-op lip dehiscence
- Timing of revisions
- Whistle deformity
- Failed:
    - Tissue expander
    - Flap
    - Skin graft
    - Web creep
    - Inadequate gynecomastia correction
- Child or family not happy with surgical plan or outcome
- Exposed bone post attempted burn reconstruction

Chapter Sixty-Seven

Cleft Lip and Palate

67
Cleft Lip and Palate

1. Identify General Problem/Diagnosis/Planning
   (Describe photo, give working diagnosis, key problems, evaluates patient)

   - Describe and classify cleft
     o Side (left or right)
     o Unilateral or bilateral
     o Complete or incomplete
     o Anatomic details
       - LAHSHAL classification (simplest)
       - (Lip/Alveolus/Hard Palate/Soft Palate/Hard Palate/Alveolus/Lip, Right to Left)
   - Note key problems caused by clefting
     o Feeding primary issue early on if palate involved (cannot form a seal to suck for feeding)
     o Airway issues present?
     o Think about: Pierre Robin Sequence
     o Speech problems
     o Aesthetic deformity
   - History
     o Family history of clefts? Genetics
     o Prenatal issues
       - Maternal medical problems
         • Seizures
         • Smoking
       - Maternal medications
     o Breathing issues in perinatal period?
     o Pierre Robin Sequence
       - Respiratory distress
       - Glossoptosis
       - Micro/retrognathia
       - Failure to thrive
       - +/- Cleft Palate
       - Can occur in isolated cleft palate or as part of syndrome
   - PE
     o Note features of:

- Lip
- Nose
  - Intact nasal sill
  - Simonart band
  - Nasal distortion
  - Posterior inferior displacement
  - Variable severity but always present
  - Splayed lower lateral cartilage
  - Buckled lateral crus
  - Septal deviation
- Alveolus
  - Is dental arch aligned?
- Palate involvement
            - What is involved?
              - Cupid's bow
              - Philtral columns
              - Tubercle
              - Vermilion
              - Orbicularis
            - Be aware of the forme fruste cleft:
              - Only muscle involved
              - Aberrant muscle
              - Microform cleft
      - Associated Congenital Anomalies
        - Most common:
          - Stickler Syndrome
          - 22q11.2 deletion (AKA Velocardiofacial syndrome, Di George syndrome)
          - Van der Woude syndrome (lip pits)
        - Over 250 associated syndrome
        - >90% of cases no associated syndrome, isolated CLP
      - CLP Incidence
        - Whites 1:700
        - Blacks 1:1300
        - Asians 1:500
      - Isolated Cleft Palate Incidence
        - 0.5 to 1:900 all comers, more frequent in females
      - Genetics
        - Increased risk of occurrence in second child
        - No family history of clefts 4% risk
        - 1 cleft in family 9% risk

- o 1 parent and 1 sibling with cleft 17%
- o Varies with severity of cleft
  - i.e. Slightly higher in bilateral clefts
- Work-up
  - o Genetics evaluation
  - o R/O cardiac defects
  - o R/O other syndromes
  - o Ophthalmology eval to R/O Stickler's

2. Consider reasonable goals in diagnosis and management *(Management and treatment, surgical indications, operative procedures and anesthesia)*

- Cleft lip and palate management
- Pre-surgical orthopedics
- Consider:
- Pre-surgical nasoalveolar molding if available
  - o Based on severity of nasal deformity
  - o Ideal candidates bilateral CLP can be used in unilateral cases
- Other Options
  - o Taping
  - o Bonnet
  - o Latham appliance
  - o Lip adhesion
- Multidisciplinary assessment and long-term management
  - o ACPA minimal components of cleft team
    - Cleft surgeon (Plastics/ENT)
    - Orthodontist
    - Speech therapist
  - o Other important subspecialists for cleft patient care:
    - Genetics
    - Oral Surgery
    - Social work
    - Pediatric dentist
    - Otolaryngology
    - Audiology
    - Child psychiatry
    - Ophthalmology- especially in isolated cleft palate
- Feeding issues
  - o Speech and swallow evaluation at birth

- Special nipple/bottle (Haberman or Pigeon)
  - Most feeding issues addressed with minimal intervention
  - If more than a special nipple required other medical issues are present
    - R/O Pierre Robin Sequence and GERD first
    - Neurologic related swallowing issues relate to other unknown medical diagnosis
- Orthodontic Intervention
  - Used if available
  - Nasoalveolar molding facilitates nasal shaping as well as facilitating cleft lip repair
  - Latham appliance
- Audiogram
  - As in every newborn
  - External ear/Tympanic membrane/Middle ear
  - Due to abnormal insertion of tensor veli palatini muscle cleft palate patients are prone to ear infections due to poor drainage secondary to kinking of eustachian canal.
  - Some patients may require myringotomy tubes, which can be done at the time of cleft lip or cleft palate repair
  - Primary indication for ENT evaluations
- Timing of surgical intervention for lip repair
- Rule of 10's
  - 10kg = 22lb
  - 10gm Hb
  - 10 weeks of age
  - Associated with decreased risk of anesthesia
- Timing of repair will be postponed if lip adhesion is used or if patient is undergoing NAM or Latham appliance
- Optimize medically prior to surgery
  - Hb 10gm
  - Verify appropriate weight gain
  - Feeding well
  - No active medical issues
  - Growing normally
- Goals of lip repair
  - Normal lip contour, i.e. Cupid's bow
  - Restoration of vertical height on philtral ridge
  - Realignment of orbicularis oris muscle

- Good muscle repair is critical to any cleft repair technique
    - Minimize the appearance of scars
    - Improve cleft nasal deformity by primary rhinoplasty
- Special Considerations In Bilateral Lip Repair
    - Pre-surgical orthopedics more likely to be needed
    - Feeding with special bottles more likely to be needed
    - Area of controversy:
        - Primary surgical pre-maxillary setback
            - Generally not recommended
            - Affects midface development
            - Risk of devascularization of premaxillary segment
    - Nasal deformity more difficult to management
        - Increased incidence of flat nose, lacks projection
    - NAM most helpful in bilateral lip
    - PE- Same as in unilateral lip repair
- Later interventions
    - Age 5 or older for VPI (sometimes younger if severe VPI)
        - Superiorly based pharyngeal flap
        - Sphincter pharyngoplasty
    - Lip and nasal revisions
        - Consider when school age
        - Ideally done in teen years
        - Individualize based on social situations and family preferences
    - Alveolar Bone Graft
    - Orthodontics
    - Orthognathic surgery (age 13-17)
        - Lefort I needed in some for midface deficiency
        - On occasion bimaxillary surgery indicated
    - Rhinoplasty (age 15-18)
        - After orthognathic surgery
- Cleft Management Protocol- varies by institution
    - Early evaluation for feeding post-birth
    - Pre-surgical orthopedics
    - Lip repair at 3-6 months

- Myrigotomy tubes at lip repair or palate repair
- Palate repair at 12 months
- Speech evaluation between 3-5 years of age
- Palate revision or pharyngoplasty for VPI
- Lip revision evaluation prior to school
- Secondary bone graft at age 6-8 years for alveolar defect
- Orthodontics
- Orthognathic surgery 13-17 years
- Rhinoplasty 15-18 years

3. Select appropriate options in diagnosis and management

- Pre-surgical molding techniques are generally used a minimum of 2-6 months prior to lip repair.
- Lip adhesion
    - Generally used if:
    - Other pre-surgical orthopedic options are not available or fail or…
    - As a first choice if lip is unusually wide or…
    - Some surgeons use lip adhesion with every case
    - When doing a lip adhesion it is critical to preserve anatomic landmarks for the ultimate lip repair
    - Advantages
        - Narrows cleft
        - Decreases tension across maxilla
        - Eases lip repair by conversion to incomplete cleft
        - Can elongate a short lip
        - Fewer secondary revisions
    - Procedure
        - Make standard marking for lip repair
        - Elevate rectangular book-like flaps, medial to lip markings for future repair
            - One on mucosal side
            - One on skin side
        - Expose the orbicularis muscle
        - Place deep muscle sutures with 3-0 prolene and suture together, wide bites
            - Sutures should be placed across the premaxillary segment in the case of bilateral clefts

- Maintain for a minimum of 2 weeks, usually 2-3 months
- Unilateral Cleft Lip Repair
    - Most widely used techniques in the U.S.
        - Millard Rotation-Advancement Repair
            - Some would go so far as to say this is the standard of care
            - Board examiners most familiar with this operation
            - Many variations
                - Mohler Repair (most common variation)
        - Tennison-Randall
        - Functional Kernahan
        - Davis (Z-plasty) repair
        - Anatomic Subunit Repair (Fisher repair)
            - Most novel repair
            - Becoming more popular
    - If lip remains short after Millard Repair:
        - Add Z-plasty at the white roll
        - Or…
        - Add triangular flap at the white roll
        - Gives a little more length to lip
    - Key Landmarks for Millard
        - High point (Cupid's bow) non-cleft side
        - Low point (Cupid's bow) non-cleft side
        - High point (Cupid's bow) of minor lip element
        - Commissures
        - Alar bases
        - Columellar midpoint
    - Flaps used in Millard Repair
        - Rotation Flap- on major lip element
            - Back cut may allow more rotation- rarely needed
            - Mohler variation
                - Incision is carried into the columella
        - Advancement Flap
        - C-flap (Columellar flap)
            - Fills upper lip defect
            - Can be used to fill nasal floor defect

- L-flap (Lateral nasal wall, lining flap)
  - Augments nasal lateral wall at vestibular incision
  - Allows more medial rotation of alar base
- M-flap (Mucosal flap)
  - Primarily lines nasal floor
- Septal flaps
  - Line nasal floor
  - o Gingivoperiosteoplasty (GGP)
    - Can be used to close alveolar defect in clefts with near edge-to-edge abutment of the alveolus.
    - May avert the need for alveolar bone graft in the future
    - Controversial procedure
- Bilateral Cleft Lip Repair
  - o Deformity of bilateral cleft lip
    - Splayed lower lateral cartilages
    - Short columella
    - Poor tip projection
    - Splayed alar bases, tethered to piriform rims
    - Loss of normal philtrum
    - Anteriorly displaced maxillary segments
    - Orbicularis oris discontinuity
      - There is no muscle in the premaxillary segment
  - o Surgical goals
    - Nasal tip reconstruction
    - Creation of columella from nasal tissue (Contemporary approach)
    - Mulliken repair stresses columellar reconstruction with like tissue- "The columella is in the nose."
    - Single stage reconstruction
    - Creation of columella from lip tissue
    - (Traditional approach)
    - Millard bilateral repair multi-stage reconstruction using:
      - Banked forked flaps
      - Columella reconstructed from lip tissue

- Mulliken repair evolved from general dissatisfaction with results from banked forked flap technique
- General consensus amongst cleft surgeons is to use Mulliken type repair or some variation of "the columella is in the nose."
  - Key Points of Reconstruction
    - Release and repositioning (overcorrection) alar bases
    - Philtral subunit reconstruction
    - Creation of philtrum from prolabial tissue
    - Creation of Cupid's bow central lip tubercle from lateral lip elements
    - Re-establish muscle sphincter
- Mulliken Technique
  - Nasal reconstruction
    - Complete alar base release and mobilization
    - Overcorrect with cinch suture
    - Rim incisions for lower lateral dissection
    - Excision of fibrofatty tissue
    - Interdomal sutures
    - Judicious excision of soft triangle
    - Columellar shaping sutures
  - Philtral reconstruction
    - "Tie-shaped" philtrum from prolabial tissue
    - Will stretch over time horizontally and vertically
    - 2-3 mm width at columellar-philtral junction
    - 6-8 mm in height
    - (The longer the better, limited by available tissue)
    - 4mm width at distal border, may curve for Cupid's bow
    - Remaining skin
      - Deepithelialized
      - Discarded (Yes, discarded)
  - Lateral lip elements
    - Mark high point on lateral lip element where vermilion begins to lose fullness
    - White roll of Cupid's bow and vermilion of central philtrum come from lateral lip elements

- Make them 1-2mm longer than the philtral "tie-flap"
- Excess tissue is excised later at closure
  - Muscle reconstruction
    - Orbicularis oris muscle is freed from skin and mucosa bilaterally
    - Released from abnormal insertion on maxilla
    - Set height of sulcus and repair mucosa
    - Attempt to bring muscle across midline and repair over premaxillary segment under "tie-flap".
  - Skin repair
    - Attempt deep subdermal closure only if possible
    - Obviates need for external sutures
    - Use fine absorb. for external repair if needed
- Cleft Palate Repair
  - Goal:
    - Radical intravelar veloplasty to optimize speech
    - Avoid fistulas
    - 10% require secondary surgery for residual velopharyngeal insufficiency
  - Techniques
    - 2 flap palatoplasty AKA Bardach repair AKA Dorrance repair
    - Von Langenbach (lateral relaxing incisions)
    - V-Y advancement AKA Veau-Wardill-Kilner Repair
      - Consensus to discontinue, excessive scarring
    - Sommerlad repair
    - Furlow (Double Z-plasty)
  - Procedure
    - Three layer repair
    - Nasal mucosa
    - Levator veli palatini muscle repair (key portion of procedure)
    - Oral mucosa repair
  - Post-op
    - No-no's

- Tongue stitch or nasopharyngeal tube
- In-patient 1 or 2 nights
- Review technique of alveolar bone grafting

4. Understand risks and benefits of various approaches

    - Know some basic differences between different lip repairs
    - Be able to discuss benefits of presurgical orthopedics and what you prefer, no wrong answers here, but must be familiar with all options.
    - Advantages or disadvantages of different lip repairs
        o Know one step for step in detail
    - Furlow slightly better speech results, higher fistula rate compared to 2 flap palatoplasty

5. Address complications and unexpected problems adequately

    - Complications of cleft lip/palate surgery
        o Bleeding
            - Usually self-limited
            - Back to OR for any significant bleeding
            - Afrin may be tried in PACU after palate repair
                - Back to OR: no improvement w/i hr.
        o Airway compromise
            - May be from tongue swelling after palate repair
                - Racemic epinephrine
                - Steroids
                - Nasopharyngeal tube
                - Close observation
                - Reintubate if necessary
                    o Use tongue stitch to minimize risk of palate dehiscence during reintubation
            - Narrowing of nasal airway after lip repair
        o Infection
            - Rare
        o Dehiscence
            - Rare
            - Etiology- most likely excessive tension

- Treat with local wound care
- Attempt re-closure after healed
- Wait for scar to soften
- Minimal wait to re-closure 3 months
- Consider presurgical interventions to narrow cleft prior to second attempt at closure
  - Hypertrophic scar
    - Massage
    - Steroids
    - Laser treatment
    - Scar revision after minimum of 9 months non-operative treatment
  - Fistula
    - Incidence 10-50%
    - Requires secondary repair in some cases
    - Management
      - Observation 9-12 months
      - Initial surgical intervention
        - 2 layer repair, re-elevate flaps
      - If fails or too wide for re-repair
        - Tongue flap
        - Buccal mucosal flap
        - FAMM flap
        - Obturator
        - Free flap- radial forearm (Rarely needed)
  - Velopharyngeal insufficiency
    - Incidence 10-15%
    - Assessed between age 3-5 years of age
      - Nasoendoscopy
      - Fluoroscopy
      - Speech evaluation
    - Management
      - Superiorly based pharyngeal flap or…
      - Sphincter pharyngoplasty
      - Based on results of nasoendoscopy

6. Demonstrate ability to structure alternative plan

- Be able to make plan based on presented patient

- Other options if NAM not available
- Delay palate repair in Pierre Robin patients due to potential airway problems, usually at 15-18 months vs. 1 year.
- What if family has no insurance?
- Family refuses care due to religious beliefs?

Chapter Sixty-Eight

Cleft Palate

68
Cleft Palate

1. Identify General Problem/Diagnosis/Planning
   (Describe photo, give working diagnosis, key problems, evaluates patient)

   - This patient has a cleft of the:
     - Primary or secondary palate
     - Incisive foramen defining anatomic landmark
     - Anterior to- primary palate (include lip)
     - Posterior to- secondary palate
     - Left or right?
     - Complete or incomplete
     - Isolated or CL also present
     - LAHSHAL or Kernahan Striped Y classification or Veau Classification
     - Consider submucosal cleft palate
   - Hx:
     - Age of patient
     - Any interference with feeding or speech
     - Weight gain
     - Inadequate suck- Tx. Specialized nipples/bottles
     - Swallowing problem reflects other pathology (GI or neurologic)
     - Associated syndrome (CLP 10%, isolated CP 30%)
     - Lip pits?
   - Cleft Palate Associated syndromes:
     - Pierre Robin Sequence
     - Sticker Syndrome (retinal pathology)
     - Van der Woude (lip pits)
     - Apert
     - Crouzon
     - Treacher Collins syndrome
     - 22q11.2 deletion syndrome (AKA Velocardiofacial syndrome, DiGeorge syndrome)
   - PE
     - Ear exam- serous otitis media
     - Audiology- if hearing problems may require myringotomy tubes

- o Hearing problems represent:
- o Eustachian tube dysfunction secondary to tensor veli palatini and levator veli palatini malposition and function
- o Extent of primary palate involvement- lip and alveolus
- o Chronic ear infection problems
  - Recurrent infections
  - Tympanic membrane perforation
  - Hearing loss
  - Cholesteatoma
- o Note arch alignment- presurgical orthopedics
- o Note lower jaw
  - Micro/retrognathia
  - Glossoptosis
  - Respiratory distress
  - Consider Pierre Robin Sequence
- o Other congenital anomalies-ear, eyelids, orbits
- o R/O cardiac, pulmonary, renal other defects
- Anatomy
  - o Tensor veli palatini
  - o Levator veli palatini
  - o Palatoglossus
  - o Palatopharyngeus
  - o Uvula
- Innervation pharyngeal branch of vagus (CN X) except Tensor Veli Palatini- Mandibular nerve Branch V3 (Trigeminal nerve)
- Blood supply
  - o Greater (Greater palatine foramen) and lesser (soft palate) palatine arteries
  - o Branches of descending palatine artery off third part of maxillary artery
- Consultations
  - o Genetics
  - o Orthodontist
  - o Speech/swallow therapist
  - o Cleft team
  - o ENT
- No formal imaging required

2. Consider reasonable goals in diagnosis and management
   (Management and treatment, surgical indications, operative procedures and anesthesia)

   - Cleft Lip and Palate Management Algorithm
     - Pre-natal consultation if diagnosed during pregnancy
     - Post-birth speech and swallow evaluation
     - Lip Repair at 3 months
     - Palate Repair at 12 months- earlier repair better speech outcomes
   - Secondary Bone graft- ball park, between 6-12 yrs of age
   - Palate repair options
     - Von Langenbeck
     - Bardach (Dorrance/two-flap palatoplasty)
       - (decreases anterior fistula rate)
     - Veau-Wardill-Kilner (V-Y)
       - (more fistulas and maxillary deficiency)
     - Sommerlad repair
     - Soft palate closure
     - Intravelar veloplasty
       - Three layer closure- levator veli palatine repositioned
       - Tensor veli palatini release improves mobility
     - Furlow double opposing Z-plasty (CHOP modification uses relaxing incisions)
       - Lower fistula rates with relaxing incisions
       - Good speech outcomes
       - Transposes levator muscle by overlap, not anatomic repair
     - Consider acellular dermis in nasal mucosa for areas that cannot be closed or in fistula repair

3. Select appropriate options in diagnosis and management

   - VPI Work-up
     - Speech pathologist
     - Soft Palate Evaluation
     - Nasoendoscopy
     - Videofluoroscopy
     - Intensive speech therapy
   - If no improvement with therapy, then surgery:

- Inadequate length:
    - Furlow Z-plasty
- Creation of partial obstruction with sphincter pharyngoplasty or pharyngeal flap
- Augmentation of posterior pharyngeal wall- mixed results
- Nonsurgical candidates
    - Consider- speech bulb prosthesis
        - Creates bulk in posterior pharynx

4. Understand risks and benefits of various approaches

    - Improvement in feeding
    - Maxillary retrusion/orthognathic surgery
    - Speech outcomes
    - Use of arm restraints
    - Pre-surgical orthopedic options
    - Choice of palate repair

5. Address complications and unexpected problems adequately

    - Postop
        - Tongue suture, eases emergent intubation by tongue traction
        - Nasopharyngeal tube to protect airway
        - Feeding- full liquid or soft diet
        - Arm restraints to prevent placing hard objects in mouth
    - Complications
        - Bleeding- edges of flap
            - Prevention
                - Use of epinephrine
                - Meticulous hemostasis
                - Surgicel or gelfoam
            - Return to OR if significant
    - Airway compromise
        - Obligate nasal breathing till age 6 months
        - Closure of palate redirects airflow and narrows posterior pharyngeal airway
        - Postop tongue swelling with mouth gag
        - (in OR time >90-120 minutes)
    - Fistulas form in areas of tension
        - Most frequently at junction of hard and soft palate

- - - Frequency 5-10%, increased in Pushback
    - Tx: observation, obturator, reoperation
      - Surgery
        - Two layer closure
        - Acellular dermis
        - Tongue flap
        - FAMM flap
        - Buccal Flap
        - Free flap (radial forearm) (rare to need this)
  - Velopharyngeal insufficiency (VPI)- nasal air loss with positive pressure consonants
    - Result of scarring postop
    - Innate problem with the muscles or surrounding anatomy
    - Causes:
      - Neuromuscular insufficiency
      - Disproportion between length of palate and depth of pharynx
      - Scar formation in palate or pharynx
      - Regression of adenoid pad
      - Maxillary advancement (post Lefort I)
      - Tonsillectomy and adenoidectomy
    - Surgical Treatment:
      - Superiorly based pharyngeal flap
      - Sphincter pharyngoplasty

6. Demonstrate ability to structure alternative plan

   - VPI management plan and workup
   - Short palate (Furlow)
   - Associated congenital problems
   - Management of Pierre Robin Sequence
   - Fistula management
   - Submucous cleft palate management (what is different?)

Chapter Sixty-Nine

Pierre Robin Sequence

———

69
Pierre Robin Sequence

1. Identify General Problem/Diagnosis/Planning
   (Describe photo, give working diagnosis, key problems, evaluates patient)

   - Describe photo
     - Note position of mandible
     - Tongue position
     - Does patient have tracheostomy?
     - Describe cleft if present
   - Pierre Robin Sequence (PRS)
     - Respiratory distress secondary to glossoptosis
     - Glossoptosis
     - Retro/micrognathia
     - +/- cleft palate (1/3 of patients)
   - IMPORTANT:
   - Isolated cleft palate is a different clinical entity than cleft lip and palate.
   - History
     - Breathing problems/Respiratory distress
       - Aggravated by supine positioning
       - Alleviated by prone positioning
       - Alleviated by nasopharyngeal tube
       - Stridor
       - Excessive inspiratory effort
       - Cyanotic attacks
       - Sternal retractions- intubate urgently
     - Feeding difficulty
       - Secondary to inadequate neuromuscular control of tongue
       - Worsened in cleft palate due to inability to suck
         - Treatment Haberman bottle
     - Monitor weight gain
     - Failure to thrive
     - Indications for surgery:
     - Unable to feed or severe airway obstruction

- PE
  - Posterior positioning of the tongue
  - Retro- or Micrognathia- lack of structural support
    - Ball-valve effect
  - Mandible
    - Typically mandibular dental arch 10mm posterior to maxillary arch
    - Measure by ruler
    - Amount of discrepancy does not necessarily correlate with disease severity
  - Glossoptosis
  - Palate
    - U-shaped cleft palate vs. V-shape cleft palate
      - U-shape associated with Pierre Robin sequence
      - Can be any shape
    - Submucous cleft palate
      - Bifid uvula (2% of population)
      - Notch in hard palate
      - Zona pellucida
  - Sternal retractions
  - Ears
    - Fluid behind tympanic membrane
    - Routine audiology examination
  - Other anomalies to check for:
    - Polydactyly
    - Club feet
    - Cardiac murmur
- Pierre Robin Sequence
  - Energy expenditure for growth used in respiratory effort
  - Leads to:
    - Chronic airway obstruction
    - Hypoxia
    - Failure to thrive
    - Cor pulmonale
    - Mortality 30% untreated
  - Etiology
    - Hypoplastic mandible
    - 7th to 8th weeks gestation
    - 25-35% of cases are in context of syndrome

- Work-Up As in Cleft/Lip and Palate (CLP)
    - Genetics evaluation
    - Speech and Swallow evaluation
    - R/O cardiac defects
    - R/O other syndromes
    - Ophthalmology evaluation to R/O Stickler's
- Associated syndrome
    - As in CLP
        - Stickler syndrome
        - 22q11.2 deletion
        - Treacher Collins syndrome
- Work-Up in Pierre Robin Sequence
    - Transcutaneous pulse oximetry
    - Polysomnography
        - Check for hypoxia
        - Check for airway obstruction
    - Complete airway assessment from ENT
        - Laryngoscopy
        - Bronchoscopy
    - Must determine exact site of obstruction prior to surgery, guides airway management
        - Tongue base obstruction (PRS)
        - Glottic/infraglottic obstruction
        - Tracheomalasia or laryngomalasia
    - CT scan head and neck
        - Coronal/Sagittal 3-D reconstruction
            - Evaluates
                - Retroglossal airway
                - Mandibular anatomy
    - Consults
        - Pulmonary
        - ENT
        - Audiology
        - Speech and swallow
        - NICU

2. Consider reasonable goals in diagnosis and management *(Management and treatment, surgical indications, operative procedures and anesthesia)*

- Pierre Robin Sequence
    - Indications for surgery:

- - - o Unable to feed or significant airway obstruction
  - Management of Pierre Robin Sequence
    - o Multidisciplinary team
      - Craniofacial plastic surgeon
      - Pediatric ENT
      - Neonatology
      - Pulmonary-sleep medicine
      - Pediatric anesthesia
      - Genetics
      - Others as needed
  - Options for management
    - o Majority of cases respond to non-operative management
      - Improves over the 1st weeks of life
      - Requires close monitoring in NICU
    - o Initial management
      - Prone positioning
      - Feeding in upright position
      - Nasogastric or feeding tube
      - Nasopharyngeal tube
    - o If stable- monitor on home pulse ox
    - o Failure of non-operative measures:
      - Inability to breath easily while resting or sleeping
      - Episodes of cyanosis
      - Failure to thrive
    - o Consider surgery if:
      - Failure to gain weight
      - No tongue control within the first weeks of life
      - Requires ETT or tracheostomy for airway management
    - o Surgical options
      - Tongue-Lip Adhesion (TLA)
      - Mandibular distraction (MD)
      - Tracheostomy
      - Orthognathic surgery
        - Adolescent with failure to have catch-up growth
        - To correct class II occlusion
  - Cleft palate repair

- Around age 9-12 months depending on severity of cleft
- May wait longer in wide clefts
- Repair all patients before age 24 months to minimize impact on speech
- Anecdotally wait longer in cases of PRS because of potential airway problems. In theory if mandibular distraction was performed timing should not need to be changed.

3. Select appropriate options in diagnosis and management

- Tongue Lip Adhesion (TLA)
    - Primary indication compromised airway in Pierre Robin Sequence (PRS)
    - Procedure
        - Anterior portion of tongue sutured to lower lip
        - Suture lip extended posteriorly and bilaterally to close denuded areas
        - Pulls tongue base anteriorly preventing glossoptosis
    - Tongue released
        - At age 6-7 months, or
        - At the time of cleft palate repair
    - Patient can feed and speak with tongue lip adhesion in place
- Mandibular distraction
    - Primary indication compromised airway in PRS either at rest or with feeding
    - Can be used for earlier decannulation in patients with prior tracheostomy
    - For use in severe PRS cases when TLA fails
    - Corrects airway by moving tongue forward relieving tongue base obstruction
    - Beneficial effects on swallowing and reflux
- Option for internal or external devices
    - Internal device
        - Easy use
        - Single vector
        - Maximum distance 25-30mm
        - (only 20-25mm needed)

- Second procedure for removal
    - External device
        - Can distract in multiple planes
        - Maximum distance up to 40mm
        - Bulky, more easily dislodged
        - Second procedure still needed for removal
- Procedure
    - Placement
    - Risdon incision- 1 finger breadth below mandibular angle, avoid marginal mandibular branch
    - Inverted L osteotomy
    - Preserve inferior alveolar nerve if possible
    - Activate device in OR to ensure that it works
    - Distract 1mm/day for 3 weeks
- Protocol
    - Activate post-op day 1, Lag period not needed
    - Distract 1.5-2.0mm/day over 3 turns per day
    - Serial x-ray may be helpful to monitor progress
    - Monitor mandibular-maxillary discrepancy
    - Goal: overcorrection of 2-3mm
- After the first week dramatic improvement in breathing and feeding
- Can generally extubate after 1 week of distraction
    - Extubate in OR
    - Monitor in OR for 1 hour to be sure airway is stable
    - Have ENT available for airway emergency
- End distraction after 10-14 days
- Consolidation for 6 weeks minimum then distractors removed
- Cleft Palate Repair
    - Goal:
        - Radical intravelar veloplasty to optimize speech
        - Avoid fistulas
        - 10% require secondary surgery for residual velopharyngeal insufficiency
    - Techniques
        - 2 flap palatoplasty AKA Bardach repair AKA Dorrance
        - Von Langenbach (relaxing incisions)
        - V-Y advancement AKA Veau-Wardill-Kilner Repair

- Sommerlad repair
            - Furlow (Double Z-plasty)
        - Procedure
            - Three layer repair
            - Nasal mucosa
            - Levator veli palatini muscle repair key portion of procedure
            - Oral mucosa repair
        - Post-op
            - No-no's
            - Tongue stitch or nasopharyngeal tube

4. Understand risks and benefits of various approaches

    - Be able to discuss risks and benefits of various management options. Discuss when you would use one approach or another.

5. Address complications and unexpected problems adequately

    - Short-term complications of tongue-lip adhesion
        - Dehiscence 10-50%
        - Injury to neurovascular or salivary structures of the tongue
        - Interference with normal tongue function
    - Long-term complication of tongue lip adhesion
        - Tongue or lip scarring
        - Interference with normal tongue function
    - Mandibular distraction complications
        - Pin site infection
            - Conservative management
            - Antibiotics
            - Local wound care
        - Osteomyelitis (Rare)
        - Dental injury
        - Inferior alveolar nerve injury
        - Premature consolidation
        - Device failure
    - Cleft Palate Repair (See also Cleft Palate Chapter 68)
        - Bleeding
        - Airway obstruction
        - Dehiscence

- Fistula
- Velopharyngeal insufficiency

6. Demonstrate ability to structure alternative plan

    - How would you manage device failure?
    - Family refuses your suggested management plan
    - What if TLA or mandibular distraction fail?

Chapter Seventy

Velopharyngeal Insufficiency

70
Velopharyngeal Insufficiency

1. Identify General Problem/Diagnosis/Planning
   (Describe photo, give working diagnosis, key problems, evaluates patient)

   - Describe photo
     - Note features of submucous cleft palate
       - Bifid uvula (seen in 2% of the population, alone meaningless)
       - Zona pellucida
       - Notch on hard palate- must palpate for this finding
       - 2 or more features present usually diagnostic
     - Note features of Treacher Collins
   - What is VPI?
     - Anomalous velopharyngeal closure secondary to velopharyngeal insufficiency or incompetence
     - Multiple causes not just cleft palate
   - PE
     - Hypernasality
     - Nasal emission
     - Facial grimacing
     - Look for and evaluate:
       - Palatal fistulae
       - Hypertrophic tonsils
       - Prominent adenoid pad
       - Palatal mobility
     - In submucosal cleft palate:
       - On visual inspection:
       - Zona pellucida (trough in midline of palate)
       - Bifid uvula
       - On palpation:
       - Notch at junction of hard and soft palate (palpate)
     - In OR:
     - Check for visibly aberrant carotid pulsations
     - Palpable carotids near midline
   - Key problem

- o Abnormal speech
- Etiology
  - o Cleft palate unrepaired
  - o Cleft palate repaired (10-20% VPI)
  - o Neurogenic
  - o Idiopathic
- Work-up
  - o Speech therapy evaluation
  - o Nasoendoscopy- most useful
  - o Fluoroscopic speech evaluation
  - o Nasometry
  - o Aerodynamics
  - o Cephalometrics
  - o Consider sleep studies preop based on history
  - o R/O 22q11.2 Deletion (AKA Velocariofacial syndrome, DiGeorge)
    - FISH studies
  - o Consultants
    - Speech and swallow
    - ENT
    - Prosthodontist
    - Genetics
    - Pulmonary

2. Consider reasonable goals in diagnosis and management *(Management and treatment, surgical indications, operative procedures and anesthesia)*

- Requires multidisciplinary team
- Multimodal evaluation
- Goal of surgery
  - o Create subtotal nasopharyngeal obstruction that improves resonance but avoids airway morbidity
- Options
  - o Prosthesis- trial if unsure if structural problem
    - For use in short scarred velum
  - o Autogenous posterior wall augmentation
    - Fat injection
  - o Lengthen palate by repositioning palate
    - Re-repair by Furlow palatoplasty
  - o Velopharyngeal narrowing

- Reduction of static opening between nasal and oral pharynges
- Surgical Options
    - Pharyngeal flap
        - Most effective in patients with:
            - Good lateral wall movement, and
            - Sagittal or circular closure pattern
        - Creates single subtotal central obstruction of velopharyngeal port
        - Two lateral open ports
    - Sphincter pharyngoplasty
        - Most effective in patients with:
            - Good velar elevation
            - Poor lateral wall motion
            - Large central gap
            - Coronal closure pattern
        - Palatopharyngeus myomucosal flaps
        - Decreases cross sectional area
        - Decreases flow through nose
- Contraindications
    - Patient declines surgery
    - High risk of airway obstruction
    - Intermittent or inconsistent closure responding to speech therapy
    - Incomplete diagnostic results
- Age
    - At any age above 5 years, after failure of speech therapy
    - Can be done in older patients
    - Can consider in younger patients if VPI is severe
- Speech therapy
    - Resumed after surgery
    - Generally 1-2 months postop
    - Significant improvement by 9-12 months post-op with therapy
- Pre-op
    - Consider tonsillectomy & adenoidectomy (T&A) if:
        - Contributing to speech dysfunction
        - History of chronic obstructive sleep apnea
    - Perform T&A 3 months prior to VPI surgery.
- Avoid T & A if no clear indication, can worsen VPI post-op!

3. Select appropriate options in diagnosis and management

   - Pharyngeal flap
     - Width of flap?
       - Make as wide as operative field will allow, approximately 2cm minimum
       - Controversial
     - Insert flap at junction of hard and soft palate
     - Reduce postop contraction by
       - Lining raw surfaces with nasal mucosa, book flaps
     - Lateral port size
       - Cannot be rigorously controlled
     - Place nasopharyngeal tubes in OR to preserve lateral ports
       - Keep in place for first 24 hours post op
     - If flap is well positioned it should not be visible post-op
   - Sphincter Pharyngoplasty
     - Elevate tissue from tonsillar pillars
     - Myomucosal flaps sutured closed to pharyngeal wall
     - Narrow nasopharyngeal space
     - Muscle gives dynamic function
   - Resume speech therapy 3-6 weeks post-op

4. Understand risks and benefits of various approaches

   - Post-op complications (bleeding, obstruction, fistulas)
   - Screen intermittently for sleep apnea
     - Questionnaire
     - Sleep study if suspicious
   - Velopharyngeal insufficiency treatment sometimes considered "more art than science".

5. Address complications and unexpected problems adequately

   - Airway obstruction
   - Bleeding
   - Sleep apnea
     - Acute
     - Chronic
     - Signs

- Tired during the day
           - More napping
           - Difficulty with schoolwork
       - Infection (Rare)
       - Inadequate correction
       - Re-operation needed in 10%
       - Dehiscence
       - Injury to internal carotids
           - Increased risk in velocardiofacial patients
           - No pre-op work up needed
               - In the past MRA was recommended
           - Hard to control potentially disastrous injury

6. Demonstrate ability to structure alternative plan

   - What if chosen surgery fails?
   - Family refuses surgery
   - Nonsurgical management options (obturator)

Chapter Seventy-One

Secondary Cleft Lip and Nasal Deformity Management

71
Secondary Cleft Lip and Nasal Deformity Management

1. Identify General Problem/Diagnosis/Planning
   (Describe photo, give working diagnosis, key problems, evaluates patient)

   - Describe all abnormalities seen in photo
   - Bilateral cleft lip and palate a common secondary cleft lip/nasal deformity scenario
   - Classify deformity whenever possible
   - Note all key problems
   - Note families have high expectations
   - History
     - Note if severe physical or mental illness is present. Give careful consideration of risks and benefits of surgery in these cases. Can make life better for parents.
     - Prior surgical interventions
     - Type of previous surgeries
   - PE
     - Careful and detailed evaluation of all deformities present
     - Note the probable cause (surgical and anatomic) and consequence of deformity present
     - Anticipate surgical options available
   - Categories of Lip Deformity
     - Poor scar
     - Mismatch of landmarks
     - Tissue distortion
     - Tissue deficiency
     - Tissue excess

2. Consider reasonable goals in diagnosis and management
   (Management and treatment, surgical indications, operative procedures and anesthesia)

   - Principles of management

- o Skeletal correction before soft-tissue correction
  - ▪ Eg. alveolar bone graft prior to definitive rhinoplasty
- o Foundation first
- o In re-repairs use old scars whenever possible
- o Be systematic
- o Correct all abnormal components
- o Open rhinoplasty for nasal corrections
  - ▪ Internal splints (cartilage grafts)
  - ▪ External splints
- o Careful handling of tissues intraop
- ▪ Indications for intervention
  - o No absolute indications or contraindications
    - ▪ Except:
    - ▪ Severe physical or mental illness can be a relative contraindication
    - ▪ Even these patients may benefit from surgery if anesthetic risk is not prohibitive
  - o Need based on patient and/or caregiver's request
  - o Ability to correct deformity
- ▪ Lip Scar Revision Principles
  - o Excise orbicularis oris muscle wider than width of scar
  - o Suture the muscle tighter than skin, minimal width of the scar
  - o Leave bulk at the white roll
  - o Loose skin can be more prominent than the white roll
  - o Depressed scar
    - ▪ Address by approximating the orbicularis muscle or by z-plasty
- ▪ Mismatch landmark principles
  - o Cupid bow medial aspect still higher than lateral aspect
  - o Options:
    - ▪ Manage with z-plasty- small discrepancy 1-2 mm
    - ▪ Re-rotation with triangular skin flap to lower Cupid's bow in larger discrepancies
      - • Important to have adequate rotation
    - ▪ Elevate lateral lip element
- ▪ Tissue distortion

- Mild elevation of Cupid's bow
    - Insert small triangle flap
- Notch in lip
    - Usually secondary to inadequate muscle positioning or orbicularis dehiscence
    - Tx: Open scar and re-repair in moderate to severe cases
- Deviation of Cupid's bow to cleft side
    - Secondary to short lateral lip horizontally
    - Treatment options:
        - Abbe flap
        - If length is okay
            - Correct by:
            - Re-opening cleft
            - Lateral lip release and re-advancement
- Tissue deficiency
    - Usually related to skeletal deficiency of maxilla
    - Managed with orthodontics, orthognathic surgery or alveolar bone grafts
- Free border deficiency
    - Vermilion deficiency can be ambiguous
    - Composed of:
        - Vermilion- generally dark, dry
        - Mucosa- lighter color, wet
        - Red line
        - Orbicularis oris muscle
- Mucosa Deficiency
    - Tight mucosa/sulcus
    - Treatment:
        - Mucosal advancement
        - Z-plasty
        - V-Y plasty
    - Will not correct deficiency of muscle but will improve lip pout
- Muscle deficiency
    - Generally characterized by notch in the free border of the lip
    - Treatment:
        - Correct by re-approximating orbicularis oris muscle, marginalis aspect
    - Other options:

- o Many cleft surgeons now avoid forked flap procedures and Cronin procedures
  - Generally result in poor scarring
- o Scar Categories for bilateral lip same as in unilateral
- o Lip Scar
  - Muscle repair critical to prevent recurrence
  - Steps
    - Raise prolabial flaps
    - Approximate muscle
    - Trim scars
    - Re-drape prolabium
- Landmarks
  - o Unnatural Cupid's bow
  - o Mismatched peak points
  - o Excise scars and realign
- Tissue Disproportion
  - o Re-repair wide central lip or short lateral lips
  - o Narrow into suitable width
  - o Re-approximate muscle
- Tissue Deficiency
  - o Vertically short central lip
  - o Central whistling deformity
  - o Tight upper lip
  - o Asymmetric free border
    - Correct by re-repair through previous incisions
    - May need Abbe flap to import tissue
    - Goals:
      - Narrow philtrum
      - Align peak points
      - Vertically stretches central lip
      - Get white roll from lateral elements
- The Abbe Flap
  - o Useful in:
    - Tight upper lip
    - Absence of Cupid's bow
  - o Lateral muscle should be attached to nasal spine
  - o Guideline:
    - 10mm wide
    - 14-15mm long
- Deficiency of skin white roll

- - o Treat with secondary advancement of white skin roll free borders of lateral lip
  - Tissue Excess
    - o Uncommon problem in bilateral clefts
    - o Usually only seen in incomplete clefts, incomplete side has increased bulk.
    - o General rule increase the volume of the smaller side with free grafts rather than trim the bulky side.

  - Nasal Deformity
    - o No silver bullets here. Difficult problem to correct.
    - o Typical finding:
      - Wide nose
      - Short columella
      - Flat, blunt nasal tip
      - Lower lateral cartilage widely separated
    - o Timing of intervention same as in unilateral cases
  - Columellar lengthening or reconstitution at primary cheiloplasty
    - o Options
      - Lip via forked flaps or central lip
      - Tends to cause big nose
      - Increased projection, nasal width remains wide
      - Poor scarring can occur
      - Vs.
      - "Columella is in the nose" now widely accepted
      - Columellar reconstitution rather than lengthening
      - From skin in the nose
  - Re-repair
    - o Open lip via previous scars
    - o Extend into open rhinoplasty exposure
    - o Reverse U incision into dome of the nose
    - o Goals:
      - Narrow central lip
      - Alar bases advance medially to reduce nasal width
      - Open rhino best chance for complete correction

- Missing columella reconstituted from bilateral U-incisions on both soft triangles
  - Incisions
    - 8-10mm apart
    - 10-12mm from alar facial groove on each side
    - Discard skin between, consider use as graft material
    - Use reverse U-incisions
  - Dissection
    - Open rhino
    - Lip columella tip one unit
- Narrow nasal width
  - Total mobilization of lateral lip elements
  - Medialize alar bases on both sides
  - May need to excise orbicularis oris muscle anterior to premaxillary segment to facilitate adequate medial advancement of lateral lip elements (if present).
  - Anchor orbicularis to septum
- Algorithm Of Correction Nasal Framework
  - Address lining deficiency
  - Cartilage strut to maintain medial crura
  - Rib graft preferred as septum often deficient
  - Liberal use of tip graft or shield graft for tip definition
  - Dorsum is usually short
  - Batten graft may push nasal tip caudally and lengthen the dorsum
  - Osteotomies
    - Narrow the width of the nose
  - Submucosal resection for septal deviation
  - Dorsal augmentation
    - Diced cartilage generally better than a single piece
  - Re-drape skin
- Principles of Re-repair
  - No new scar on lip and columella except for reversed U-incisions
  - Final scar in alar rim
  - Blood supply to prolabial skin should remain intact
  - Surgery can be repeated

- - -
        - No need for additional tissue to increase columellar length with this approach
        - Alternative
            - Forked flaps
            - Cronin
        - No scar at nasolabial junction
    - Cleft Rhinoplasty
    - In the case of cleft rhinoplasty open approach is recommended
        - Excellent exposure
        - Flexible approach
        - General Steps and Techniques
            - Stair-step incision at narrowest part of columella
            - Dissection
                - Loose areolar space b/w medial crura
                - Separate fibro fatty tissue from lower lateral cartilage
            - Correct any lining deficiency
                - Release nasalis muscle laterally on piriform adequate for mild deficiency
                - Z-plasty or V-Y plasty for moderate deficiency
                - Inferior turbinate flap may be needed in severe lining deficiency
            - Correct any soft tissue deficiency
            - Cleft side lower lateral cartilage should be advanced to match non-cleft side
            - Columellar strut useful to maintain position of lower lateral cartilage
                - Septal cartilage
                - Rib cartilage if septal cartilage deficient
            - Osteotomy for nasal bone deviation
                - Dorsum
                    - Non-cleft side in-fracture
                    - Cleft side out-fracture
            - Submucosal resection
                - For nasal obstruction due to displaced vomer or septal cartilage

- Reposition septum
- Cartilage grafts may be needed
- Reshape nasal tip and ala
  - Defat fibrofatty tissue in tip
  - Cartilage grafts as needed for
    - Projection- shield or umbrella grafts
    - Extended spreader
    - Beware batten grafts can push tip caudally
- Dorsal augmentation
  - Useful adjunct
  - Autogenous tissue preferred
    - Cranial bone- high resorption, may result in asymmetry
    - Rib- decreased resorption, can have warping
      - K-wire
      - Carve as needed
    - Turkish delight
      - Diced cartilage wrapped in surgicel
- Re-draping soft tissue
- Re-drape skin over grafts
  - Carefully trim webbing at soft triangle
- Balance nostrils
  - Cleft side alar base typically displaced laterally, wider nostril
  - Advance alar base medially
    - Simple V-Y plasty
    - Advancement with lip revision
  - Small nostril on cleft side
    - Try to avoid at initial repair- difficult problem to correct
  - Tissue deficiency
    - Nasal floor- Tx: z-plasty on nasal floor
    - Columella- wedge shaped skin-fat composite graft

- Alar rim- composite earlobe graft
- Weir excision- normal alar base as composite graft to cleft side ala or composite graft of helical rim
- Prominent alar dome non-cleft side
  - Cephalad resection of lower lateral cartilage
- Increase alar rim non-cleft side
  - Composite graft (cartilage skin) from concha
  - Graft placed in infra-cartilaginous incision line on non-cleft side
- Weir excision on the non-cleft side
  - Decreased alar rim prominence
  - Narrows nasal floor
- Absence of nasal sill- difficult to reconstruct
  - Secondary to excess excision of nasal tissue during primary repair
  - Z-plasty if remnant cartilage present
  - Composite graft from non-cleft side to nasal sill
- Bone deficiency of nasal floor
  - Alveolar bone graft
  - Rib graft if still deficient

4. Understand risks and benefits of various approaches

- Be able to defend your suggested management plan and discuss the risks and benefits of various options based on presented clinical scenario.
- What are the downsides of early revisions and/or multiple surgeries? Increased scarring, midface deficiency, more difficult revision in the future, other
- Additional post-op measures
  - Scar massage
  - Silicone
  - Micropore tape on suture line 3-6 months
  - Silicone nasal conformers
  - 80% of patients have some improvement

5. Address complications and unexpected problems adequately

    - Potential complications
        - Scarring (hypertrophic/keloid)
        - Uneven free border
        - Persistent deformity/nasal deviation
        - Relapse of original deformity
        - Under correction

6. Demonstrate ability to structure alternative plan

    - Have back up plan if planned intervention fails
        - Did you miss something in your assessment?
    - What if insurance declines coverage due to "cosmetic" surgery?
    - Patient has no visible deformity
    - Family doesn't agree with your management plan
    - Patient not satisfied with outcome but you are?

Chapter Seventy-Two

Giant Congenital Nevus

72
Giant Congenital Nevus

1. Identify General Problem/Diagnosis/Planning
   (Describe photo, give working diagnosis, key problems, evaluates patient)

   - Describe photo
     - Detail most pertinent clinical concerns
     - Give details of involved anatomic areas and clinical concerns
     - What is the distribution? Describe in detail.
       - Bathing suit nevus
       - Vest-like nevus
       - Garment nevus
       - Cape-like nevus
       - Panda-like nevus
       - Other
     - Note how many lesions are present and size, satellite lesions
     - Note key problems related to the location of the nevus
   - Establish the diagnosis prior to planning intervention
     - History and physical generally adequate
     - If concerning clinical features or suspicious areas
       - Consider biopsy
       - Biopsy not always practical in large nevi
     - Pigmented lesion with hair in an otherwise healthy patient is most likely giant hairy nevus, i.e. congenital melanocytic nevus
   - History
     - Present at birth
     - Incidence of giant congenital nevus 1 in 20K
     - Change in nevus or increase in size
       - Expect growth in proportion to child's natural growth
     - Family history
       - Most cases are sporadic
       - May be clusters in congenital melanocytic nevus

- o Signs of CNS Involvement, neurocutaneous melanosis
  - Lethargy
  - Seizures
  - Vomiting
  - Signs of increased intracranial pressure
  - These signs usually manifest by age 5
  - Grave prognosis if CNS is involved
  - Death within 2-3 years of diagnosis of CNS involvement
- PE
  - o Features of giant congenital nevi:
    - Face, Torso, Extremities
      - Typically- Superficial, well differentiated, epidermis to upper dermis, lighter in color
    - Back, Scalp, Buttocks
      - Typically- Thick, irregular lesions
  - o Classification
    - Small nevus- <1.5cm in greatest diameter
    - Medium nevus between 1.5cm and 20cm in greatest diameter
    - Large or Giant > 20cm in greatest diameter in adolescents or adults. 9cm on child's head, 6cm on child's body. (Guide in infants and children lesions >1%TBSA [size of patient's palm] considered giant)
  - o Suspicious findings of any skin lesion:
    - Rapid growth
    - Pain
    - Bleeding
    - Ulceration
    - Change in color
- Work-up
  - o Goal to rule out associated lesions:
    - Overlying vertebrae/posterior scalp
    - Ocular manifestations
    - Spina bifida occulta
    - Neurofibromatosis
    - **Neurocutaneous melanosis**
    - Tumors
      - Schwannomas

- Neurofibromas
- Hemangiomas
- Wilm's tumors
    - If lesion is unusual biopsy, multiple punches may be needed
    - MRI may be needed if CNS involvement suspected
    - Important to r/o and consider neurocutaneous melanosis.
    - Melanoma can be visceral in these cases, risk 6.3%, 17x increase in incidence of visceral melanoma
- Consultations
    - Dermatology- for long-term follow-up, differential diagnosis
    - Neurology
    - Neurosurgery
    - Genetics
    - Ophthalmology
    - Multidisciplinary treatment
- Differential Diagnosis
    - Epidermal nevus
    - Café-au-lait spots (neurofibromatosis type I)
    - Mongolian spot
    - Nevus sebaceous
    - MELANOMA
- Melanoma
    - General risk of melanoma 6-9%
        - 70% of cases in giant congenital nevi before age 3
        - Incidence is much higher than expected for pediatric population
    - Risk factors
        - 3 or more lesions
        - Size >20cm^2
        - Age 3-5
- Neurocutaneous melanosis
    - Hydrocephalus
    - Seizure
    - Developmental delay
    - CN palsy
    - Tethered cord
    - Intracranial hemorrhage
    - Two peaks of presentation

- Age 2-3 years
- Age 20-30 years

2. Consider reasonable goals in diagnosis and management *(Management and treatment, surgical indications, operative procedures and anesthesia)*

- Indications for treatment
    o Suspicion of melanoma
    o Reduce risk of melanoma
    o Family anxiety regarding risk of melanoma
    o Melanoma
    o Aesthetics
    o To decrease and control associated symptoms
        - Pruritus
        - Bleeding
        - Ulceration
    o Psychological well-being
        - Bullying
        - Self-esteem regarding appearance
    o Maintenance of function
- Options
    o Vigilant observation with biopsies as indicated
    o Surgical excision with reconstruction
- Goals of surgical treatment
    o Remove lesion with as few operative procedures as possible
    o Negative margins if possible- lesions can extend to the fascia
        - Fascial excision is more disfiguring
    o Atypical lesions warrant immediate excision to r/o melanoma
    o Prophylactic excision of small lesions is controversial
        - Risk of melanoma probably exceeding low in small lesions
- Surgical principles
    o Resect into subcutaneous tissue to optimize chances of complete resection
- Long-term follow-up is needed to monitor for melanoma
    o Routine follow-up lifetime of patient
- Tissue expander management

- o Remote port
- o Fill 2 weeks after placement
- o Weekly expansion ideal
- o Inflate to 2x capacity ideal
- o Score capsule at removal of expander
- o Delay reinsertion minimum of 3 months

3. Select appropriate options in diagnosis and management

    - Reconstructive options for congenital melanocytic nevi
        - o Simple serial excision if can be completed within 3 procedures
        - o Tissue expansion for large lesions
            - Workhorse for large lesions
            - Always consider tissue expansion, as it is the only technique that replaces like tissue with defect
            - Best anatomic regions:
                - Scalp
                - Face
                - Trunk
                - Increased risk, but possible in extremities
            - Increased risk of complications in pediatric population
        - o Wide excision and split thickness skin graft
            - Generally not a first choice option
            - Significant post-op contracture
            - Benefit
                - Potential single stage reconstruction
        - o Wide excision and full thickness skin graft
            - May require pre-excision tissue expansion to have adequate skin for coverage in large lesions
        - o Pre-expanded free-flap
            - Useful in large lesions
            - TRAM free flap
            - ALT
            - Benefit- minimal secondary contracture
        - o Integra plus thin split thickness skin graft
            - Useful in large lesions
            - Good aesthetics

- Less contracture than STSG alone
- Requires two stages
- Cultured epithelial autograft
  - Consideration in large congenital nevi
  - Very expensive
  - Friable, poor long-term durability
- Dermabrasion, chemical peels, laser, curettage
  - Minimally invasive
  - Improves appearance
  - Does not decrease risk of malignancy
- Typical timing of intervention
  - Age 6 months to school age
    - Why?
    - 70% of melanoma occurs in the first 3 years of life
- Anatomic site management
  - Trunk
    - Use advancement flaps with minimal back cuts
  - Breast
    - Beware the breast bud!
    - Serial excision of skin may be best option
  - Extremity
    - Use proximally expanded transposition flaps

4. Understand risks and benefits of various approaches

- Complications of giant congenital nevus
  - Hyperpigmentation
  - Color variation
  - Hypertrichosis
  - Ulcerations
  - Nodularity
  - Bleeding
  - Erosions
  - Pruritus
  - Malignant melanoma increased incidence (6-9%, most cases >70% by age 5)
- What is your protocol of management in pediatric patients?
  - Tissue expanders

- Placement
- Injection
    - Skin grafts
        - Immobilization
        - Dressing changes
        - Splints
    - Integra
    - Timing for serial excision?
        - Every 3 months
- Be familiar with risks and benefits of various interventions and the common associated complications

5. Address complications and unexpected problems adequately

- Typical tissue expander complications
    - Post-op of skin ischemia
        - Decompress expander
        - Nitro paste
        - +/- antibiotics
    - Wound dehiscence/Exposure
        - Removal with advancement
        - Reattempt expansion in 3 months
    - Infection
        - Early antibiotics, removal with failure
        - Delayed flap advancement
    - Pain during expansion
    - Seroma
    - Scar widening
    - Altered aesthetics/appearance during expansion
    - Hematoma
    - Flap ischemia
    - Extrusion
    - Device failure
- Complications of minimally invasive techniques
    - Difficult to monitor
    - Excision is surgical mainstay of treatment
- Skin graft complications
    - Graft loss
    - Infection
    - Hematoma

- Your management including your donor site and graft management protocol (eg. VAC therapy, donor site coverage, scar management)

6. Demonstrate ability to structure alternative plan

    - If lesion so extensive no good donor site present or surgery will cause significant physical deformity or functional deficit?
        - Monitor annually with photos
        - Biopsy suspicious lesions
        - Further surgery based on biopsy results
        - E.g.
            - Eyelid lesions
            - Nevus covering entire hand
    - Patient/family desires may guide surgical management
    - Family refuses your surgical recommendations?

Chapter Seventy-Three

Syndactyly

Refer to Chapter 63

Chapter Seventy-Four

Hemangioma and Vascular Malformations

74
Hemangiomas and Vascular Malformations

1. Identify General Problem/Diagnosis/Planning
   (Describe photo, give working diagnosis, key problems, evaluates patient)

   - Differentiate hemangiomas and vascular malformations by presentation:
     - History
     - Physical exam findings
   - Hemangiomas- benign vascular tumors, true neoplasms of endothelial cells
   - May be high flow, low flow or no flow depending on growth phase (Early proliferation, involuting, involuted)
   - Types
     - Infantile- Glut-1 positive
     - Congenital- Fully formed hemangioma, present at birth, Glut-1 negative
       - RICH- rapidly involuting congenital hemangioma
       - NICH- non-involuting congenital hemangioma
   - Vascular malformations- remnants of embryonic tissue, abnormal vasculature, Glut-1 negative lesions
   - Types
     - Arterial- (AV malformations) high flow
     - Venous- low flow
     - Capillary- low flow
     - Lymphatic- low flow
       - Microcystic
       - Macrocystic
       - Mixed
   - History
     - When first noted?
       - Hemangiomas
       - Typically noted at 2 weeks to 2 months after birth

- Sometimes red papule noted at birth
- Vascular malformation
- Although present at birth not generally clinically noted till much later. Adolescence is when they become clinically apparent.
- Slow steady enlargement into puberty then pronounced expansion with sex hormones
- Lymphatic malformations may present infancy especially head and neck with viral illness
  - Growth pattern
    - Vascular malformation commensurate to patient
    - Hemangioma rapid early growth followed by stabilization within a year then involution.
  - Recurrent infections
    - Lymphatic malformations- treat with antibiotics
    - May swell and enlarge with viral illness
  - Family history
    - Some syndromes associated with vascular lesions
    - 10% of hemangiomas family history
    - Venous and AV malformations
      - Autosomal dominant in minority of cases
      - Sporadic in most
  - Venous malformations
    - May cause:
      - Hypertension
      - Airway obstruction
      - Speech abnormalities
      - Dentition abnormalities
      - Aesthetic problems
  - AV Malformations
    - High output cardiac failure is a risk
- PE
- Describe what is seen
  - Vascular lesion
  - Raised

- Anatomic distribution
- Clinical concerns based on location
- Color
- Flat vs. elevated
- Ulceration
- Visual obstruction- amblyopia
- If more than 3-5 hemangiomas consider disseminated hemangiomatosis
  - R/O Visceral hemangioma, primarily liver- very morbid
- Distribution
  - V1, V2 port-wine stain-capillary malformation
    - Consider Sturge-Weber
      - Port-wine stain
      - Ipsilateral brain vascular anomalies
      - Ocular anomalies (retinal detachment, glaucoma)
- PHACE syndrome
  - Posterior cranial fossa malformation (Dandy-Walker)
  - Hemangioma (large segmental facial hemangioma)
  - Arterial abnormalities
  - Coarctation aorta
  - Eye anomalies
- Extremities
  - Bony abnormalities more frequently associated with vascular anomalies
- Venous malformations
  - Pain
  - Skeletal and muscle deformations
  - Thrombosis/bleeding
  - Phlebolith
  - General Findings
  - Compression of lesion
    - Partial emptying more likely hemangioma
    - Flattens with compression more likely venous malformation
  - Flat patch
    - Venous or other vascular malformation
  - Firm mass
    - AV malformation
- Specific findings

- Capillary Malformations
    - Flat, macular vascular stain
    - Early difficult to differentiate from hemangioma or early
- AVM
    - Can cause soft tissue or bone hypertrophy
- Venous Malformation
    - Bluish discoloration
    - Compressible swelling
    - In head and neck valsalva maneuver may accentuate lesion
- Lymphatic Malformation
    - May have small vesicles in overlying skin
- AV Malformation
    - Fast-flow lesion
    - Palpable thrill, audible bruit
    - Classification (4 stages) worsens at puberty
        - I- Quiescence- erythema, warmth, macular stain
        - II- Expansion-pulsation, bruit, thrill, tortuous vessels
        - III- Destruction- pain, bleeding, ulceration
        - IV- Decompensation- CHF
- Work-up Hemangiomas and Vascular Malformations
- Imaging not always needed
    - Ultrasound (US) differentiates high vs. low flow
        - Check for visceral hemangiomas
        - Useful in defining extent of venous malformations
    - MRI
        - If uncertain of diagnosis from US
        - Critical for pre-op work-up in AV malformation
            - Always more extensive than clinically apparent
            - Abnormal vasculature not yet physically active
    - X-ray may be needed in extremities to check for bony abnormalities
        - Especially useful in vascular anomalies
    - CT scan
- Generally further work-up not necessary unless affecting the following:

- Airway
  - ENT consultation
  - Imaging
- Visual field
  - Ophthalmology consultation
- Pre-op embolization for AV-malformations
  - Interventional radiology
- Differential Diagnosis
  - Kaposiform Hemangioendothelioma
    - Associated with respiratory compromise
    - Failure to thrive
    - Fatigue
    - DIC, platelet consumption
    - Congestive heart failure
- Syndromes
  - Blue rubber bleb syndrome
    - Associated with GI bleed
  - Proteus syndrome
    - Vascular malformation and asymptomatic gigantism
  - Klippel-Trenauny Syndrome
    - Venous malformation and limb hypertrophy
  - Maffucci syndrome
    - Venous malformation and Enchondromas
  - Parkes-Weber
    - AV malformation and soft tissue hypertrophy
  - Disseminated hemangiomatosis
  - Benign hemangiomatosis

2. Consider reasonable goals in diagnosis and management *(Management and treatment, surgical indications, operative procedures and anesthesia)*

- Indications for treatment in hemangiomas
  - Ulceration
  - Infection
  - Bleeding
  - Anatomic destruction or deformation
  - Local skin issues (excess skin post-involution, telangiectasia's, abnormal pigmentation)
  - Obstruction

- - - Airway
    - Visual field
    - Auditory canal
  - Psychological distress
    - Parental
    - Patient-self-esteem issues
  - Large destructive lesion
  - Life threatening lesions (Rare)
- Indications for treatment in venous malformations
  - Hypertension
  - Airway obstruction
  - Speech abnormalities
  - Dentition abnormalities
  - Aesthetic problems
  - Pain
  - Bleeding
- Indications for treatment in AV malformation
  - High output cardiac failure
  - Bleeding
  - Tissue ulceration and or destruction
  - Pain
- Indications for treatment in lymphatic malformations
  - Airway obstruction
  - Functional limitations
- Other Indications
  - Treat secondary deformities
    - Bone hypertrophy
    - Soft tissue hypertrophy
- Early intervention in the case of bleeding, ulceration, visual obstruction, airway obstruction.
- Goals of intervention
  - Restore normal contour
  - Eliminate scarred skin from ulcer
  - Prevent repeat episodes of bleeding
  - Restore damaged/distorted anatomy
  - Optimize psychological and social development
  - Improve functional deficits
- May require multidisciplinary management
  - Plastic Surgery
  - Pediatrics
  - Hem/Onc
  - Dermatology

- Interventional radiology
- Ophthalmology
- Orthopedics
- ENT
- Cardiology
- Psychiatry
- Support groups
- Hemangioma Management Options
    - Observation
        - Regular exams first 3 months check for complications
        - If no complications or significant cosmetic deformity Then observe
        - After involuted years down the line address residual changes with surgery PRN
    - Medical therapy
        - Steroids
            - Intralesional 3-5mg/kg up to 5 treatments 6-8 week intervals
            - Systemic prednisolone- treatment course lasts upwards of a year before taper can be done
        - Propranolol
            - IV then switched to oral
            - Requires cardiology for monitoring
        - Timolol topical gel
        - Vincristine for kaposiform hemangioendothelioma
    - Laser therapy
        - Yellow light
        - Pulsed dye
        - Nd:YAG
        - IPL
    - Surgical excision
        - Primary indication cosmetically deforming lesions
        - Purse string technique minimizes scarring
- Management Vascular Malformations
    - Pharmacologic
        - Sclerotherapy
    - Surgery

- - - Resect well-circumscribed, limited lesions when easily removed with minimal morbidity
    - Embolization
  - Venous Malformations
    - Pain
      - Elastic compression
        - Pressure support garments
      - Low dose aspirin
    - Sclerotherapy
      - Interventional radiology
    - Laser therapy
      - Pulsed-dye, most useful in superficial lesions
    - Excision
      - Ortho may be needed to excise bony overgrowth
      - Areas of hypertrophy can be surgically recontoured
  - Capillary Malformation
    - Laser therapy- Pulse-dye
      - Intervene early prior to cobble stoning which may begin in adolescence/adulthood
      - 15% complete resolution
      - 65% considerable resolution
      - 20% no improvement
      - Face better response than extremities
    - In the case of soft tissue or bone hypertrophy
      - Mandible can be affected
        - Resection and recontouring can be needed
        - Orthognathic surgery
      - Extremities
        - Leg length discrepancies may need orthopedic intervention
  - Arteriovenous (AV) Malformation
    - Embolization
      - Alone
        - Palliation for unresectable symptomatic lesions
        - Repeat embolization will be needed
      - Combination with surgery

- - - Prior to surgical debulking
  - Surgical resection
    - Usually wait until severely symptomatic due to very high recurrence rate
    - Super selective embolization w/i 24 hours of surgical resection
      - Decreases blood loss during surgery
    - High blood loss cases, frequent transfusions needed
    - Easier to resect at younger age but high risk of bleeding
    - High-risk cases require radical resections
  - Treat symptomatic lesions
  - Observe asymptomatic ones
    - Serial MRI useful to monitor progression or decide on timing of intervention
  - Routine type and cross pre-op
    - Pre-op sclerotherapy or embolization to decrease blood loss
- Lymphatic malformation
  - Sclerotherapy
    - OKT3
    - Bleomycin
  - Special areas
    - Lips
      - MRI for extent of lesion
    - Buccal fat
      - Frequent extension to parotid
- Treatment kaposiform hemangioendothelioma
  - Medical first:
    - Steroids
    - Vincristine
  - Surgery if chemotherapy fails
- Contraindications to treatment
  - Resection asymptomatic lesion solely for parental desire
  - Debulking not desired by parents and no immediate threat to patient
  - AV malformations
    - If resection of entire lesion impossible
    - Resection will cause morbidity worse than original lesion

3. Select appropriate options in diagnosis and management
    - Hemangiomas
        - Eyelid
            - Medical treatment 1st choice in most cases
                - Propranolol
                - Steroids
                    - Avoid intralesional injection on oral exam
                    - Risk of retinal embolization
                - Laser
            - Surgery
                - Failure of medical therapy
                - Can be first choice
                - Pedunculated
                    - Lesion excise and close primarily
                - Broad
                    - Leave some skin for primary closure even if hemangioma involved primary closure less morbid than skin graft
        - Nasal tip
            - If intervention needed
            - Medical treatment 1st choice in most cases
            - Propranolol
            - Steroids
            - Surgical resection early at age 2-3
                - Debulk via standard open rhino approach
                - Intradomal sutures
                - Resect excess skin
        - Lip
            - High risk for ulceration
                - Ulceration may result in scarring
            - Medical treatment okay initially
                - Steroids
                - Propranolol
            - Avoid over resection

- Can always take more later
            - Bilobed wedge excision
                - Preserves central fullness
            - Re-approximate orbicularis oris muscle
        - Ear and Cheek
            - Parotid and cheek respond well to steroids
            - Surgery for damaged or redundant skin
            - Do not resect parotid during proliferative phase
            - Otoplasty may be needed if ear distorted by malpositioning
    - No cure for AV malformations
        - Adjacent tissue is abnormal but quiescent
        - Vessels are recruited and reform malformation after resection
    - Not all vascular malformations require treatment
        - Treatment generally indicated for symptomatic lesions
        - Asymptomatic lesions may be observed
        - All types of vascular malformations are challenging to cure
    - Sclerotherapy and embolization
        - May manage symptoms, alleviate pain
        - Can be repeated as needed
        - Used in the case of extensive, unresectable venous malformations
        - Maintenance program of sclerotherapy at repeated intervals
    - Laser therapy generally requires minimum of 3-5 treatments
    - Pressure Support Garments
        - Useful in low-flow lesions such as lymphatic or venous malformations
    - Surgery good option if:
        - Resection easy to achieve with minimal morbidity
        - When sclerotherapy and embolization fail
        - Irreversible tissue damage
        - In extensive lesions not amenable to complete resection
            - Surgery may be palliative only
    - Airway obstruction
        - May require tracheostomy +/- surgical resection

- o Especially in lymphatic malformations
- Weigh aesthetic/functional deformity vs. benefits of removal
- No cure guarantee in most vascular malformations
- AV Malformations
- Treatment of Stage I and II most successful
- BUT no guarantee of cure without recurrence
- Generally follow Stage I and II expectantly
  - o Surgery can traumatize the lesion and cause progression or worsening unacceptable deformity
- Routine Post-op management
  - o Local hygiene
  - o Soap and water
  - o Bacitracin
  - o No-no's if concerned about scratching at surgical site
  - o No strenuous activity
  - o Sun avoidance
- Venous Malformation
  - o Frequently no clear capsule at surgery
    - Invades surrounding tissue not apparent at surgery
    - Complete resection not usually possible
  - o Closure based on reconstructive ladder
  - o Pre-op sclerotherapy or embolization in large lesions
  - o Hemostasis
    - Bovie
    - Bipolar
    - Ligature
    - Argon laser
  - o Consider drains post-op
  - o Preserve normal skin if possible
- Mixed lesions/Lymphatic malformations in Lower Extremity
  - o Operate one side per operation
  - o Use longitudinal incisions
    - Medial or lateral
  - o Perform resection
  - o Excess skin trimmed
  - o Skin closure
  - o Drain
  - o Allow 3 months healing before attempting 2nd side

4. Understand risks and benefits of various approaches

- Risks of intervention
    - Bleeding
    - Infection
    - Poor scarring
    - Inability to completely resect lesion
    - Injury of nerves and other adjacent structures
    - Disfigurement
    - Functional impairment
- In hemangioma
    - Lesion may not be fully manifest at time of excision
    - More growth may occur in periphery of lesion
    - Timing important
        - Less likely to have further growth if excision can be delayed
- Long-term follow-up needed to monitor for recurrences
- Be aware of side effects of scleropthery and medical interventions (steroids cause growth delay, catch up over 2 years)
- What is your algorithm of management for various vascular lesions? Medical vs. surgical treatment, timing of intervention

5. Address complications and unexpected problems adequately

- Complications of steroid therapy
    - Hypopigmentation
    - Ulceration
    - Systemic effects
    - Adrenal suppression and growth retardation
    - Rebound effect when stopped
- Complications of sclerotherapy
    - Allergic reactions
    - Cerebral intoxication
    - Skin necrosis and ulceration
    - Neuropraxia
    - Recurrence
- Complications of laser therapy
    - Delayed healing of ulcerations
    - Skin slough
    - Hyperpigmentation (10-20%)
        - May resolve spontaneously

- ▪ If no resolution 4% hydroquinone may help
  - o Chronic hypopigmentation
- ▪ Complications of surgical resection in AV
  - o Bleeding
  - o Death from blood loss
  - o High recurrence
- ▪ Complications of lymphatic malformation treatment
  - o High recurrence rate around 50%
  - o Anecdotally less in localized lesions and with post op VAC therapy
- ▪ Facial nerve injuries in treatment of facial vascular malformations especially lymphatic
- ▪ Post-op Complications
  - o Bleeding
  - o Poor scarring
  - o Over resection- later atrophy of hemangiomas
  - o Recurrence

6. Demonstrate ability to structure alternative plan

- ▪ Plan for recurrence of lesion
- ▪ Failed resection
- ▪ Management of uncontrollable bleeding during any vascular lesion resection

Chapter Seventy-Five

Prominent Ear Deformity

75
Prominent Ear Deformity

1. Identify General Problem/Diagnosis/Planning
   (Describe photo, give working diagnosis, key problems, evaluates patient)

   - Describe deformity
   - Three most common features of prominent ear deformity
     - Effacement of scapho-fossa
     - Enlarged conchal bowl
     - Prominent lobule
   - Note key problems
     - Is patient self-conscious regarding ears?
     - Teasing and/or bullying from peers or others
   - Prominent ear deformity in 5% of population
     - If not self-conscious or teased/bullied surgery not necessary
     - No surgery on prophylactic basis unless severe deformity
       - Even then consider waiting until psychosocial issues arise unless patient too immature or incapacitated to make a decision and the deformity is impacting the care giver's life
   - Embryology
     - Anterior hillocks (helical root and tragus)
     - Posterior hillocks (helix, antitragus, triangular fossa, scapha, concha cymba, concha cavum, lobule)
   - About the ear
     - Growth
       - 90% adult size in width at 1 year of age
       - 85% adult size in length at 3 years of age
   - Deformity is generally present at birth
     - Splinting is a viable option in infancy
     - Most effective up to 4 months of age
     - Dependent on parental desire
   - History
     - Associated hearing problems?
     - Teasing at school or other psychosocial problems

- o Concomitant congenital anomalies
  - Fragile X
  - VATER
- PE
  - o Etiology
    - Unfurling of antehelical fold resulting in effacement of scapho-fossa
    - Scaphoconchal angle 90 degrees or >
    - Deepening of conchal bowl, large concha, >1.5cm
    - Obtuse scapho-mastoid angle
    - Prominent lobule
    - Combination
  - o Objective measurements that can be used
    - Auriculocephalic angle
    - Scaphaconchal angle
    - Antehelix to helix
    - Depth of conchal bowl >1.5cm
    - Horizontal distance of helix to skull/scalp (good guide)
    - Normal projection of ear
      - Superior pole 10-12mm (10mm)
      - Middle pole 16-18mm (15mm)
      - Inferior pole 20-22mm (20mm)
      - Useful for positioning ear during otoplasty
  - o Judge ear subjectively
    - Patient or family perceptive
  - o Size
    - Ear length 5.5-6.5 cm in adult
    - Width 50-60% of length
    - Height generally 2x width
  - o Position
    - Superior aspect corresponds to brow
      - Usually at or a little below
    - Inferior border at base of columella
    - Low-set ear may indicate genetic syndrome
    - Vertical axis in profile
      - Normal projection 15-30 degrees posteriorly
  - o Other anomalies
    - Overprojected lobule

- Excess antitragal protection
- Insufficient helical curl
- Cup ear (microtia variant)
- Macrotia
- Prominent mastoid may contribute to deformity
            - Be sure ear canal is patent
            - Note feel of cartilage
                - Floppy- often in younger patients under 3
                - Limber- responds well to manipulation
                - Stiff- often in older patients teens and adults
                - Floppy and stiff cartilage harder to shape and maintain long-term result
            - Summary of Inspection
                - Topographical features of ear
                - Mechanical characteristics of cartilage
                    - Prognostic of outcome risk of revision/relapse
                - Dimensions and projection
                - Bilateral asymmetries
    - Work-up
        - No specific work-up needed

    - Genetics evaluation if suspicious of syndrome
        - Renal US for microtia

2. Consider reasonable goals in diagnosis and management *(Management and treatment, surgical indications, operative procedures and anesthesia)*

    - Pre-op photos in all cases
        - Frontal/Lateral/Oblique/Posterior view
    - Ear Aesthetics
        - Helix- ideally free edge in full view just beyond rim of antehelix
        - Often partially hidden in attractive ears
        - Antehelix asymmetric "Y"
        - Concha hemispherical bowl with defined rim
    - Corrective measures
        - Splinting is a viable option in infancy
            - Most effective up to 4 months of age
            - Dependent on parents

- Maternal estrogen keeps cartilage soft and pliable
    - Cartilage sparing (suture techniques)
        - Bends and shapes cartilage
        - Generally preferred techniques for otoplasty
    - Cartilage excision
        - Avoid excision techniques if possible
    - Scoring cartilage (Stenstrom technique)
        - Gibson's principle
            - Cartilage bends away from scored surface
            - Usually anterior scoring done to get posterior bending
        - Age under 4 scoring not usually needed
        - Above age 6 scoring generally needed due to stiffening of cartilage
        - Scoring decreases recurrence and assists in correction of antehelical fold
        - Posterior scoring can be effective in assiting bending of cartilage when sutures are placed
            - Useful and practical clinically, but, may not be a "safe" answer on boards. Violates Gibson's principle regarding direction of bending.
    - Repositioning of cartilage
    - Lobule often overlooked, various techniques:
        - Reposition helical tail to concha cavum (Webster procedure)
        - Skin excision and dermal plication
        - Posterior skin excision
    - Address specific deformities, combined approach often best
- Address
    - Antehelical fold
        - Mustarde sutures
        - Fossa-fascial sutures
    - Deep conchal bowl
        - Furnas sutures (concha-mastoid)
        - Cartilage excision
    - Earlobe reposition
- Timing
    - Maturity of patient important

- When patient asking for surgery good indicator of cooperation
  - Reasons for wanting surgery
  - Patient expectations
  - Consider individual circumstances
    - Patient's today earlier exposure to peers and caretakers due to day care
- Relative indication
  - Teasing
  - Earliest age 3
  - Controversial
    - Some advice surgery before age of socialization
    - Others wait until patient asks for surgery
  - Safe answer wait until ear growth complete, age 5
  - Earlier if family experiencing severe bullying with higher risk of relapse/recurrence requiring revision
- Sequence of surgery
  - Correct more defined ear first
  - Mustarde suture placement
    - Scapho-fossa first, then conchal cartilage
- Technique
  - Furnas
    - Conchal-Mastoid Sutures for set back
    - Expose posterior aspect of concha
    - Push back and place sutures at contact point
  - Elliott Maneuver
    - Division of postauricular muscle
    - Expose mastoid fascia 2cm
    - 3-0 horizontal mattress sutures
    - Full thickness bites of cartilage needed
  - Excision of postauricular muscle and fibrofatty tissue may assist in setback
  - Cartilage excision can be done via anterior or posterior incision
    - Reapproximate cartilage
  - Mustarde sutures
    - Scaphoconchal sutures
    - 4-5 horizontally placed
    - Wide 4mm intervals
  - Scoring
    - Done anteriorly traditionally

- - - Posterior scoring weakens cartilage decreases recurrence of Mustarde sutures
      - Skin excision generally not necessary but conservative excision acceptable (5-10mm)
  - Macrotia (large ear)
    - Treat by crescent shaped excision for ear reduction
  - Postop Management
    - Headband minimum 6 weeks as long as 6 months
  - Primary surgical goal
    - Improve self-confidence
    - Natural ear shape and contour- somewhat subjective
    - Correct all upper pole protrusion
    - Reduce ear prominence not necessarily perfect form
    - Match ears within 3mm acceptable
  - Anatomic goals of surgery
    - Helix visible beyond antehelix
    - Helix and antehelix anatomically correct
    - Posterior sulcus maintained
    - Helical rim projects beyond lobule
    - Standard projection at superior, middle, inferior poles (10mm-15mm-20mm)
    - At end of procedure ear should look natural
    - No more than 3mm difference between ears

3. Select appropriate options in diagnosis and management

   - Management of conchal prominence
     - Normal 1.5cm
     - 2.5cm set back with Furnas (conchal-mastoid sutures)
     - >2.5cm requires conchal excision to set back
   - Consider general anesthesia vs. local with sedation in older patients
   - Delineate your operative plan based on presented anatomy of auricular deformity and mechanical characteristics of ear.
   - Judge appearance based on front and lateral views of ear

4. Understand risks and benefits of various approaches

   - Stunting of growth with early surgery- controversial
     - Gosain published studies growth disturbance does not occur with early surgery

- - Note on exam you have considered this possibility
    - Safer to operate later on oral exam age 5 or older so ear almost adult size
  - Early surgery more likely to require revision (?)

5. Address complications and unexpected problems adequately

    - Recurrence (10%)
      - 1.8% with Mustard sutures in age <6
      - Significant increase in relapse with Mustarde sutures alone age >6. Add scoring to minimize recurrence.
      - Prevention
        - Headband 6weeks to 6 months
        - Splinting with mold 6 weeks to 6 months (Pick your number for exam purposes)
        - Use combination of techniques
        - Scoring important
        - Avoid excess skin excision of post-auricular skin
        - Non-cutting round taper needles
        - Preserve perichondrium
        - Correct more severe ear 1st
    - Bleeding/Hematoma (2-3%)
      - Early evacuation of hematoma
      - Asymmetric pain clinical sign
      - Cauliflower ear in undrained hematoma
    - Infection (5%)
      - Can be a devastating event, but rare
      - Total ear loss can occur
      - Treat aggressively (IV antibiotics/debridement)
      - Topical sulfamylon
      - Bacteria (pseudomonas/Strep/Staph)
    - Malposition
      - Redo otoplasty
    - Obliteration/Kinking of external auditory canal with Furnas sutures
      - Redo otoplasty
    - Telephone ear deformity
      - Overcorrected middle ear
      - Recurrent upper or lower pole only
      - Middle pole correction with inadequate superior and inferior pole correction

- - -
          - Correct by redo Otoplasty
      - Reverse telephone ear deformity
          - Middle ear protrusion compared to superior and inferior pole
          - Correction by treating concha
      - Chondritis
      - Chronic pain
      - Suture related complications
          - Sinus tracts
              - Complication of permanent suture
          - Granuloma
              - Higher with braided suture (?)
          - Extrusion
          - Visible sutures
          - Preventative measures
              - Fascial flap to cover sutures (Gault flap)
              - Minimize skin tension
      - Hypertrophic scar or keloid
          - 11% African-Americans
          - 2.1% Caucasians
      - Deformation
          - Sharp rigid antehelical fold
          - Abnormal curvature to superior crus
          - Irregular contouring
          - Malposition antehelical fold
          - Narrow ear
          - Large scapha
      - Constricted post-auricular sulcus
      - Stuck-on appearance
      - Very acute auriculocephalic angle
          - Difficult to correct
              - Associated tissue deficiency
              - May require skin grafting
      - Post-surgical appearance
      - Obscured helix
      - Unnatural kinks in ear

6. Demonstrate ability to structure alternative plan

    - What if family does not agree with your proposed timing?
    - What if insurance will not cover the procedure?
    - Do you bill for revision surgery?

- Initial otoplasty does not correct deformity, consider if you missed something in diagnosis
- How would you manage a recurrence? (Consider cartilage excision if not performed in initial surgery)

Chapter Seventy-Six

Gynecomastia

Refer to Chapter 5

Chapter Seventy-Seven

Meningomyelocele

77
Meningomyelocele

1. Identify General Problem/Diagnosis/Planning
   (Describe photo, give working diagnosis, key problems, evaluates patient)

   - Describe photo, detail size of defect, what is exposed, what is missing
   - Classify defect
     o Neural tube anomaly (incidence 1 in 400 live births)
       - Spina bifida occulta
       - Spina bifida- developmental dorsal defect in vertebral column
       - Spina bifida cystica
         - Meningocele- no neural involvement
         - Myelomeningocele- variable neural involvement
         - Syringomyelocele- variable neural involvement
         - Myelocele- variable neural involvement
     o What happens?
       - Paralysis of lower limbs and perineal sphincters
     o Defect
       - All lesions involve open dysplasia of spinal cord and meninges
       - No overlying skin, muscle and/or vertebral column
       - May have an associated lipoma
   - Work-up
     o Imaging
       - MRI
     o Consultation
       - Neurosurgery
       - Urology- associated urologic deformities, neurogenic bladder

- 90% of spina bifida cystica die from:
  - Meningitis
  - Progressive hydrocephalus
  - Complications related to paralysis
- Early mortality rate 40%
- Progressive hydrocephalus in 50%
- Prognosis: Guarded in all cases

2. Consider reasonable goals in diagnosis and management *(Management and treatment, surgical indications, operative procedures and anesthesia)*

- Initial management
  - Keep moist with topical antibiotic
  - Goal prevent infection, prevent desiccation
  - Prevention of desiccation- prevents further loss of function
    - Options
      - Silvadene dressings
      - Normal saline dressings
- Wound closure ASAP
- Algorithm
  - Simple meningocele with skin coverage
    - May defer surgery until 3 months of age
- Surgical/Medical goals
  - Coverage of spinal cord
  - Decompress hydrocephalus
    - Temporary followed by permanent VP shunt
  - Physical therapy
    - Render patients as ambulatory as possible
    - Ambulation prevents later pressure sore formation
  - Urology evaluation
    - Optimize urinary function/prevent renal infections
- Multidisciplinary team management long-term
  - Neurosurgery
  - Orthopedics
  - Urology
  - Plastic Surgery
  - Pediatrics
  - Genetics

- Social work

3. Select appropriate options in diagnosis and management

    - General Management
        - Tailor to each individual defect
        - No treatment for bony defect
        - Overlying hair bearing skin
            - Excise for cosmesis
        - Thin or atrophic skin
            - Excise and cover with well-vascularized tissue
    - Sequence of Management
        - Neural repair
        - Followed by skin closure
    - Closure options
        - Primary closure
        - Wide undermining and skin advancement
        - Cutaneous flaps
            - Rhomboid
            - Rotation advancement (single or double) +/- back grafting
            - Transposition flap (single or double)
        - Split thickness skin graft (STSG)
        - Muscle flap with STSG
            - Latissimus dorsi
            - Gluteus maximus
            - Trapezius
        - Musculocutaneous flap with STSG of donor defect
        - Vertical bipedicled latissimus-gluteus maximus
        - Vertical bipedicled latissimus-gluteus fasciocutaneous
        - Reverse latissimus island flap
        - Bilateral sliding muscle flap
            - Latissimus dorsi
            - Latissimus dorsi-gluteus maximus combined flap
        - Paraspinous osteomuscular flap
    - Management
        - Primary closure first choice if tensionless repair possible
            - Smaller defects

- Simple undermining of skin edges and tension-free approximation
- Larger defects are more difficult to repair
  - Primary complications
    - Wound breakdown
    - Infection
- Primary healing is a significant determinant of neurologic outcome
  - Good healing preserves functioning neural tissue

- Options based on anatomic site
  - General category: Posterior Trunk Defects
  - Cervical region
    - Trapezius flap or musculocutaneous flap (latissimus)
  - Upper Thoracic
    - Trapezius or musculocutaneous flap
    - Latissimus dorsi
  - Mid-thoracic region
    - Trapezius or musculocutaneous flap
    - Latissimus dorsi
    - Reverse latissimus dorsi
    - Paraspinous turnover
  - Lower Thoracic region
    - Latissimus dorsi musculocutaneous flaps
    - Reverse latissimus dorsi
    - Paraspinous turnover flap
  - Lumbosacral area
    - Latissimus dorsi musculocutaneous flaps
    - Reverse latissimus dorsi
    - Gluteus maximus
    - Greater omental free flap (adults)
    - Latissimus dorsi with vein graft elongation of pedicle
  - Sacral area
    - Gluteus maximus musculocutaneous flap
    - Latissimus dorsi flap with vein graft elongation of pedicle

4. Understand risks and benefits of various approaches

    - Skin grafts
        - No longer favored poor long-term durability and coverage
        - Vulnerable to injury
        - Can be used as a temporary cover or bridge to more permanent coverage
    - Fasciocutaneous or muscle flaps preferred especially in larger defects
    - Rhomboid flaps useful for defects up to 8cm diameter
        - Preserve perforating vessels if possible
        - Decreased tension
    - Muscle and musculocutaneous flaps
        - More durable coverage
        - Paraspinous osteomuscular flap
            - Complex
            - Increased blood loss
        - Latissimus dorsi musculocutaneous flaps for thoracolumbar defects
            - Ideal flap
            - Broad muscle
                - Blood supply- thorcodorsal artery

5. Address complications and unexpected problems adequately

    - Management of wound complications
    - Seroma management
    - Wound breakdown- anticipate why wound breakdown occurred
    - Any preventative measures?

6. Demonstrate ability to structure alternative plan

    - Management of failed flap
    - Alternatives if wound breaks down

Chapter Seventy-Eight

Ptosis

78
Ptosis

1. Identify General Problem/Diagnosis/Planning
   (Describe photo, give working diagnosis, key problems, evaluates patient)

   - Hx:
     - Inability to fully open one or both eyes
     - Difficulty holding eyes open
     - Was this present at birth? Congenital ptosis, maldevelopment of levator muscle
     - Age of patient
       - Disinsertion or laxity of levator aponeurosis most common cause of ptosis seen with increasing age
         - Progressive rather than acute
     - What are the specific patient complaints?
       - Aesthetic concerns (adults)
         - Excess skin from aging
         - Consider concurrent bleph at time of ptosis repair
       - Interference of vision (neonates, infants, children)
     - Does eyelid position change over the course of the day?
       - High in morning
       - Low in evening
       - Ptosis may be secondary to myasthenia gravis, muscle fatigue
     - Associated symptoms:
       - Miosis of pupil
       - Anhydrosis of skin
       - Ptosis of eyelid
       - Think Horner's syndrome
         - Disruption of sympathetic nervous system
         - Causes
         - Defect in pre- or postganglionic neuron

- Tumor apex of lung
- Trauma
- CVA
  - Previous surgery of eyelids
- PE
  - Sagging of upper eyelid
  - Is visual axis obstructed?
  - Is patient using frontalis for eyelid elevation?
    - Compensated brow ptosis
    - Brow returns to normal low position after bleph
  - Eyebrow position
    - Normal 22mm to central eyelid
    - 10mm from temporal and nasal areas
    - Position higher in females than males
  - Opening of upper lid controlled by:
    - Levator palpebrae superioris muscle
    - Innervation: CNIII (Oculomotor nerve)
    - Originates at apical cone of orbit
    - Runs anteriorly to become an aponeurosis
      - Superior transverse ligament runs from lacrimal gland fossa laterally to trochlea medially
      - Acts as a clothesline and levator hangs over this.
    - Aponeurosis divides into an anterior and posterior portion
      - Anterior inserts into lower third of anterior surface of tarsal plate
      - Posterior portion inserts into superior edge of tarsal plate as Muller's muscle
      - Muscle fibers are replaced with fibrous tissue and fat in congenital ptosis
  - Levator excursion
    - Block brow movement
    - Check levator palpebrae superioris function
    - Pt looks down with ruler measuring position

- Looks upward measure excursion
  - \>8mm good
  - 5-7mm moderate
  - <4mm poor
- At rest
  - Eyelid 1-2mm below superior limbus
  - Eyelid closure facilitated by facial nerve innervation of orbicularis
- Eyelid position in ptosis
  - Mild 1-2mm over upper limbus
  - Moderate 3mm
  - More severe 4mm
- Does pupil dilate and constrict appropriately if not? Consider Horner Syndrome
- Position of eyelid crease measured from lash line
  - Normal 9-12mm
  - Laterally 5-6mm above lateral canthus
  - Medially 6-7mm above punctum
- Margin Reflex Distance (MRD)
  - Accurate assessment of presence and degree of eyelid ptosis
  - Distance b/w eyelid margin and light reflex on forward gaze
  - MRD less than 4-5mm consider ptosis as diagnosis
- Margin Crease Distance
  - Distance of upper eyelid margin to lid crease normal central measurement
    - 10-11mm women
    - 8-10mm men
- Check for palpable tumor in eyelid- mechanical ptosis
- Lacrimal gland position
- Important to assess contralateral eye
  - Herring's test to reveal ptosis on other eye
  - Herring's law- equal innervation bilaterally, may mask mild ptosis on contralateral eye
  - Immobilize brow, elevate affected lid with q-tip, check opposite eye
- Work up:
  - No specific studies
  - MRI if brain tumor suspected

- 10% phenylephrine can be used to stimulate Mueller's muscle
  - Ptosis caused by myasthenia gravis should be improved by this
- Preop- Ophthalmology consultation mandatory

2. Consider reasonable goals in diagnosis and management *(Management and treatment, surgical indications, operative procedures and anesthesia)*

- Treatment depends on etiology:
  - Neurogenic- Myasthenia gravis medical treatment
  - Mechanical ptosis- tumor excision
  - Involutional (senile)- myogenic from stretching or dehiscence or levator aponeurosis
  - Traumatic (second most common)
    - Allow myoneuronal recovery
    - Resolution of edema
    - Softening of scar
    - Minimum 6 months
    - After cataract surgery-dehiscence
- General surgical principles
  - Rearrangement of levator mechanism if possible
  - Replacement if not
- Awake anesthesia, best technique if possible
  - Patient can cooperate with lid opening
- Postop care
  - Ice packs
  - Liberal lubricating drops for lagophthalmos

3. Select appropriate options in diagnosis and management

- Select procedure by excursion of levator:
  - 8-12mm good- levator advancement
    - Without dividing muscle inferior edge of levator aponeurosis is sutured to superior border of tarsal plate
    - Always overcorrect
  - 5-7mm moderate- levator resection and resuspension
    - Also done if more than 4mm of aponeurosis must be advanced over tarsal plate

- - - 0-4mm poor warrants suspension of levator mechanism from frontalis muscle
          - Autogenous or Alloplastic material
          - Eye then opens with frontalis contraction
    - Levator advancement
      - Mark incision at lid crease
      - Can use local but should try to overcorrect
      - Incise skin and orbicularis, keep levator aponeurosis intact
      - Skin muscle flap until preaponeurotic fat pad
      - Button hole septum and incise horizontally
      - Id aponeurosis
      - Elevate pretarsal orbicularis, expose tarsal plate
      - Suture aponeurosis to tarsal plate 2-3mm below superior margin
      - Adjust to correction then tie down
      - Aponeurotic sutures should be placed at junction of aponeurosis and levator muscle
      - Plication sutures or muscle excision can be done in addition to adjust height
    - Frontalis Sling
      - Be familiar with one technique in detail
      - Autogenous sling likely preferred technique for exam purposes
      - What tissue do you harvest and how?
      - How do you perform the procedure?
      - What are the key steps?
      - General or Local with sedation
      - Postop management

4. Understand risks and benefits of various approaches

    - Be familiar with the indications for various ptosis techniques
    - What are the risks and benefits of different procedures?
    - Preventative measures for complications
    - High revision rates, ptosis correction is difficult to get precise

5. Address complications and unexpected problems adequately

    - Complications
      - Bleeding

- Infection
- Mild lagophthalmos- lubricating drops
- Exposure keratitis
- Overcorrection
  - Responds to massage
  - Early can release sutures
- Undercorrection
  - Less than 2mm observe until edema resolution
  - More than 2mm reoperate early in first postop week
  - Repeat suspension of aponeurosis

6. Demonstrate ability to structure alternative plan

- Alternative procedure for 5-7mm excursion:
    - Muller's muscle-conjunctival resection in patients whose eyelids respond to phenylephrine
        - Upper lid everted
        - Clamp conjunctiva and Muller's muscle preset distance from superior tarsal border (6.5-9mm) sparing anterior levator mechanism
        - Resection:
        - 4mm for 1mm ptosis
        - 6mm for 1.5mm
        - 10mm for 2.0mm
        - 11-12 for >3mm
        - Intervening tissue excised and wound closed

Chapter Seventy-Nine

Microtia Hemifacial Microsomia

79
Microtia/Hemifacial Microsomia

1. Identify General Problem/Diagnosis/Planning
   (Describe photo, give working diagnosis, key problems, evaluates patient)

   - What is the psychological impact on the patient? Teasing or bullying?
     - Microtia anecdotally less than prominent ear deformity

   - Hx:
     - Status of hearing?
       - Anticipate if middle ear reconstruction or BAHA will be needed
       - Problematic if no canal present
       - Bone vs. air conduction of sound
     - Problems associated with monaural hearing
       - Increased risk for delayed speech
       - Poor school performance
       - Require close monitoring without hearing aid
         - Early intervention with external hearing aid if needed
       - Latest philosophy improve hearing early with implant (BAHA or other) or middle ear reconstruction
       - Many centers starting to stop offering middle ear reconstruction due to poor outcomes. Germany no more middle ear recon, implants only.
     - Ear infections can occur in patients without a patent canal
     - Family history
     - Maternal drug use
     - Medical history:
       - Medications

- Allergies
- Other medical problems
  - Breathing issues?
    - Hypoplastic mandible may present with respiratory distress or difficulty feeding (i.e. aspiration with feeds)

- PE
  - Classify defect and describe what is missing
    - Nagata classification, simplest surgical classification
      - Lobule type- most common, sausage like remnant
      - Conchal type- may have lobule, conchal remnant present
      - Small concha type- small conchal remnant present
      - Anotia- no ear structures
    - Note which parts of the ear are present which parts are missing
      - Dictates plan for framework (total vs. subtotal)
      - Canal?
      - Middle ear involvement
        - Middle ear involvement in 10%
    - Associated auricular findings
      - Preauricular tags
      - Pits- risk of infection
      - Sinus tracts- risk of infection
      - Chondrocutaneous remnants
      - Actively draining mass or sinus?
    - Position of hairline
      - Favorable
      - Unfavorable- if you anticipate > 50% of framework will be covered by hair
        - Consider coverage with TPF flap primarily
    - Check eyelid margins
    - Colobomas (lid, iris, retina)

- - - Abnormalities seen in Treacher-Collins
  - Epibulbar dermoids- Goldenhar
  - Orbitozygomatic contour or projection
  - Hypoplastic?
    - Think:
      - Treacher-Collins Syndrome
      - Nager Syndrome
  - Syndromes can present with microophthalmia to anophthalmia
    - Temporal bone and/or soft tissue hypoplasia
    - Check for bilateral microtia (10-15% bilateral)
  - Mandible
    - Hypoplasia?
    - Occlusal slant
    - Distraction vs. conventional orthognathic surgery
    - Monitor for speech/feeding difficulties
    - Chin position midline?
  - Kaban/Mulliken Classification modification of Pruzansky
    - Type I- mandible/TMJ normal shape but small
    - Type IIa- mandible/TMJ present, hypoplastic and malformed
    - Type IIb- ramus and TMJ severely hypoplastic, TMJ inferiorly displaced
    - Type III- absent ramus and glenoid fossa, no TMJ
  - Macrostomia (Tessier No.7)
    - Treacher Collins (Tessier No. 6,7,8)
    - May cause feeding difficulty
    - Drooling
  - Facial nerve (VII) function
    - Adequate corneal protection?
    - Asymmetry
    - Document pre-op

- Management individualized
- Infrequently symptomatic other than minor asymmetry
- Torticollis
- C-spine anomalies?
- Hands- malformed or absent thumbs, clinodactyly, syndactyly, foreshortened radius- Think Nager syndrome
- Cardiac
  - Check for murmur (ASD, VSD, Tetralogy of Fallot)
- Oculoauricular vertebral syndrome
- Work-up
  - Audiology
  - ENT evaluation
  - CT scan for middle ear evaluation if indicated
    - Not before age 3
  - Oral surgery evaluation if mandibular involvement present, orthognathic work-up
  - R/O associated anomalies
    - C-spine
      - Plain x-ray, CT scan- Goldenhar screen
      - Can affect positioning in OR, injuries can occur
    - Cardiovascular anomalies
      - Echocardiogram
    - Renal (ectopic kidney, reflux, obstruction, duplication)
      - Ultrasound
  - Multidisciplinary Care
    - Geneticist
    - Pediatric ENT
    - Audiology
    - Oral Surgery
    - Orthodontist
    - Plastic surgeon
    - Cardiology/Urology/Nephrology as needed
  - Pre-op Work up for Mandible
    - Detailed assessment of affected structures
    - Panorex
    - Lateral and AP cephalograms

- 3-D Reconstruction CT scans +/- models for surgical planning: Dental models

2. Consider reasonable goals in diagnosis and management *(Management and treatment, surgical indications, operative procedures and anesthesia)*

  - Goal of management
    - Reconstruction of external framework
    - Optimization of hearing
  - Template for ear framework
    - X-ray tracing of normal ear or family member ear
    - Or…
    - Prefabricated template
    - Note relation of normal ear to:
      - Nose
      - Oral commissure
      - Lateral canthus
      - Critical to pocket placement
  - Age for reconstruction
    - Autologous
      - Earliest age 5-6 years of age (Brent)
        - Have to wait for adequate cartilage volume
      - Firmin and Nagata wait till age 10, more cartilage available. They use larger frameworks.
    - Alloplastic
      - Can be done as early as age 3-5
    - Prosthesis age depends on thickness of mastoid bone
      - Age 5?
  - Stage rib reconstruction two options
    - Traditional Brent 4 Stage Recon
    - Fabrication and insertion of framework
      - Harvest
        - Oblique incision 6-8cm
        - Contralateral costal margin
        - Preserve rim of 6th and 7th ribs
        - Preserve synchondrosis
        - Check for pneumothorax, valsalva at closure

- - -
        - Layered closure (rectus fascia, deep dermis, skin)
        - Preserves perichondrium
      - Carve base block from 6th and 7th ribs
      - Add helical rim from 8th rib
      - Construct with 4-0 clear nylon
      - Excise remnant cartilage
      - Always leave drain for tissue adherence
    - Lobular transposition by z-plasty
      - 3 months later
    - Framework elevation and full thickness skin graft
      - 3 months later, elevation always minimum 6 months from framework placement. Optimizes blood supply to skin overlying framework.
    - Tragal reconstruction, conchal bowl excavation
      - 3 months later
      - Composite chondrocutaneous graft from contralateral ear
    - Contemporary Nagata/Firmin 2 Stage Recon
      - Fabrication and insertion of framework, simultaneous lobule transposition and tragal reconstruction.
        - Harvest Nagata
          - 2cm transverse incision, split rectus, preserve perichondrium, place remaining cartilage in perichondrial pocket
          - Ipsilateral cartilage, does not preserve perichondrium, leaves in situ
          - Goal decrease chest wall morbidity
          - Increased anesthesia time
          - Harvest 6th, 7th, 8th, 9th ribs
          - Check for pneumothorax, valsalva
          - Layered closure
        - Harvest Firmin

- Oblique incision 6-8cm
- Ipsilateral costal margin
- Harvests 6th-9th ribs
- Check for pneumothorax, valsalva at closure
- Layered closure (rectus fascia, deep dermis, skin)
- Nagata and Firmin similar frameworks differing skin approaches
    - Base block
    - Helical rim
    - Antihelix
    - Tragus
    - Excise remnant cartilage
    - Constructed with wire
    - Always drain for tissue adherence
    - Goal increased detail in framework, increased risk of soft tissue complications
- Elevation 6 months later
    - Nagata: Routinely uses cartilage chock and TPF flap
    - Firmin: Type of elevation dependent on amount of elevation needed
        - TPF flap with cartilage chock
        - Chock only in subcutaneous tunnel
        - Elevation with skin graft
- Alloplastic Reconstruction
    - John Reinisch (Medpore)
    - Two stages
- Medpore wrapped under TPF flap
    - Prefabricated antihelix, triangular fossa, tragus and antitragus, second component helical rim
    - Covered with FTSG or STSG
- Projection and refinement

- o Disadvantage of Medpore
- o Unknown long-term performance compared to cartilage
- o Foreign material
- Osseointegrated prosthesis as alternative option
    - o Generally discouraged in children, but a perfectly feasible option
    - o Disadvantage cost, need for new implant(s) every 3-5 years
- Important to manage family expectations
    - o No option truly duplicates a native ear at this time
    - o The ear will not be soft or flexible
    - o Show photos, links, give direct contacts
    - o Operate when family is ready and comfortable
- Mandibular management (no full consensus on management)
    - o Type I and IIa
        - If no maxillary deformity observe initially till full growth and reassess in adolescence
        - If maxillary deformity
            - Treat at age 7-8 with mandibular osteotomy and lengthening or distraction
    - o Type IIb
        - Reestablish facial/maxillary/mandibular midlines
        - Costochondral graft for condylar head
        - Center mandibular midline
        - Distraction
        - +/- Lefort I maxillary advancement
    - o Type III
        - Reconstruct TMJ with rib graft
        - Reconstruct zygomatic arch and glenoid fossa
        - Costochondral rib graft
        - +/- Lefort I maxillary advancement

3. Select appropriate options in diagnosis and management

- Ear reconstruction options
    - o No intervention
    - o Autologous cartilage reconstruction (gold standard)- rib cartilage

- - -
    - - Alloplastic reconstruction (Medpore)
      - Prosthesis with osseointegrated titanium stud
  - Selection based on:
    - Family wishes
    - Surgeon's experience
    - Available tissues for reconstruction

4. Understand risks and benefits of various approaches

   - 50% of ears grow with patient as per Brent
   - Autogenous reconstruction
     - Advantages
       - Patient's own tissue
       - Low long-term complication rate
       - Lower cost compared to other options
       - "Tried and true"
     - Disadvantages
       - High learning curve
       - Prosthesis better aesthetics
       - Poor outcome ear looks horrible
   - Alloplastic reconstruction
     - Advantages
       - Consistent aesthetic results
       - Lower learning curve
     - Disadvantages
       - Foreign material
       - Unknown long-term outcomes
   - Prosthesis
     - Advantages
       - Best aesthetic results
     - Disadvantages
       - Not integrated into patient
       - High cost long term
       - Requires replacement every 3-5 years
       - High maintenance must maintain excellent hygiene of studs
         - Inflammation from poor hygiene results in periods of not being able to wear prosthesis

5. Address complications and unexpected problems adequately

- Beware airway issues in infancy
    - Treat like Pierre Robin sequence due to potentially hypoplastic mandible
- If pleural tear at rib harvest
    - Evacuate air with small red rubber catheter, suture defect with figure of eight or purse string suture
    - If lung injury chest tube must be placed
- Residual hair
    - Electrolysis
    - Laser therapy
    - Thinning of skin flaps
- Infection
    - IV antibiotics
    - I & D early if needed
    - Possible graft loss
- Exposure of framework
    - Treatment:
        - Conservative
        - Topical 10% sulfamylon
        - Small exposure will heal, risk of framework loss
        - 2-3cm exposure requires local flap or TPF flap for salvage
- Warping
    - May require revision or second graft or Medpore as salvage procedure
- Costochondral rib grafts have unpredictable growth
    - Rule of thirds
        - 1/3 no growth
        - 1/3 overgrowth
        - 1/3 normal growth

6. Demonstrate ability to structure alternative plan

- Backup plan for failed cartilage reconstruction- prosthesis
- What if family refuses reconstruction?
- What is your management plan for hearing issues?
- Your timing of middle ear reconstruction vs. external ear recon?

Chapter Eighty

Treacher-Collins Syndrome

80
Treacher-Collins Syndrome

1. Identify General Problem/Diagnosis/Planning
   (Describe photo, give working diagnosis, key problems, evaluates patient)

   - Describe physical findings in photo
     o Physical appearance of patient will suggest the diagnosis
     o Classic features
       - Microtia
       - Colobomas
       - Mid-face deficiency in area of Tessier 6-8, sometimes 9
       - Flat malar region
       - Micrognathia
     o Note
       - Midfacial structures
       - Eyes
       - Ears
       - Cheeks
       - Shape of nose
       - Cranial vault usually normal
       - Skeletal deficiency
         - Zygoma
         - Maxilla
         - Mandible
           o TMJ
           o Condyle
           o Ramus
       - Oral symmetry
       - Facial nerve function
       - Check for cleft palate (isolated secondary or submucosal)
   - History
     o Problems with breathing
     o Problems with feeding
     o Dry eye or signs of corneal exposure
   - Family history

- o Treacher Collins- autosomal dominant
- Potential ocular problems
  - o Amblyopia
  - o Strabismus
  - o Ptosis
- Other associated anomalies
  - o Parotid gland
  - o Cryptorchidism
  - o Congenital heart
- May have developmental issues
- Differential Diagnosis
  - o Hemifacial microsomia- no colobomas, less severe cheek and mandibular involvement
  - o Goldenhar syndrome- Epibulbar dermoids
  - o Nager syndrome- hand anomalies; absent thumbs, clinodactyly, syndactyly, short radius
- Work-up
  - o Ophthalmology evaluation
  - o Audiology evaluation
  - o ENT
    - BAHA
    - Tracheostomy?
    - R/O tracheomalasia
  - o Genetics
    - Treacle gene, Chromosome 5q
  - o Oral surgery and/or orthognathic surgery evaluation
    - When planning surgery:
      - AP and lateral cephalograms
      - 3-D CT scan
  - o Panorex
  - o Echocardiogram
  - o Renal U/S

2. Consider reasonable goals in diagnosis and management *(Management and treatment, surgical indications, operative procedures and anesthesia)*

- Management of airway/feeding problems same as Pierre Robin Sequence
  - o Prone positioning
  - o Nasopharyngeal tube
  - o Tongue lip adhesion

- ETT
- Tracheostomy
- Mandibular distraction
- Feeding interventions
  - Orogastric tube
  - G-tube with Nissen fundoplication
- Dry eye/Corneal exposure
  - Tx: Initial medical management with lubrication followed by repair of coloboma based on size of defect as in any eyelid reconstruction case (skin and muscle flaps)
- Early intervention for hearing loss
  - Early hearing aid in infancy enhances development of speech and language
- Manage family expectations
  - Discuss
    - Outcomes and expectations
    - Staged nature of intervention
    - Need for repeat surgeries
    - Patient will never look completely normal

3. Select appropriate options in diagnosis and management

- Choice of airway management in Pierre Robin sequence
  - Depends on:
    - Clinical presentation
    - Surgeon experience
- Algorithm of Management
- @3-6 months
  - Repair macrostomia (Tessier No.7)
    - Superior and inferior vermilion flaps
    - Reconstruct orbicularis oris muscle at the commissure
    - Skin can be managed with straight line repair or z-plasty
    - Muscle repair should be performed as a z-plasty
- @12-24 months
  - Cleft palate repair
    - Timing dependent on width of cleft, some advantage to waiting in wide clefts

- Observe submucosal cleft until it becomes symptomatic
- Will know if intervention needed usually by age 5
- Based on speech therapy evaluation for presence of VPI
- @ 2 years of age
  - If type III Pruzansky rib graft for ramus
  - Consider distraction osteogenesis
  - Will still need conventional orthognathic procedure in adolescence
- @ 6-10 years of age
  - Ear reconstruction for microtia if present
  - Gold standard:
    - Autogenous cartilage reconstruction
      - Costochondral cartilage framework
      - Lobule transposition
      - Secondary elevation procedure of framework
      - Tragal reconstruction
      - (See Chapter 79 Microtia-Hemifacial Microsomia for full details)
    - Other options
      - Medpore and TPF flap
      - Prosthesis
      - No intervention
- @7-8 years of age
  - Can start bony reconstruction at the same time as ear reconstruction
  - Grafts vs. Medpore implants for cheek bone reconstruction
    - Graft options:
      - Cranial bone
      - Rib
      - Iliac crest
- @ Adolescence (after completion of facial growth)
  - Orthodontics followed by orthognathic surgery
  - Lefort I +/- sagittal split, bimaxillary surgery often needed in these cases
  - Address the nose, rhinoplasty after definitive orthognathic surgery

4. Understand risks and benefits of various approaches

    - Consider what you would choose as first choice procedures
    - What factors would make you decide on one procedure vs. another?

5. Address complications and unexpected problems adequately

    - Bleeding
    - Infection
    - Poor scarring
    - Consider procedure specific complications:
        - Macrotomia repair
        - Palate repair
        - Mandibular reconstruction
        - Malar reconstruction
        - Orthognathic complications
        - Rhinoplasty

6. Demonstrate ability to structure alternative plan

    - Need to be familiar with general needs of Treacher-Collins patients
    - Timing of interventions important
    - Be able to plan and stage surgeries
    - What if insurance will not cover certain procedures?

BURNS

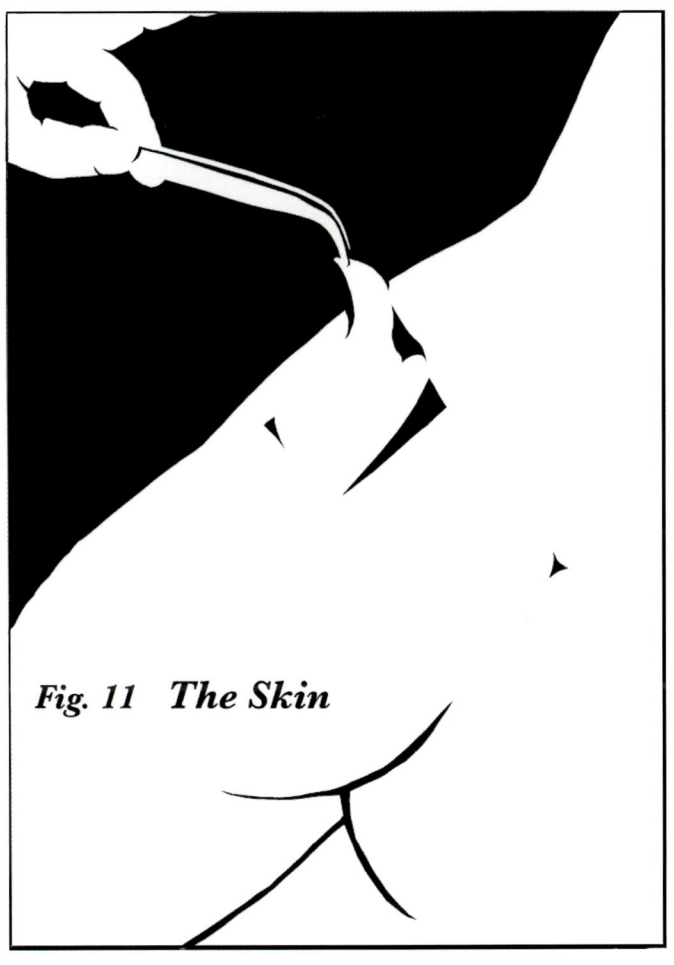

Fig. 11 The Skin

Section Twelve
Burns

Chapter Eighty-One

Burns Overview

81
Burns Overview

1. Identify General Problem

   - Describe photo; Give working diagnosis
   - Key problems; Evaluate patient
   - Go through ABC's of trauma management
   - Resuscitation- Modified Parkland
   - Estimate size of burn
   - Classify depth of burn
   - Prognosis based on extent of injury, age of patient
   - Need for escharotomy, fasciotomy, compartment syndrome?
   - ATLS protocol and secondary survey?
   - R/O other injuries CNS, abdominal trauma, orthopedic
   - Need for further work-up or consultations?

2. Consider reasonable goals in diagnosis and management

   - Management and treatment
   - Surgical indications
   - Operative procedures and anesthesia
   - Resuscitation
   - Topical antibiotics
   - Temporary closure modalities
   - Specifically mention availability of donor sites
   - Goal:
     - Definitive closure with STSG
     - Staged closure?
       - Trunk, Extremities, Hands/Feet, Face
   - What are your surgical goals?
   - Early skin closure and prevention of functional deficits
   - What is your timing of intervention?
   - Indications for transfer to burn unit

3. Select appropriate options in diagnosis and management

   - Closure planning options for coverage
     - Staging
       - Trunk, Extremities, Feet, Hands, Face

- Specify your closure plan
    - Cadaver
    - Xenograft
    - STSG or FTSG
    - Integra
    - CEA
    - Flaps (local, regional, free)
- PT/OT, nutrition, social work, rehab
- Preventative measures of skin graft failure?
- When would you use meshed vs. sheet grafts? Specify:
    - Donor sites you will use
    - Mesh width
    - Graft thickness at time of harvest (Range for STSG 0.008-0.018 inch depending on donor site)
- Extent of surgery per operative session? How do you determine length of surgery and end point? Time by clock, blood loss, temperature of patient, other.
- Indications for early termination of surgical procedure?
- Estimated timing to closure based on burn size
- How is procedure performed?
- Key steps of surgery
- Markings and relevant anatomy

4. Understand risks and benefits of various approaches

- What are the risks, benefits of various closure modalities?
- Describe timing for intervention and closure plan?

5. Address complications and unexpected problems adequately

- Hypertrophic scar/keloid scar management
- Burn scar contracture management (joints, neck, axilla)
- Facial scarring
- Chronic open wound
- Exposed bone management

6. Demonstrate ability to structure alternative plan

- Failed skin graft
- Chronic wound
- Contracture development
- Management of keloid and hypertrophic scars

Chapter Eighty-Two

Burns
———

82
Burns

1. Identify General Problem/Diagnosis/Planning
   (Describe photo, give working diagnosis, key problems, evaluates patient)

   - CLASSIFY BURN
     - Estimate size of injury (Rule of 9's, Palmar Method)
       - Mention Lund-Browder Chart would ultimately be used specially in children, more precise in determining size of injury
       - Primary reasons for determining size: resuscitation, prognosis, determining need for transfer to burn unit
     - Classify depth of burn, your best guess
       - Superficial
       - Superficial partial thickness
       - Deep partial thickness
       - Full thickness
     - Note that demarcation may change for better or worse over first 3-5 days.
     - Surgeon's estimate of burn depth 50% accuracy.
     - Give your best estimate based on photo.
     - Mention pertinent features to back up your assessment (white leathery area, mottled skin= full thickness)
     - Quantify extent of burn (dictates resuscitation requirements)
     - Note key problems that will need to be addressed
     - Note if toxic chemicals were present or if this was a chemical burn, affects management.
   - Anticipate:
     - Management of airway
       - IV access
       - Fluid resuscitation
       - Timing for debridement and closure
       - Long-term rehab issues
     - Consider risk of compartment syndrome
       - Palpate the compartments

- Any suspicion check pressures Stryker or CVP or A-line transducer
                - Pressure >18mmHG fasciotomy
            - Potential for arrhythmias in electrical injury
                - Need for escharotomies or fasciotomies
                - Circumferential eschar on chest wall?
        - After stabilizing the patient do secondary survey:
            - Diagnose and treat any potentially life-threatening injuries:
                - Blunt or penetrating trauma
                - Head injury
                - C-spine
                - Brain injury
                - Thoracic injuries
                    - Pneumo or hemothorax
                    - Mediastinal injuries
                    - Aortic rupture
                - Abdominal injuries
                - Hemorrhage
                - Pelvis and long bone fractures
                - Lower extremity injury
                - Blood loss in the field?
        - TETANUS status important
        - Medical history/medications/allergies
        - WORK-UP
            - X-ray
                - CXR
                - C-spine
                - Pelvis
            - LABS
                - CBC
                - Lytes
                - ABG + Carboxyhemoglobin
                - Glucose
        - REVIEW ABA CRITERIA FOR TRANSFER TO BURN UNIT
            - Basic Criteria
                - Second or third degree burn > 10% TBSA
                    - In patient <10 yo or >50 yo
                - Second or third degree burn > 20% TBSA
                    - In patient age 10-49

- Serious threat to function/cosmesis (hands/face/feet/genitalia/perineum/joints)
- Third degree > 5% TBSA any age
- Electrical or chemical burn with threat to function or cosmesis
- ELECTRICAL INJURY
    - Classify
        - Low Voltage <1000 Volts (household injury)
            - If no loss of consciousness, then no telemetry
            - Can discharge from ER in minor burns
        - High voltage >1000 Volts
            - Mandates telemetry and EKG check for arrhythmias
            - Long-term risk for cataracts
            - Seizures risk of long bone fractures
- RISK FACTORS FOR MORTALITY
    - Inhalation injury
    - Age <2 or >60
    - Burns >40% TBSA
    - Significant full thickness burn injury
    - Pre-existing illnesses
        - Diabetes
        - Coronary artery disease
        - Smoker
        - Alcohol abuse
- NUTSHELL PATHOPHYSIOLOGY OF BURN INJURY
    - Fluid and electrolyte imbalance
    - Impaired host resistance to wound infection
    - Hypermetabolic state with increased resting oxygen demand
    - Large burns high risk for multisystem organ failure (pulmonary, renal, GI, cardiac)
- Zones of injury
    - Hyperemia
        - Recover with minimal effort (superficial to superficial partial thickness injury)
    - Stasis
        - Potential to recover with adequate resuscitation

- Cell death with inadequate resuscitation (superficial partial thickness and deep partial thickness burn injury)
  - Coagulation
    - Dead cells
    - Necrotic tissue (deep partial thickness to full thickness burn injury)

2. Consider reasonable goals in diagnosis and management *(Management and treatment, surgical indications, operative procedures and anesthesia)*

   - BROAD GOALS AFTER BURN INJURY
     - Survival of patient (life over limb)
     - Pain Control
     - Wound Closure
     - Recovery of optimal function, motion and activity
     - Restoration of normal appearance
     - Treat as a trauma patient: ATLS Protocol
       - A= Airway
         - Early intubation?
         - Signs of inhalation injury
         - Avoid compromised airway
         - PE Signs
           - Stridor
           - Singed nasal hair
           - Facial or oropharyngeal burn
           - Carbonaceous sputum
           - Hoarse voice
           - Air hunger
         - Combination of stridor/hoarse voice/air hunger = INTUBATE
         - At time of intubation note presence of soot, edema, signs of airway injury
       - B= Breathing
         - Ventilation, oxygenation
         - Consider if circumferential or even non-circumferential chest wall burn is affecting ventilation
         - Management: Escharotomy

- Chevron incision over costal margin
- High-flow percussive ventilation
- Inhalation Injury
  - Work-up
  - Bronchoscopy gold standard
- CO poisoning
  - Must check ABG and specifically request carboxyhemoglobin level
  - Management:
  - Carboxyhgb >10%
  - Treatment: 100% Oxygen Non-rebreather mask (decreases CO washout time from half-life of 250 minutes to 50 minutes)
  - Carboxyhgb >20% neurotoxic
    - Indication for hyperbaric chamber
- C= Circulation
  - Palpate distal pulses
  - Check capillary refill
  - Warm the patient (warmed IV fluids, blankets, Bair hugger)
  - Think about compartment syndrome
- WOUND CARE
  - Topical antibiotics until ready for surgery
  - Topical antibiotics single most important factor in minimizing infection
  - Deep Wounds
    - Colonized in 24 hours by gram (+)
    - Colonized in 3-7 days by gram (-)
  - CHOICES
    - Silver sulfadiazine (Silvadene)
    - Mafenide acetate (sulfamylon) cream or solution
    - Collagenase/Polysporin powder or ointment
    - Nystatin power
- EXTREMITY ESCHAROTOMY
  - Incise along mid-lateral line of affected extremity

- Escharotomy should extend from normal skin through the eschar to normal skin on the opposite side.
- Avoid:
  - Ulnar nerve in upper extremity
  - Common peroneal nerve in lower extremity
- Include the fingers if severely burned
  - Mid-lateral line of fingers
    - Ulnar aspect of 2nd, 3rd, 4th
    - Radial aspect thumb and 5th
    - Minimizes scar on primary working surfaces of digits
- Escharotomies can be performed at the bedside
- Consider decompressive fasciotomy of thenar and hypothenar muscle compartments.

- **DEEP HAND BURNS**
  - Dorsal escharotomies with interosseous compartment fasciotomies may be needed
- **FLUID INITIAL MANAGEMENT**
  - IV access in unburned skin if possible
    - 18 gauge catheters x2
  - Initiate fluid resuscitation in TBSA:
    - >10% in peds
    - >20% in adults
  - Modified Parkland 4ml/kg x TBSA %
    - First 24 hours
      - 1/2 volume in 1st 8 hours
      - 2nd 1/2 over the next 16 hours
    - Clock starts from time of injury
    - Second 24 hours
      - Add albumin to resuscitation fluids
  - Monitor resuscitation by urine output
    - Foley mandatory
    - Goal
      - 0.5ml/kg/hr minimum urine output in adults
      - 1ml/kg/hr minimum urine output in children
- **NUTRITIONAL SUPPORT**
  - Critical in large burns
  - Use gut if available
  - NGT for feeding if necessary

- Goal 30-40 kcal/kg/day
- Follow prealbumin levels bi-weekly
- H2 Blockers (antiulcer prophylaxis) if unable to feed via GI tract
- PAIN MANAGEMENT
  - Liberal use of analgesics and sedation
- WOUND MANAGEMENT
  - After stabilization and resuscitation wound management decisions must be made on the need for and timing of surgical intervention for wound closure.
  - Decisions are based on depth of burn, and available options are based on extent of injury
  - Xenograft, cadaver or integra may be used to temporize wounds until complete closure
  - CEA may be needed in large wounds in which adequate amount of skin for grafting is not available

3. Select appropriate options in diagnosis and management

- Prompt excision and grafting in all burns unlikely to heal spontaneously within 10-14 days.
  - Start grafting after fluid resuscitation and stabilization of patient at around 48 hours in large burns >10% peds, 20% adults.
  - Early excision of inflammatory load of burn eschar, decreases SIRS reaction, quicker recovery and healing, better outcomes.
- OPTIONS FOR EXCISION
  - Traditional:
    - Tangential excision
      - High blood loss, avoid excising more than 20% TBSA at the time of each debridement to control blood loss.
    - Excision to level of fascia:
      - More reliable wound bed
      - Decreased blood loss compared to tangential excision
      - More aesthetic deformity down the road (debatable)
    - Contemporary:

- Versajet (works by Venturi effect)
- Preserves viable dermis
- Decreases blood loss
- May take more operative time
- May improve functional and aesthetic outcome long-term
- GRAFTING
  - Immediate autograft if adequate skin is available, otherwise temporize closure with xenograft, cadaver skin or integra.
  - Large areas for grafting may require staging.
  - Consider cultured epidermal autografts (CEA)
    - Friable skin, poor coverage, but necessary in large burns >80%
  - Priorities for staging:
    - Trunk
    - Extremities
    - Hands
    - Feet
    - Face
  - Most grafts 0.010 to 0.012 inches
  - Sheet graft whenever possible and practical
    - Especially face/hand- better aesthetics
  - If meshing needed keep to 1:1.5 if possible and practical.
    - 1:2 will cover most large burns.
    - 1:4 if very large >70%
    - Meshing more than 1:4 grafts themselves are difficult to handle
      - "like linguine"
  - Flap coverage may be needed in hand and extremity burns especially if bone or tendon exposure present.
  - See Chapter 84 Hand and Frostbite
- BURNS OF THE FACE
  - Delay grafting in deep partial thickness burns, may get more healing than anticipated.
  - Full thickness burns can consider early grafting.
  - Ideal color match scalp donor site
  - Sheet graft if practical and possible
  - Scar management:
    - Massage
    - Silicone

- Steroids
- Laser therapy
- Facemask
- INDICATIONS FOR INTEGRA
  - Designed for use in large burns
  - Can be used over poorly vascularized structures
  - Will generally give better contour

4. Understand risks and benefits of various approaches

- Consider individual clinical scenario
  - Depth of burn, size, anatomic region involved will dictate management
  - Might avoid integra as a first choice on board exam although it is designed for use in burns
  - Understand timing of intervention
  - Your algorithm for:
    - Initial management
    - Surgical intervention
    - Specific goals for closure
    - Long-term therapy scar management
    - PT/OT plan
  - How do you secure your skin grafts?
  - What is your post-op management regimen?
  - When do you take dressings down? Start ROM? Scar management?

5. Address complications and unexpected problems adequately

- Hypovolemia
- Myocardial depression common in >40% TBSA burn injury
- Inhalation injury (risk factor for mortality)
- CO inhalation
- Direct thermal injury to airway (Rare- except in steam injury)
- Systemic sepsis (most commonly secondary to pneumonia!)
- Wound infection
  - Management: Wound biopsy for quantification $>10^5$ organism/gram of tissue
    - Topical antibiotics- sulfamylon
    - Re-excise burn wounds if wound biopsy positive!

- Graft loss
- Compartment syndrome
- Myoglobinuria
- Early scar contracture
- RARE CONDITIONS
    - Stevens Johnson Syndrome- <10% epidermal skin loss
    - Toxic epidermal necrosis (TEN) >10% epidermal skin loss
    - Management:
        - Same as burn injury, primarily topical antibiotics
        - Grafting rarely needed, usually superficial partial thickness skin loss, but graft if indicated.

6. Demonstrate ability to structure alternative plan

- Closure options and plan in >60% burn injury
- What if you run out of donor site prior to complete closure of wounds?
- Grafted area sloughs with resultant tendon or bone exposure
- Large graft loss- work-up causes
- Scar management
- Contracture management
- Wound infection management

Chapter Eighty-Three

Burn Reconstruction

83
Burn Reconstruction

1. Identify General Problem/Diagnosis/Planning
   (Describe photo, give working diagnosis, key problems, evaluates patient)

   - Describe details of scar
     - Note potential problems based on anatomic location
     - Give detailed description of what you see
     - What are the problems at hand? Functional? Aesthetics?
   - Hypertrophic Scar (HTS)
     - Common after burn injuries
     - Typically worsen for 4-6 months and improves over 2-3 years
     - Delayed wound closure contributes to HTS formation.
   - Pathophysiology- exaggerated healing response
   - Contractures
   - Poor aesthetics?

2. Consider reasonable goals in diagnosis and management
   (Management and treatment, surgical indications, operative procedures and anesthesia)

   - Treatment goal:
     - Optimize function and aesthetics
     - Minimize risk of recurrence
   - Small-localized HTS:
     - Serial excision
     - Local z-plasties or w-plasties
     - Other local tissue rearrangements
   - Massive areas HTS:
     - Scar release followed by grafting or integra + graft
     - Full thickness grafting preferable if available
     - Can increase area of full thickness grafting by tissue expansion
   - Tissue expansion
   - Complex reconstruction (flaps, free tissue transfer)

- Graft Choice
    - Based on location
    - Donor sites available
    - Consider integra, good option for burn reconstruction
- INDICATIONS FOR SURGICAL MANAGEMENT
    - Prevention of HTS
        - Early debridement and wound closure
        - Excision of burned skin
        - Wound closure with grafts
    - Stalled recovery
    - Stiffness and limited motion
    - Abnormal appearance of wounds and grafts
    - Aggressive PT should be initiated prior to surgery.
    - Failure of PT to improve scars over 3-6 months minimum, surgical intervention should be considered.
- Classify Patient Needs
    - Urgent/Essential/Desirable
- Specify your surgical goals
- TISSUE EXPANSION IN BURN RECONSTRUCTION
    - Plan for more tissue than anticipated for coverage
    - Use multiple expanders
    - Plan incisions carefully
    - Avoid incision in scar tissue or expander under scar tissue
    - Use EMLA over needle entry site
    - Plan for weekly injections when possible

3. Select appropriate options in diagnosis and management

- Choose what you believe to be the best option based on clinical scenario
    - Choice based on:
    - Normal or unburned tissue available
    - Reconstruction goals
    - Plan for recovery
- Urgent Procedures
    - After acute injury in order to preserve function and/or tissue
    - Exposed ear cartilage

- - - o Exposed cornea (eyelid loss)
      - o Severely injured hands
    - Essential Procedures
      - o Restore function
      - o Contracture release
    - Desirable Procedures
      - o Restore appearance
        - Primarily facial reconstruction
        - Correction of scalp alopecia
  - TO OPTIMIZE OUTCOME
      - o Diagnose anatomic cause of deformity (specify to examiners)
      - o Consider management in specific patient (eg, peds vs. adult)
      - o Fully release all contractures
      - o When grafting, always overgraft
      - o Initiate early motion in postop period (w/i 5-7 days)
  - What is your post-op management?
      - o Periop antibiotics
        - Potential bacterial nidus in scar
      - o Splinting method for stabilizing grafts
        - Traditional bolster vs. V.A.C. (what settings?)
      - o Early mobilization protocols
      - o Scar management
        - Scar massage
        - Silicone
        - Pressure garments
        - Steroid injections
        - Laser therapy
  - FACE
      - o Indications for intervention
        - Scars
        - Abnormal appearance
        - Corneal protection
        - Mouth contractures
      - o Intervention
        - Early debridement and graft in full thickness injuries
        - Graft donor site (scalp ideal color match, supraclavicular skin)
      - o Options

- Skin grafting and/or integra
- Z-plasties
- Local flaps
- Tissue expansion
- Post-op
  - Scar massage
  - Steroids
  - Silicone
  - Facemask
  - Splinting (especially oral commissure reconstruction)
- Reconstruction of the Face
  - Break down into units
  - Options
  - Grafts (full thickness if possible)- upper lip, forehead
  - Tissue expansion may increase available full thickness skin (eg. abdominal expansion)
  - Ideal
    - 1 large full thickness skin graft
    - Integra + thin split thickness skin graft (0.008 inches)
  - Flaps or tissue expansion- cheeks, chin
    - Scapular free flaps
  - Circumoral contracture of the mouth
    - Release skin lateral to the commissure
    - Mobilize oral mucosa
    - Motion and stretching at 7-10 days post-op
- Nose
  - Indications
    - Airway obstruction
    - Aesthetics
  - Use standard reconstructive techniques if available
  - Local flap advancement
  - Postauricular FTSG
  - Forehead flap
  - Reposition/reconstruct underlying structures
  - Rhinoplasty techniques
  - Total nasal skin turndown flap with STSG

- Neck
  - Indications
    - Limited or painful motion
    - Severe contractures
    - Drooling
    - Dental deterioration
    - Folliculitis
    - Significant deformity, loss of contour
    - Obstacle for intubation for general anesthesia
  - Pre-op
    - Note potential anesthetic difficulty in airway management
    - Selected cases may benefit from tracheotomy
  - Options
    - Moderate contracture or linear scar band
    - Local flaps
    - Z-plasties
    - Convert vertical scar to transverse scar
  - Severe contracture
    - Need shoulder roll and doughnut
    - Stabilize with stacked towels
    - Release at base of neck
    - Dissect to subplatysmal level
    - Be sure to do COMPLETE release- most important aspect of reconstruction, most common error
    - Release all bands
  - If lateral neck and upper chest NOT BURNED:
    - Tissue expansion maybe used
    - Tissue expansion is safe in the neck even in light of tracheostomy, theoretical compression of IJ and carotid not seen clinically
  - If lateral neck and upper chest BURNED:

- Must use grafts and/or free tissue transfer
- Choose: FTSG vs. Integra + thin STSG
- Integra a good option especially if free flap fails or as first choice
- Board acceptable answer for neck recon
- Standard free flap options (fasciocutaneous flaps- radial forearm, ALT, parascapular)
- Postop Bolster (Foam dressing vs.VAC [Note your settings])
- Your immobilization technique?
    - Post op in Neck Reconstruction
        - Immobilize 10 days
        - Splint
        - C-spine immobilization
        - 89% recurrence of contracture w/o splinting
        - 17% recurrence of contracture with splint
- o Eyelid Reconstruction
    - Indications
        - Tissue deficits
        - Ectropion of upper and lower lids
        - Contractures across concavities (medial and lateral orbit)
    - Critical function
        - Protect cornea from exposure keratopathy
- o Ectropion
    - Can be a persistent problem
    - See Ectropion Chapter 21
    - Prevention
        - Conformers
        - Splints
    - Evaluate for extrinsic contracture transmitting forces
        - Face
        - Neck

- Forehead
    - Pre-op Hx and Management
        - Topical ointment
        - Protective eye shields
            - For chronic eye irritation, corneal damage
    - History & PE Findings
        - Difficulty closing eyes while sleeping or opening the mouth
    - Corneal exposure in burn injury
        - Usually results from tissue deficiency
    - To correct exposure keratitis and ectropion
        - Generally need to replace lost or contracted skin
        - Grafting is treatment of choice
    - Operative Techniques
        - Tarsorrhaphy
            - Useful first few weeks post injury to prevent exposure keratopathy while addressing life-threatening problems in large burn injuries.
        - Eyelid Release and Skin Graft
            - Wide over-correction
            - Place releasing incision as close to eyelashes as possible
            - Preserve rim of tissue for suture placement
            - Extend release beyond medial and lateral canthal areas
            - Elevate tissue 15 degrees above horizontal plane and extend 15 mm beyond canthus.
            - FTSG ideal, postauricular if available

- Thick STSG acceptable for upper eyelids, more mobility
- Web deformity of medial canthus
  - Manage with z-plasties
- Eyebrow
  - Indication for intervention
    - Eyebrow destruction or distortion
    - Important anatomic landmark for aesthetics
  - Options
    - Free scalp composite grafts
    - Micrografts- effective for partial destruction
    - Island flaps based on superficial temporal artery and vein
- Scalp
  - Clinical Challenges
    - Wound closure for exposed calvarium
    - Burn scar alopecia
  - Management of open scalp wound
    - Approach based on defect size
      - Small to moderate defects
      - Scalp advancement or rotation advancement flaps with back grafting of resultant underlying pericranium.
      - Pericranial flap with skin graft
      - Burring of bone, VAC and graft of subsequent granulation tissue
    - Extensive injury
      - Free flap- omentum or latissimus
      - Burr to diploe and STSG or integra
  - Management of scalp alopecia
    - Small area (<5% of scalp)
      - Advancement flap

- Rotation advancement
- Rhomboid flap
- Galeal scoring may be needed to assist mobilization
- Large defects (up to 50% of scalp)
  - Tissue expansion
  - Consider orientation of hair prior to cutting flaps
  - > 50% defects tissue expansion may be used but hair may thin out
- Hand and Upper Extremity
  - Indications for intervention
    - Any scar or contracture that limits motion and function
    - Dorsal claw deformity- incomplete MCP flexion, hyperextension MCP joints
    - Palmar contracture- primarily in children
    - Web space deformity- may occur despite grafting esp. in syndactyly
    - Nail bed deformity
    - Axillary contracture- decreased mobility and function
    - Nerve compression
  - Pre-op question?
    - Do symptoms warrant surgical intervention?
  - Surgical options
    - Z-plasty
    - Grafting- thick STSG best
    - Glabrous grafts for palmar defects
    - Integra
  - Dorsal claw deformity
    - Complete release of contracture and resurface with STSG, FTSG, or integra
    - In severe deformity PIP joint may be destroyed

- If MCP motion cannot be restored fuse PIP joint
          - Post-op Management
            - Early range of motion
            - Splinting
          - Web space deformity
            - Z-plasty
            - Jumping man flap
          - Palmar contracture
            - Scar release
            - FTSG vs. glabrous skin grafting
            - Glabrous graft ideal in patients with dark skin
            - High risk of recurrence
            - Prolonged splinting
        - Breast
          - Indication for intervention- chest burn
          - Initial conservative debridement
          - Avoid injury of breast bud in pediatric population if possible
            - Monitor growth through puberty
            - Delay surgery until after scar maturation and breast development
          - Operative technique
            - Release constricting overlying skin envelope
            - Resulting defect managed with FTSG, STSG or integra
            - Can pre-operatively expand abdominal skin if available for FTSG
            - In the event of complete breast destruction use standard breast reconstruction techniques- autologous tissue usually best choice if available

4. Understand risks and benefits of various approaches
   - Timing of intervention is important

- Discuss risks and benefits of various procedures based on presented scenario, there are "best answers"
- Burn reconstruction should positively impact quality of life
    - Improve impaired physical function
    - Improve body image
    - Improve sexual life
- Most burn survivors have a good quality of life, hand function is important.
- Consider affected anatomic region: See above details
- ALL BURN RECONSTRUCTION PROCEDURES REQUIRE HIGH PATIENT COMPLIANCE IN THE POST-OP PERIOD FOR 12-18 MONTHS!

5. Address complications and unexpected problems adequately

   - Inadequate or incomplete reconstruction common
   - Early scar contracture
   - Graft or integra infection
   - Graft or integra loss
   - Failed flap or flap loss
   - Tissue expanders- exposure, infection, deflation
   - Consider anatomic region specific complications
   - Your management of each of these problems

6. Demonstrate ability to structure alternative plan

   - Consider back up plan if reconstruction fails or initial choice of intervention not available
   - How will you stage the patient if multiple areas involved?
   - How will you manage burned stiff extremity from shoulder to digits?
   - What if patient unwilling to follow therapy protocols?
   - What if patient not insured?

Chapter Eighty-Four

Hand: Burns and Frostbite

84
Hand: Burn and Frostbite

1. Identify General Problem/Diagnosis/Planning
   (Describe photo, give working diagnosis, key problems, evaluates patient)

   - Hand Burn
   - Describe photo, your clinical guess of burn depth
   - Classification of burn injury:
     o Superficial (1st degree)
     o Superficial partial thickness (superficial 2nd degree)
     o Deep partial thickness (deep 2nd degree)
     o Full-thickness (3rd degree)
     o Full-thickness involving underlying tissues muscle/bone (4th degree)
     o Can elaborate on depth of injury based on type of burn (scald vs. flame vs. electrical)
   - Note primary concerns
     o ABC's
     o LOC
     o Trauma evaluation
     o Fractures in electrical injury
     o Other trauma
     o Ophthalmologic involvement in electrical injuries
     o Myonecrosis
   - Note risk of compartment syndrome
   - Does this patient need escharotomies?
   - Etiology of injury important in management and prognosis
   - Scald vs. grease burn vs. flame vs. chemical vs. electrical vs. frostbite vs. contact
   - Location of burn
   - Appearance of injured hand
   - Characteristic position is INTRINSIC MINUS
     o Wrist flexion
     o Hyperextension MCP joints (tightness)
     o Flexion of proximal and distal IP's (Claw deformity)
   - FROST BITE
     o Old Classification:
       - 1°- (Superficial)

899

- Erythema, edema, hyperemia
- No blisters or tissue loss
- 2°- (Full thickness skin)
  - Erythema, vesicle formation, superficial skin slough, no deep necrosis
- 3°- (Full thickness + Subcutaneous tissue)
  - Local edema, grayish-blue discoloration, skin loss to subcutaneous level
- 4°- (Full thickness, subcutaneous tissue down to bone)
  - Deep cyanosis without vesiculation or local edema but necrosis of deep tissue to muscle, tendon, bone
    - New Classification
      - Superficial- minimal to no tissue loss
      - Deep- significant tissue loss
    - Pertinent Hx: duration of time in cold
  - PE: assess depth and degree of injury
  - PATHOPHYSIOLOGY
    - Ice crystals within extracellular fluid, direct cellular injury

2. Consider reasonable goals in diagnosis and management *(Management and treatment, surgical indications, operative procedures and anesthesia)*

- Take photographs for documentation
- Initial basic wound care
  - Debridement
  - Daily cleaning
  - Topical antibiotics (silvadene gold standard)
  - Dressings
- Options to obviate need for daily dressings:
  - Debridement followed by
  - Application of biobrane, xenograft or mepilex (silver impregnated silicone foam)
- Edema control
  - Cool the burn for 1st 30 minutes maximum (5-10 minutes of cooling adequate)

- Apply moist towels no more than 20% TBSA at a time to avoid hypothermia
- Splinting- position of safety
  - SPLINT IMMEDIATELY
  - Intrinsic plus
  - Wrist 30 degrees of extension
  - MP'S flexed 40 degrees
  - IP'S 0 degrees
  - Thermoplast
- Avoid INTRINSIC MINUS
  - Wrist flexion
  - Hyperextension MCP joints (tightness)
  - Flexion of proximal and distal IP's (Claw deformity)
- Early PT/OT evaluation
  - Critical component to all hand burn injuries
  - General burn principle definitive skin closure in <3 weeks
  - ASAP after depth of burn determined to be full thickness or unlikely to heal in under three weeks
- Maintain perfusion by fluid resuscitation
- Maintain circulating volume
- Remove mechanical obstruction to blood flow
  - Escharotomy- Where would you do this? Bedside, in the office, OR?
- Electrical Injury
- Attempt salvage in electrical injuries but note high amputation rates 40-70%
- Tissue decompression is the key to salvage
  - Early escharotomy and/or fasciotomy
    - 1000 Volts mandates decompression fasciotomy
- Attempt to:
  - Preserve function
  - Avoid infection
  - Debride necrotic tissue
  - Tissue decompression within 6-8 hours of injury
- Temporary coverage until definitive coverage, allow demarcation time
  - Options- Cadaver/xenograft/integra
- Amputation may be needed:
- In cases of extensive soft tissue injury or…
- If a severely injured extremity jeopardizes patient's life

- Remember palmar skin is thicker than dorsal skin
  - Consider glabrous skin grafting
- Monitor for occurrence of compartment syndrome in extremities
  - Hands and digits
- Indications for Surgery
  - Escharotomy
    - Pain
    - Resistance to passive straightening of fingers
    - Disappearance of capillary refill in nail beds
  - Fasciotomy (Decompression)
    - Dorsal interossei
    - Severe edema of hand
    - Decreased finger flexion
- Excision and grafting
  - EARLY in deep partial thickness and full thickness burns
  - EXCEPTION- Frostbite
    - Avoid early excision and grafting
    - Extent of damage is difficult to assess
    - High capacity for healing in this clinical situation
  - Treatment overall is based on the depth of burn and TBSA which dictates extent of resuscitation.
- Basic Principles
  - Wound healing as soon as possible, ideally complete closure in 3 weeks or less.
- Goals Major Principles
  - Avoid additional injury
  - Early closure to decrease ongoing catabolic reaction and decrease risk of infection
  - Maintain active and passive range of motion
  - Prevent infection or loss of soft tissue coverage
  - Early functional rehabilitation
- FROST BITE
  - Work-up
    - Technetium (Tc)-99 Bone Scan- standard study within first several days
    - Can assess tissue viability
    - Predicts amputation level in 84% of cases
  - Avoid early excision and grafting

- Management
- Restore core body heat
- Rapid rewarming of frozen extremity 40-44°C water bath
- 15-30 minute bath
- Sedation and analgesia
- Triple phase Tc-99 Bone Scan
- Tetanus prophylaxis
- Open dressings with topical antibiotics
- NSAIDS- Oral Ibuprofen
- Antibiotics for confirmed infection ONLY
- Amputation or debridement only after full demarcation
  - ➢ May take weeks
- Physical therapy, splinting

3. Select appropriate options in diagnosis and management

- What is your prognosis?
- Timing of interventions
- How long do you do dressings before grafting?
- What is you post op protocol?
- Parameters for excision and debridement
- Principles of treatment
  - Evaluation of size (Lund-Browder chart most accurate, palmar method, Rule of 9's)
  - Evaluation of burn depth
  - Wound care and dressings (silvadene gold standard other collagenase/polysporin power)
  - Decide operative or non-operative therapy
  - Escharotomy if indicated
  - Early hand therapy and splinting
  - Surgical management (escharotomy/skin grafting/flap options)
  - Early post-op treatment
  - Functional rehabilitation
  - Secondary and tertiary correction of contractures/scars if necessary
  - PT/OT is critical in ultimate long-term functional outcome.

- OPERATIVE APPROACH

- Deep partial thickness and full thickness burn injuries
    - Early excision and grafting within first five days
    - Tangential excision or versajet
- About the versajet
    - Less blood loss, more tissue preservation
    - Works by Venturi Effect
        - High-speed stream of water pulverizes tissue
    - Sheet graft when possible in smaller burns better aesthetics otherwise mesh based on size of burn larger burn > mesh (1:1.5, 1:2, 1:3; 1:4, > 1:4 skin difficult to handle)
- Full thickness burns
    - May extend to tendons, bone or joint (Indication for flap for soft tissue coverage)
    - Workhorse flap reverse radial forearm or groin flap
    - Free flap if neither available (Fascial flap radial forearm, TPF, ALT)
- IMMOBILIZE GRAFTS (minimum 5 days then start OT)
- SPECIAL CLINICAL SCENARIOS
    - Young Women and Children
        - Conventional groin flap
        - Multiple procedures needed
        - Keep donor site hidden
    - Palmar Burns
        - Skin graft rarely needed
        - Flap coverage may be needed
        - Full-thickness skin grafts generally adequate
        - Consider interga or glabrous STSG from foot
        - Deep sensation return in 12-15 months
- FROST BITE INJURY
- NO EARLY EXCISION AND GRAFTING
    - Conservative surgical management
    - First 9-15 days in serious injuries
        - Black, hard, leathery eschar forms
        - Overtime eschar separates revealing healthy underlying skin

- Those who do not heal over this time proceed to complete mummification within 3-6 weeks.
- In cases of mummification primary amputation often the most expeditious and least morbid method of restoring function.

4. Understand risks and benefits of various approaches

   - Be able to discuss the differences between local wound care, skin grafting or using flaps based on different clinical scenarios such as depth of injury, extent of injury and timing.
   - Be able to make a plan of management based on the same scenarios.

5. Address complications and unexpected problems adequately

   - Complications and Side Effects
   - Graft loss secondary to infection
     - Treat infection topical and systemic antibiotics
     - Get control of wound and restart the process
   - Graft Loss
     - Inadequate debridement
     - Hematoma
     - Shearing
     - Poor bolster
     - Infection
   - Early hypergranulation
   - Early contracture

6. Demonstrate ability to structure alternative plan

   - Patient noncompliant with PT/OT
   - How would you manage limited donor site availability?
   - Full-thickness hand burn with exposed bone?
   - No improvement with nonoperative therapy, timing of intervention
   - General timing of various management options

Chapter Eighty-Five

Keloids and Hypertrophic Scars

85
Keloids and Hypertrophic Scars

1. Identify General Problem/Diagnosis/Planning
   (Describe photo, give working diagnosis, key problems, evaluates patient)

   - Hypertrophic scars (HTS) usually secondary to excessive tension.
     - Raised, but, do not overgrow boundary or original wound.
   - Most common locations:
     - Flexor surfaces
     - Extremities
     - Neck
     - Shoulder
     - Breast
     - Sternum
     - Lower face
   - Keloids
     - Overgrow original wound edges
     - More common in dark pigmented individuals (6-16% incidence in African-Americans)
     - Genetic predisposition- autosomal dominant
     - High recurrence with excision and closure alone.

2. Consider reasonable goals in diagnosis and management
   (Management and treatment, surgical indications, operative procedures and anesthesia)

   - Nonoperative treatment first:
     - PT- Range of motion exercises in extremities
     - Scar massage
     - Steroids (Your algorithm for injection)
     - Silicone sheets
     - Pressure garments
     - Laser treatment
     - May regress with time
   - Failed nonoperative therapy (minimum 12-18 months)
     - Re-excision with linear closure

- Most useful in cases of: infection or dehiscence
  - Z-plasty
  - Skin grafting
  - Local flaps
  - Tissue expansion
  - Consider Integra
    - Anecdotal reports of decreased recurrence rates
    - Risk donor site keloid
  - Radiation in adults in severe cases (what is your protocol?)
    - First dose immediately post-op or within 24 hours followed by 3-4 additional doses.
    - Consult radiation-oncologist pre-op and arrange radiation treatment

3. Select appropriate options in diagnosis and management

    - Making incisions in natural lines of skin tension may minimize risk of abnormal scars, parallel to skin crease
      - Why? Decreased tension
    - Avoid tension
    - Excision and closure 50% recurrence
    - Excision and closure + steroids 35% recurrence
    - Steroid beneficial early on for recurrent keloid. Base dose on size of lesion.
    - Small keloids
      - 10mg at 1st injection
      - 40mg at 2nd injection if no response
    - Long standing keloid
      - Can monitor and do nothing
      - Consider excision plus adjunct therapy
      - (steroids, PT, radiation)
    - What is the best surgical option based on presented scenario?
    - How do you decide which surgical approach you use on a case by case basis?

4. Understand risks and benefits of various approaches

    - Consider implications of different therapies:
      - Surgery

- Steroids
- Radiation
- Base intervention on:
    - Etiology of lesion
    - Duration of lesion
    - Functional/aesthetic impact
    - Previous surgery
    - Age of patient and previous history of interventions
- Minimize extent of surgery if possible
- Patient compliance with post-op therapy important

5. Address complications and unexpected problems adequately

- Infection or wound dehiscence increases the risk of abnormal scar formation
- Management of common post-op wound problems
    - Hematoma
    - Dehiscence
    - Infection
    - Flap loss
    - Graft loss
    - Common tissue expander complications
- Early recurrence

6. Demonstrate ability to structure alternative plan

- What is your plan for recurrent keloids? Time frames for intervention.
- Backup plan?
- Radiation last resort, but, never in children, growth issues especially in the face (condyles)
- Noncompliant patient
- Angry patient